AF333198

CATTLE

DOMESTICATION, DISEASES AND THE ENVIRONMENT

ANIMAL SCIENCE, ISSUES AND PROFESSIONS

CATTLE

DOMESTICATION, DISEASES AND THE ENVIRONMENT

GEORGE LIU
EDITOR

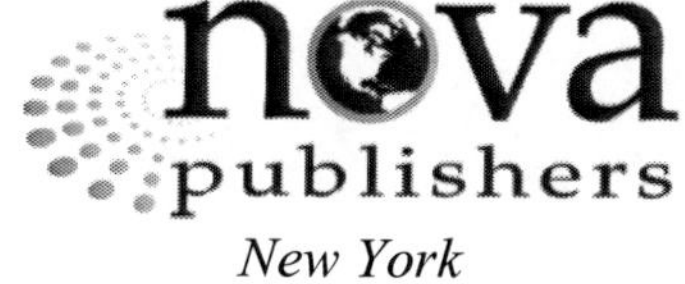

Library of Congress Cataloging-in-Publication Data

ISBN: 978-1-62417-820-7

Published by Nova Science Publishers, Inc. † New York

CONTENTS

Preface   vii

Chapter 1   Novel Perspective on Antibody Diversification from Bovine Immunoglobulin Genetics   1
Yfke Pasman, Rashpal K. Bhogal and Azad K. Kaushik

Chapter 2   The Trappin Gene Family: Structure, Function and Evolution   25
George E. Liu and Derek M. Bickhart

Chapter 3   Body Fat and Plasma Leptin Involvement in the Voluntary Feed Intake of Cattle   39
Renato S. A. Vega, Hong-Gu Lee, Hideto Kuwayama and Hisashi Hidari

Chapter 4   Epigenetics and Environmental Impacts in Cattle   59
Cong-jun Li and Robert W. Li

Chapter 5   Endocrine Control of Bull Fertility   83
Katherine L. Gilbert, Eric A. Gilbert, Aruna Govindaraju, Lyndi L. Jury, Melissa C. Mason, Kathryn E. Pfeiffer, Tricia M. Rowlison, Lori Ward, Abdullah Kaya, Jamie Larson and Erdogan Memili

Chapter 6   Ozone as a Novel Treatment Modality for Urovagina, Endometritis and Retained Placenta in Cattle   109
R. Zobel and Z. Tuček

Chapter 7   The Use of Clinoptilolite as Feed Additive for the Prevention and Treatment of Certain Diseases in Cattle   115
P. D. Katsoulos, M. A. Karatzia and H. Karatzias

Chapter 8   Occurrence, Etiology and Prevention of Abomasal Displacement in Dairy Cattle   127
H. Karatzias, M. A. Karatzia and P. D. Katsoulos

Chapter 9   Adaptations of Cattle to Stressful Environments   **139**
                  Concepta McManus, Samuel Paiva, Luiza Seixas,
                  José Braccini Neto, Júlio Otavio Jardim Barcellos,
                  Maria Eugênia Andrighetto Canozzi,
                  Bruno Stefano Lima Dallago,
                  Cristiano Barros de Melo and Michiel Scholtz

Chapter 10   Native Cattle Genetic Resources in China   **159**
                  Dongxiao Sun, Yali Hou, Qin Chu, Yi Zhang
                   and Yuan Zhang

Chapter 11   Economic Evaluation of Performance and Functional Traits
                   in Dual-purpose Hungarian Fleckvieh Cattle   **175**
                  I. Komlósi and B. Húth

Index   **189**

PREFACE

The availability of bovine genome sequences has opened new research avenues for cattle biodiversity and diseases. Cattle also have a critical role in climate change, land degradation and water shortage. This new book presents current research in the immunity, nutrition, fertility and diseases of cattle. Topics include innate and acquired immunity; epigenetics, nutrogenomics and metagenomics; hormone regulation of bull fertility; diseases like abomasal displacement; and ozone and clinoptilolit as disease treatments. This book also presents information about local adaptation, selection and biodiversity of native species and breeds of domesticated cattle in South America, East Asia and East Europe. This book was written by experts in each area, from institutions located in Brazil, Canada, China, Croatia, Greece, Hungary, South Korea and the United States.

Chapter 1 – Limited germline sequence divergence and combinatorial diversity in cattle, similar to species like sheep, swine, rabbit and chicken but unlike rodents and humans, enforce constraints on the diversification of neonatal antibody repertoire. Hence, Cattle have developed additional antibody diversification strategies involving generation of exceptionally long CDR3H and somatic hypermutations without exposure to external antigen during B cell ontogeny. About 8-10% of peripheral B-cells in adult cattle express IgM with long CDR3H ($\geq$50 amino acids) some of which are polyspecific. Such atypical CDR3H (up to 61 amino acids) in antibodies, not yet seen in other species, is encoded by the single long germline DH2 gene capable of encoding up to 49 codons. Remarkably, insertion of conserved short nucleotide sequences (CSNS) specifically at V_H-D_H junctions in the adult V_H-D_H-J_H recombinations, by an unknown mechanism, increases CDR3H size subsequent to antigen exposure. Three allotypic IgM isotypes are defined where some structural variants originate via alternate splicing. Four allotypes of IgG1 are identified where unique presence of Pro-Ala-Ser-Ser in Cγ1 domain seems to be involved in cell adhesion and migration function. The λ-light chain is predominantly expressed in bovine antibodies where most of λ-light chain repertoire is encoded by the Vλ1-Jλ3-Cλ3 recombinations. Restricted Vλ+V_H pairings occur in IgM antibodies with exceptionally long CDR3H where λ-light chain essentially seems to provide a structural support. To conclude, generation of exceptionally long CDR3H, with or without CSNS insertions, and somatic hypermutations without prior antigen exposure compensate for limited germline divergence and contribute to antibody diversification in cattle.

Chapter 2 – Trappins are a family of small secretary host-defense peptides that have many functions. Most members exhibit antiprotease and antimicrobial activities, while others influence inflammation, immunity and the promotion of tissue repair. Considered to be important guardians of mucosal surfaces, trappins possess an N-terminal transglutaminase substrate (TGS) domain and a C-terminal whey acidic protein (WAP) four-disulphide core (WFDC) domain. The numbers and compositions of trappin genes vary among eutherian mammalian species. While there is a single trappin-2 gene in human and sheep, no trappin gene was found in mouse and rat. By contrast, multiple duplicated trappin paralogs were found in pig, cattle, guinea pig, armadillo and Afrotherian species (elephant, tenrec, and hyrax). Trappin duplication events appear to have occurred independently in these mammalian lineages over a long time period, suggesting their potential roles in species formation and animal domestication. Recent duplication and accelerated evolution of trappin genes in pig, cattle and armadillo demonstrate that mammalian genomes have the capability to form trappin multigenes to acquire antimicrobial activities for niche-specific pathogens.

Chapter 3 – The involvement of adipose derived leptin in feed intake regulation remains elusive. Hence, the purpose of this chapter is to clarify the involvement of body fat measures and endogenous leptin in feed intake of cattle. In *study one*, 6 16-month old Holstein steers were offered *ad libitum* feed for seven months.

Feed intake, body weight and backfat thickness (BFT) between 6th to 7th and 12th to 13[th]rib were measured at selected monthly ages from day 1 to 8. On day 8, pre-prandial blood was sampled to measure leptin, insulin, glucose, NEFA, triglyceride and total cholesterol, then ultrasound BFT was taken. In *study two*, eight heads of finishing (n=4) and growing (n=4) steers were used for cross-over experimental design to know the effects of 2-hour interval of physiological dose intravenous insulin administration (6 mU per kg $BW^{0.75}$) on plasma leptin and TDN intake per kg $BW^{0.75}$ from 08:00 until 22:00 hours. Blood was sampled 15 minutes before and after insulin administration to measure plasma metabolites and hormones of growing and finishing Holstein steers.

In *study one*, the inter-relationship of BFT, plasma leptin and TDN intake for the period of seven months, revealed significant positive relationship between backfat thickness and plasma leptin. Negative relationship of TDN intake to plasma leptin (P≤0.004; r=0.49) and backfat thickness (P≤0.005; r=0.048) was also observed. The reduction of TDN intake from 16 to 23 months was 25%.

This inter-relationship between backfat thickness, plasma leptin and TDN intake implies strongly that 12th to 13th rib backfat, an indicator of adiposity reflects correlated elevation of plasma leptin and TDN intake reduction per kg $BW^{0.75}$ of finishing steers. In *study two*, no daytime plasma leptin variation was observed for growing and finishing steers. Plasma glucose was depressed in growing, while depression was observed only at certain period after insulin administration for finishing steers.

Plasma leptin was not elevated significantly in growing steers, whereas significant plasma leptin elevation was observed among finishing steers at 11:45 and 15:45. At this period of plasma leptin elevation, insulin administration caused 25% reduction in short-term TDN intake of finishing steers (P<0.07), whereas no short-term TDN reduction was observed in growing steers. Both growing and finishing steers did not show reduction in the 24 hour feed intake. Briefly, the over-all results revealed that leptin elevation is necessary for feed intake reduction; hence leptin is involved only in long-term feed intake regulation in cattle.

Chapter 4 – This chapter reviews the major advances in the field of epigenetics as well as the environmental impacts of cattle. Many findings from the authors' own research endeavors related to the topic are also introduced. The phenotypic characterization of an animal can be changed through epigenetic mechanisms such as histone posttranslational modification, microRNA (miRNA), and other mechanisms. The interaction between genetics and epigenetics provides transcription regulation in cattle development and growth. The multiple layers of regulatory control of gene expression provide a multitude of paths by which cells can control their responses to external stimuli or environmental stresses. The number of research efforts to discover general molecular mechanisms fundamental to epigenetic phenomena has recently exploded.

Chapter 5 – Male fertility—the ability to produce viable sperm that are able to support fertilization and oocyte activation and to sustain development during embryogenesis and beyond—is essential for success of mammalian reproduction and development. Production of quality semen depends on the existence of an effective male reproduction system that is consistently able to produce viable gametes. This requires a male with a fertility phenotype that has evolved under the influence of its genetics, environment, and epistasis to a high degree of efficacy. As the sperm from one bull can be used to inseminate tens of thousands of cows, bull fertility has an enormous influence on the efficiency and success of the cattle breeding and reproduction. Even among bulls that produce ample amounts of sperm having apparent normal morphology, some of these animals will still not exhibit high fertility. Despite large investments to study the causes of low fertility as well as research on methods to prevent, diagnose, and treat subpar male fertility, only limited success has been achieved, and the problem remains poorly defined. The objectives of this paper are to review the male reproductive system and the endocrine regulation of male fertility. It will explore the functions of specific hormones regulating male fertility, hormonal control of sperm viability, as well as environmental factors influencing male fertility. The bovine will be the species of focus, but key aspects of male fertility of other mammals (pigs, goats, horses, monkeys and humans) will be included. This review is intended to be a useful source of information for both basic and applied research, as well as for animal production and human andrologists.

Chapter 6 – Urovagina, endometritis and retained placenta are detrimental to the health and fertility of cows worldwide. Different treatment options for urovagina, so far, included only surgical modifications of vaginal tissue. Treatments of endometritis and retained placenta included antibiotics applied parenteraly and/or into the uterus as well as prostaglandin and oxytocin analogues administered parenteraly. Recently, infusion of collagenase into the umbilical arteries in animals with retained placenta was introduced. Efficacy of many of these treatments is questionable and others are too expensive and inappropriate for daily field practice. Urovagina, endometritis and retained placenta can be successfully treated by the ozone flush applied into the uterus and vagina. The ozone flush was found to be the most effective treatment modality for investigated fertility issues in cattle with an advantage of no milk and meat withdrawal period.

Chapter 7 – Clinoptilolite is a natural clay mineral that is part of the zeolite group. Zeolites are crystalline, hydrated aluminosilicates of alkali and alkaline earth cations that have infinite structures which are three-dimensional. These materials have unique properties and are characterized by their ability to lose and gain water reversibly, to absorb molecules of appropriate diameter (adsorption property or acting as molecule sieves) and to exchange their constituent cations without major change of their structure (ion-exchange property). Because of these properties, zeolites are used as feed additives, mainly in order to improve performance traits. In the last decade a there has been much interest in the investigation of whether the unique properties of clinoptilolite can be used for the prevention of certain diseases in dairy cattle. A series of experiments has been conducted in this direction. The results indicated that the dietary administration of clinoptilolite at a rate of 2.5% in the concentrate mixture during the last month of the dry period is effective in preventing milk fever and ketosis after calving. It was further proved that the daily addition of 200gr clinoptilolite in the ration enhances the immune response of cattle vaccinated against E. coli and prevents the reduction of ruminal pH in cattle that are fed high concentrate diets. As far as calves are concerned, the results of many experiments concluded that the addition of clinoptilolite in the colostrum of newborn animals increases the intestinal absorption of immunoglobulins and reduces the incidence and the duration of diarrhea syndrome. The objective of this chapter is to review the experimental results that concern the efficacy of clinoptilolite on the prevention of the aforementioned diseases in dairy cattle and calves and to suggest possible focus topics for further research.

Chapter 8 – Displaced abomasum (DA), either to the left (LDA) or to the right (RDA) side of the abdomen, is one of the most important diseases that are commonly observed in dairy cattle. It is encountered worldwide and represents the most common reason for abdominal surgery in dairy cattle, especially in cows of high-producing dairy breeds, such as Holstein. The incidence rate of DA in dairy herds varies between 1 and 15%, with LDA being more frequent than RDA. The peak of DA occurrence is during the first 4-6 weeks post partum and is commonly observed in first-calf heifers. DA is a multifactorial disease and its exact causes are still unclear. Nutritional factors, such as rations with high quantities of concentrates and reduced forage to concentrate ratio, seem to be of great importance. Metabolic diseases such as hypocalcaemia and ketosis, as well as other concomitant diseases or situations like retained placenta, metritis, mastitis or high body condition score, fatty liver and endotoxaemia can cause abomasal hypomobility, increased gas production within the abomasum and displacement. Another important factor for the development of DA is the increased stress due to calving and the beginning of lactation. Certain anatomical and physiological factors, such as location and loose wall structure promote gas collection, distention and finally, displacement of the abomasum. In the last thirty years (1981-2011) the etiological factors of DA were investigated in about 10, 000 cows. DA prevention is based on administering sufficient quantities of roughage in the ratio, avoiding abrupt ratio changes-particularly puerperium and on prevention or early treatment of postpartum diseases.

Chapter 9 – Local cattle breeds in South America originated from cattle that escaped from or were left behind by the colonizers in expeditions through the region in the 16th century. These animals were isolated by rivers and forests and became adapted to specific local conditions such as high temperatures (savannah (cerrado), sertão and Pantanal), as well as extremely low (savannah and sertão) or high (Pantanal) humidity. Disease challenges in these regions are unique and survival has meant that these animals have acquired traits that will be important in the face of future climate challenges with changes in rainfall and temperature patterns. Recent importations of Zebu and European cattle have led to the survival of these animals becoming threatened, but recently, studies have shown that the adaptation to the environment and *Bos taurus* origin have given these animals a unique combination of high heat tolerance and disease resistance combined with high carcass quality. The behaviour of these animals is such that they can walk up to 20km per day in search of water and food, and their social behaviour is more primitive than modern cattle breeds. These breeds are still reared in highly extensive systems and give us an insight into behaviour and adaptation mechanisms needed for survival in highly stressful environments. On the other hand, these changes determine the configuration of new production systems which should be linked to new Technologies, to the economic outcome and consumer demand.

Chapter 10 – China has abundant cattle breed resources, including 92 local breeds, 9 developed and 13 introduced breeds. The local breeds are comprised of Chinese Yellow cattle, water buffalo, Yak, as well as Gayal. Chinese Yellow cattle are the major breeds with high genetic divergence, and can be categorized into Northern group (*Bos taurus* like Yanbian), Southern group (*Bos indicus* like Zhaotong) and Central group (*Bos taurus* and *indicus*, like Qinchuan, Nanyang, Jinnan, Luxi) with the Yellow River, the Qinling mountain and Yangtze River as boundaries. Water buffalo in China are mostly swamp rather than river type, consisted of two clades from *Yangtze Valley* and the *South of China* respectively, present three divergent mitochondrial DNA lineages (A, B1 and B2). There are also multiple introduced breeds mainly for the breed improvement purpose. Chinese Holstein is the most dominant dairy cattle (approximately 80%), which has the most complete genetic improvement system for the last 30 years, including breed registration, dairy herd improvement, progeny testing, genetic evaluation, and recently genomic selection.

Chapter 11 – A bio-economic model was used to estimate economic values of 14 milk production, functional, growth and carcass traits for Hungarian Fleckvieh (Simmental). The highest relative economic importance was obtained for milk yield (29%), followed by productive lifetime of cows (20%) and daily gain in the rearing period (11%). Other functional traits (calving difficulty score, still birth, total conception rate of heifers, cows and calf mortality) reached a relative economic importance of 15%. Based on these results, the inclusion of productive lifetime and cow fertility in the breeding program for Hungarian Fleckvieh is advisable.

In: Cattle: Domestication, Diseases and the Environment
Editor: George Liu

ISBN: 978-1-62417-820-7
© 2013 Nova Science Publishers, Inc.

Chapter 1

NOVEL PERSPECTIVE ON ANTIBODY DIVERSIFICATION FROM BOVINE IMMUNOGLOBULIN GENETICS

Yfke Pasman, Rashpal K. Bhogal
and Azad K. Kaushik[*]
Department of Molecular and Cellular Biology, University of Guelph, Guelph, Ontario, Canada

ABSTRACT

Limited germline sequence divergence and combinatorial diversity in cattle, similar to species like sheep, swine, rabbit and chicken but unlike rodents and humans, enforce constraints on the diversification of neonatal antibody repertoire. Hence, Cattle have developed additional antibody diversification strategies involving generation of exceptionally long CDR3H and somatic hypermutations without exposure to external antigen during B cell ontogeny. About 8-10% of peripheral B-cells in adult cattle express IgM with long CDR3H ($\geq$50 amino acids) some of which are polyspecific. Such atypical CDR3H (up to 61 amino acids) in antibodies, not yet seen in other species, is encoded by the single long germline DH2 gene capable of encoding up to 49 codons. Remarkably, insertion of conserved short nucleotide sequences (CSNS) specifically at VH-DH junctions in the adult VH-DH-JH recombinations, by an unknown mechanism, increases CDR3H size subsequent to antigen exposure. Three allotypic IgM isotypes are defined where some structural variants originate via alternate splicing. Four allotypes of IgG1 are identified where unique presence of Pro-Ala-Ser-Ser in Cγ1 domain seems to be involved in cell adhesion and migration function. The λ-light chain is predominantly expressed in bovine antibodies where most of λ-light chain repertoire is encoded by the Vλ1-Jλ3-Cλ3 recombinations. Restricted Vλ+VH pairings occur in IgM antibodies with exceptionally long CDR3H where λ-light chain essentially seems to provide a structural support. To conclude, generation of exceptionally long CDR3H, with or without CSNS insertions,

---

[*] Address for correspondence: Azad K. Kaushik, DVM, DSc (Paris). Department of Molecular and Cellular Biology. University of Guelph, Guelph, Ontario, N1G 2W1 Canada. E-mail: akaushik@uoguelph.ca.

and somatic hypermutations without prior antigen exposure compensate for limited germline divergence and contribute to antibody diversification in cattle.

Keywords: Bovine Immunoglobulin, CDR3, VDJ, VJ, Antibody repertoire

1. INTRODUCTION

1.1. Evolution of the Adaptive Immune System

The adaptive immune system, based on clonally diverse receptors, finds its origin at the dawn of vertebrate evolution approximately 550 million years ago (Figure 1). However, the mechanisms to generate diverse lymphocyte receptors are radically different between jawed and jawless vertebrates [1-3]. The jawless vertebrates, lamprey and hagfish, generate diversity by assembling variable lymphocyte receptors (VLRs) from leucine rich repeat (LRR) modules by gene conversion. Such a multistep assembly of LRR modules randomly selected from a large library of flanking cassettes is likely capable of generating a repertoire of about 10^{14} antigen receptors, reminiscent of clonal selection in jawed vertebrates [3]. No evidence of major histocompatibility complex (MHC) class I and II molecules, T cell antigen receptors (TCR) and immunoglobulins (Ig) is found in invertebrates and jawless vertebrates. Nevertheless, members of the immunoglobulin superfamily are found throughout species, for example, in the innate protein response in insects, fibrinogen related proteins in snails and V-region chitin–binding protein in amphioxus [2, 4]. Whether the agnathan LRR containing VLRs were forerunners of vertebrate immune receptors or rearranging VLRs and Igs arose independently remains an open question [5].

While there is an increasing complexity of the adaptive immune system during vertebrate evolution, basic elements are relatively conserved. The innate immune system is heritable and able to recognize conserved molecular patterns to trigger an inflammatory response. The diverse specific adaptive immunity develops, in concert with the innate immunity, where lymphocytes expressing immune effector molecules, Ig and TCR, undergo clonal selection upon antigen encounter in the periphery (reviewed in [8]). Essentially, B- and T-lymphocytes expressing Ig and TCR, encoded by RAG-based recombination of variable (V), diversity (D) and joining (J) and constant (C) region genes, form the core of the adaptive immunity. A spectrum of evolutionary characteristics of RAG-based Ig and TCR recombination is evident from lower (cartilaginous) fish to higher order jawed vertebrates including humans, for example, an abundance of clan III and II genes of immunoglobulin heavy variable region (IGHV) across species in contrast to clan I genes that are either missing in most species or are present in small numbers [9]. The IGHV locus continues to evolve in a species-specific manner consistent with the 'birth and death' model. The vertebrate light-chains are categorized into four isotypes ((σ, σ-cart, κ and λ) that originated 450 million years ago prior to the emergence of cartilaginous fish [10]. Three isotypes, kappa, lambda, and sigma are classified where all of these exist in amphibians but only two (kappa and lambda) are found in reptiles and some mammals [11]. Various species differ in germline potential and their ability to use it, suggesting that through evolution different strategies for post-recombination diversification have developed to ensure host defense.

Mya	Vertebrate class	Organs of Diversification	Rearrangement, hypermutation	Immunoglobulin Isotype	Class switch	Germinal-Center formation
100	Placental mammals	GALT, Peyers Patches Thymus, Spleen, Bone marrow Lymph nodes	+	IgM, IgD*, IgG** IgE**, IgA	+	+
200	Birds	Bursa,GALT Thymus Spleen Bone marrow Lymph nodes?	+	IgM, IgY, IgA	+	+
360	Amphibians	GALT, Thymus Spleen, Bone marrow	+	IgM, IgY, IgX	+	-
400	Bony Fish	GALT, Head Kidney Thymus, Spleen	+	IgM, IgD	-	-
460	Cartilaginous fish	GALT Epigonal (Leydig) Thymus, Spleen	+	IgM, IgW, IgNAR	-	-
550	Jawless fish	GALT	?	No Ig LRRs	-	-

Figure 1. Evolutionary features of the adaptive immune system in vertebrates [modified from [6, 7]]. *IgD has one less constant domain in mice than in humans and is not expressed in species other than primates and rodents. **Both IgG and IgE are believed to be derived from an IgY like ancestor. IgNAR - immunoglobulin new antigen receptor; Mya - millions of years ago; LRR - leucine rich repeats.

1.2. Adaptive Immune System in Mammals

The Ig heavy (IgH) variable region is encoded by programmed recombination of germline V, D and J gene segments, whereas light (IgL) chain, kappa (κ) or lambda (λ) variable region originate from rearranged germline V and J genes [12-14]. The V(D)J recombination generates extensive combinatorial diversity apart from enzymatic addition of non-templated nucleotides at the recombining junctions. After antigenic stimulation and exposure to specific cytokines, responding mature B cells undergo class switch recombination (CSR) and/or somatic hypermutations (SHM), effected by AID enzyme, [15, 16] during affinity maturation in the periphery.

In species such as mice and humans where both placental and colostral transfer of Ig occurs, extensive germline sequence divergence and combinatorial diversity is evident in B-cells that develop in fetal liver and bone marrow [17]. In those species where no placental transfer of Ig occurs, diverse mechanisms to compensate for restricted germline combinatorial diversity are evident in B-cells that may also develop in other lymphoid organs, e.g., ileal Peyer's patches (PP), appendix and Bursa of Fabricius [18]. For example, gene conversion in developing chicken B cells [19] and extensive junctional flexibility in VDJ recombinations of B cells of swine [20] contribute to antibody diversification. Rabbit is an exception where despite placental and colostral Ig transfer, gene conversion and antigen-dependent SHM generate extensive diversity in developing B-cells in the appendix [21, 22]. Nevertheless, extensive junctional flexibility (N or P nucleotide addition) and SHMs provide a general antibody diversification mechanism, upon encounter with antigen in the periphery across species.

2. THE BOVINE IMMUNE SYSTEM

2.1. Maternal Antibody Transfer to Offspring

In cattle, the presence of a syndesmochorial type of placenta prevents the transfer of maternal antibodies during gestation [23, 24]. Passive transfer of maternal antibodies via colostrum is important to provide immunity during early neonatal life (reviewed in [25, 26]). Concentrations of IgG1 are the highest in the colostrum of ruminant species as compared to other species (Table 1). Bovine colostrum IgG1 levels can exceed 100mg/ml [27] and are usually present at levels up to ten times that of the other Ig classes [26]. IgG1 is the major class of antibody in milk and is abundant in serum of cattle [26, 28]. This is in contrast to humans where IgA is the major class of antibody found in colostrum and milk, and IgG is predominantly present in the serum. This suggests that there are different mechanisms responsible for transport of Igs in the mammary gland and those across the placenta, and these vary across species. Ruminant IgG1 is known to transfer passive immunity via colostrum and also protects mucosal surfaces (similar to IgA) being resistant to proteolysis [29]. The neonatal Fc receptor (FcRn) in some mammals is known to provide a transport mechanism for IgG across the placental barrier [30]. In ruminants, however, FcRn contributes to transfer and secretion of IgG on mucosal surfaces but not across syndesmochorial type placentation [31]. The Igs and other macromolecules in colostrum cross the intestinal barrier in the first 12-24 hours of newborn suckling bovine calves. Upon IgG1 uptake, 68% IgG1 clearance occurs via transfer to intestinal lumen where it protects against pathogens [32]. The relative high occurrence of IgA, IgM and IgG in colostrum as compared to serum in most species suggests that the presence of these antibodies is either to protect the mammary gland, the gut lumen of the neonate, or both. IgG is most predominant in serum present in the monomeric form [26] whereas IgA and IgM are present in polymeric forms both in blood and milk [28]. IgA is present in di-or tetrameric form when secreted on mucosal surfaces where secretory component protects it from proteolytic degradation [28]. Binding of IgG to FcRn contributes to its long serum half-life [33], consistent with the suggested role of FcRn in bovine IgG metabolism to maintain homeostasis [32-34]. Recently, it has been shown that FcRn has a similar role for albumin protecting both of these important serum proteins against endothelial intracellular degradation [35]. The predominant Ig in colostrum depends on a species and particularly on the route of transfer of passive immunity from mother to offspring. The FcRn receptors have not been detected in duodenal enterocytes of lamb [36], a species phylogenetically close to cattle. However, FcRn receptors occur in crypt epithelial cells of the large and small intestine of bull [32]. Different haplotypes of bovine FcRn genes are associated with varying serum IgG levels in newborn calves indicating that bovine FcRns may play a role in colostral immunoglobulin transport and increased IgG half-life [37]. Since ruminant FcRn is detected in multiple mucosal tissues (mammary gland, intestines and lung) [36, 38], it seems that ruminant IgG1 secretion is an FcRn-dependent process. Consistent with this prediction, an IgG transport receptor (FcRn) has been characterized in the human placenta [39] and the ovine mammary gland [31]. FcRns have been found in bovine mammary epithelial cells in combination with a change in distribution pattern before and after parturition, indicating important role in IgG transport during colostrum formation in ruminants [32].

In general, IgG predominates in the colostrum of carnivores and ungulates whereas IgA is main Ig in the colostrum of rodents and primates. In cattle IgG1 exceeds the level of IgA >10:1 in colostrum, even though IgA levels are also increased by 10-fold as compared to serum [27, 28, 44]. This supports the argument that both IgG and IgA are transported actively into mammary gland of cattle. It has been suggested that IgG is important for systemic transfer of passive immunity from mother to neonate while IgA transfer provides protection at mucosal surfaces [45]. A comparison of absolute amounts of Ig in serum and colostrum across species is difficult as the timing of sampling (especially with colostrum) and the method used, influences the measured quantity [28, 44, 46].

2.2. Bovine Lymphogenesis

Factors such as placental permeability and developing immune repertoire *per se* at birth across species, unlike T lymphocytes, have resulted in two different pathways for B-cell lymphogenesis. In mice and humans, post-natal B-cell development occurs in the bone marrow throughout life via continued VDJ recombination. By contrast, in cattle, similar to sheep, chicken, rabbit and swine, Ig diversification does not occur throughout life but only during perinatal life in the ileal Peyer's patches. The removal of ileal Peyer's patches (PP) in sheep affected Ig$^+$ cells in lymphoid organs and peripheral blood and, hence, it is considered primary lymphoid organ in ruminants [47]. Subsequent Ig diversification occurs via somatic hypermutations or other mechanisms in gut-associated lymphoid tissue. Such a variation across species is an example of divergent evolution [48, 49] and does not exclude co-existence of alternative development pathways. This is consistent with 'cross over' observed in T and B cell development, e.g., intra-thymic and extra-thymic production of B and T cells, respectively. In this context, *de novo* synthesis of IgA in bovine thymic tissue culture has been noted earlier [50]. The emergence of IgM$^+$ B cells is detectable in cattle fetus at 59 days of gestation (Table II) [51]. The ileal PP develop subsequent to jejunal PP and involute at sexual maturity. The jejunal PP appear first at mid gestation but these metamorphose into secondary lymphoid tissue with characteristic germinal centers around one month post-birth [47] and persist throughout life. The lymphoid follicles of both PP consist mostly of IgM$^+$ cells with very few IgG$^+$ cells. B cells develop and expand oligoclonally in the ileal PP [52] similar to reported development of bursal follicles in chicken. This is evidenced by a high rate of bovine B cell proliferation in PP around the time of birth that helps attain a relative stability in lymphoid cell population [53].

By day 100 of gestation in cattle, little diversity is seen in the light chain variable region repertoire outside the spleen [57, 58]. The VDJ and/or VJ rearrangements are detectable in B-splenocytes of125-day-old bovine fetus [56]. The cattle antibody diversity increases with age and becomes detectable in peripheral lymphoid tissue after 1-2 weeks post birth [49]. Bovine colostrum IgG1, in addition to providing protective immunity, may also have immunomodulatory influences on the development of the pre-immune repertoire. Colostral Igs are known to suppress the endogenous capacity of the neonate to respond immunologically, for example, via down-regulation of IgG expression at B-cell surfaces. The mechanism of such a phenomenon is unclear, but it might contribute to unknown factors that might trigger diversification of bovine antibodies in ileal PP [59]. The percentage of peripheral blood B lymphocytes in neonatal calves (<1 week) is approximately 5% of the total mononuclear cell population and reaches adult levels (approximately 19%) around 20 weeks of age [60]. It has been suggested that B-lymphocyte development declines with age as surrogate light chain (Vpreb1; IGLL1), RAG1 and RAG2 are not observed to be expressed in adult tissues (Ekman *et al.* 2012 In press).

Table 1. Transmission of immunoglobulins from the mother to the circulation of the offspring in various animal species including humans

Animal order	Transmission of Immunoglobulins			Ratio of Colostral Igs	Ratio of Milk Igs	Ratio of Serum Igs
	Prenatal transfer of Igs	Postnatal transfer of Igs	Duration of postnatal transfer			
Primates	Placenta via Fcγ-receptor	Trace amounts (small intestine)	?	IgA:IgM: IgG	IgA:IgM: IgG	IgG:IgA:IgM
Lagomorphs	Yolk sac via Fcγ-receptor	Small intestine (Minor route)	?	IgA:IgG: IgM	IgA:IgG: IgM	IgG:IgA:IgM
marsupials	None or minor	Gut, from colostrum and milk	Up to leaving the teat/pouch	IgA:IgG:?	IgG: IgA:?	NA
rodents	Yolk sac via Fcγ-receptor (minor route)	Proximal small intestine via Fcγ-receptor from milk	IgG specific 21 days	IgA:IgG: IgM	IgG:IgA: IgM	IgG:IgM:IgA
carnivores	Placenta/yolk sac Fcγ-receptor	gut	Non selective; brief to variable	IgG:IgA: IgM	IgA:IgG: IgM	IgG:IgM:IgA
ungulates	none	Entire small intestine all Ig isotypes from colostrum	Extensive, non selective 12-24 hours	IgG1:IgM: IgA	IgG1:IgA: IgM	IgG:IgM:IgA
	none	Entire small intestine IgG from colostrum	Extensive Selective 36 hours	IgG:IgA: IgM	IgA:IgG: IgM	IgG:IgM:IgA
	none	Entire small intestine IgG from colostrum	Extensive Selective 36 hours	IgG:IgA :IgM	IgA:IgG: IgM	IgG:IgM:IgA
Avian	Yolk sac	none	-	-	-	IgG:IgM:IgA

[28, 40-43]; NA=not available.

Table 2. Development of organs and cells during bovine gestation

Cells or organs of the immune system	Age of fetus in days
Thymus	42 [a]
Blood lymphocytes	45 [b]
Bone marrow/spleen	55 [a]
IgM$^+$ B lymphocytes	59 [b]
Peripheral lymph nodes	60 [a]
B and T cells in peripheral blood	70 [e]
Serum complement components	90 [c]
IgM$^+$ B ells in lymph nodes	90 [e]
TdT$^+$ cells in thymus	90 [e]
Mesenteric lymph nodes	100 [a]
VDJ and/or VJ recombination in splenocytes	125 [d]
Serum IgM	130 [a]
Blood granulocytes	130 [c]
IgG$^+$ B lymphocytes	145 [b]
Serum IgG	145 [a]
IgA$^+$ B lymphocytes	180 [e]
Ig$^+$ B lymphocytes in Peyer's Patches	180 [e]
IgM$^+$ and IgG$^+$ B Lymphocytes in tonsils	240 [e]

[a][54] ; [b][51]; [c][55]; [d][56]; [e][57].

2.3. Heavy Chain Immunogenetics

2.3.1. Limited Germline Sequence Divergence Exists at the Variable Heavy Chain Locus

The cattle variable Ig heavy chain locus on chromosome 21 [61] spans approximately 250kb. Three research groups [62-64] have demonstrated that a single bovine V_H1-gene family (BovV_H1), is mainly expressed in the cattle antibody repertoire. V_H-genes are found on chromosome 7 and 21 (unpublished data) in current Bos Taurus genome assembly UMD 3.1 of Hereford [65]. Though heavy chain locus was previously mapped to chromosome 21 [61]. The presence of V_H and D_H segments on multiple chromosomes is also found in humans [66] and is not surprising given two rounds of whole genome duplication events in the evolution of mammals [67].

2.3.3. Existence of Unusually Long Diversity Heavy Chain Genes

Given that some cattle antibodies have an exceptionally long CDR3H, there was an interest to identify the bovine D_H (BovV_H) genes that could help explain such atypical CDR3H. Characterization of BovD_H gene locus in Holstein cattle, together with the observations made in cow genome project, a total of 10 BovD_H genes have been identified [91-93]. The J_H-proximal BovD_H Q52 gene, conserved during evolution, is structurally distinct from other BovD_H gene elements that characteristically have repetitive GGT and TAT codons. These BovD_H gene elements are flanked by a classical recombination signal sequence (RSS) comprising 9 bp nonamer and 7 bp heptamer sequences. Our analysis that suggested 13 bp spacer on the 5'RSS and 12bp spacer on the 3'RSS [92] but more refined analysis [94] suggests 12 bp spacer on both 5' and 3' RSS. The $BovD_H$ gene segments, in contrast to other species, are organized in distinct subclusters where 1 to 4 $BovD_H$ gene elements are present separated by 338 to 355 bp. The sequence alignment between $BovD_H$ gene subclusters shows >79% nucleotide identity suggesting that gene duplication events led to expansion of the $BovD_H$ gene locus [91, 93]. A single unusually long D_H-element, $BovD_H2$, exists at the Holstein bovine D_H-locus that has the potential to encode up to 49 codons. The closest D_H2 gene segment in Hereford breed (UMD 3.1 [65]) has the potential to encode 51 codons (unpublished data). The $BovD_H$ Q52 gene is the shortest composed of 14 bp, whereas other $BovD_H$ genes range from 36-148 bp in size. Thus, the $BovD_H$ genes are potentially capable of encoding 3 to 49 codons. Phylogenetically three D_H gene segments, $BovD_H1$, $BovD_H6$ and $BovD_H7$, are closest to chicken DY and D6 genes. The $BovD_H2$, $BovD_H4$, $BovD_H5$ and $BovD_H8$, are closest to rabbit D2B and D5 genes. However. As would be expected, the conserved $BovD_H$ Q52 gene is closest to shark H01 gene. Based on degree of sequence divergence, $BovD_H$ genes are classified into 4 D_H gene families: $BovD_HA$ ($BovD_H1$ and $BovD_H6$), $BovD_HB$ ($BovD_H2$, $BovD_H3$, $BovD_H$ 5, $BovD_H7$ and $BovD_H8$), $BovD_HC$ ($BovD_H4$) and $BovD_HD$ ($BovD_HQ52$). Similar to other species, polymorphism is evident at the $BovD_H$ gene locus remarkable across various cattle breeds [65].

2.3.4. Presence of Two functional J_H Gene Elements

The bovine J_H ($BovJ_H$) genes are located 7 kb upstream of the $C\mu$ exons and span 18 kb. Of the six $BovJ_H$ genes identified in cattle, that lay 130-500 bp apart, only two J_H genes, $BovJ_H1$ and $BovJ_H2$, are expressed as other four $BovJ_H$ genes either lack recombination signal sequence or splice site [94]. The bovine J_H1 gene (pB7S2) has highest nucleotide identity with human J_H4 (87.2%). But $BovJ_H2$ (pB8S1) shows highest nucleotide identity to human J_H5 (84.7%) and mouse J_H1 (79.5%) with relatively lower identity to sheep J_HBr15-gene (82%) [62]. Similar to other mammalian species the $BovJ_H$ genes characteristically encode VTVSS motifs at the 3' end. In contrast to other species, the $BovJ_H$ genes are found duplicated on chromosome 11 [95], reassigned to chromosome 8 [65], in addition to chromosome 21. Nevertheless, this needs to be investigated whether the complete variable heavy chain locus is duplicated or if it reflects partial duplication. It would be useful to elucidate how, if at all, it contributes to antibody repertoire in cattle in the context of allelic exclusion.

2.3.5. Bovine Immunoglobulin Heavy Chain Constant Region

The bovine Ig heavy chain locus is organized similar to mouse [96, 97]. The organization of constant region gene locus - 5'-JH-7kb-μ-5kb-δ-33kb-$\gamma3$-20kb-$\gamma1$-34kb-$\gamma2$-20kb-ϵ-13kb-$\alpha3$-3' - spans approximately 150kb DNA on chromosome 21 [98, 99] [100].

The IgM heavy-chain constant gene ($C\mu$) comprises four constant exons ($C\mu1$-4) and two exons encoding the transmembrane domains (TM1, TM2) . The TM1 exon is spliced to the $C\mu4$ exon, as in other species [101]. Restriction fragment length polymorphism (RFLP) analysis has shown four allelic variants of the $C\mu$ gene. However, three allotypes of bovine IgM have been defined (IgMa, IgMb and IgMc) [102] where nucleotide substitutions in all $C\mu$ exons result in amino acid replacements. Additional bovine IgM variants are derived from cleavage of pre-mRNA at an alternate cryptic 5' splice donor site. This is evidenced by insertion of three in-frame codons at the Cμ1 and Cμ2 junction (e.g., B5D8 IgM) from the intervening intron [102]. Bovine IgM has the lowest number of proline residues in the Cμ2 domain when compared to other species. The relative inflexibility in the bovine Cμ2 domain, may allow for required exposure of C1q-binding site subsequent to antigen binding that may influence its complement fixing ability [102].

Transcriptionally active germline bovine IgD gene has been demonstrated in cattle [96], but definitive evidence for IgD expression [103] is awaited. Interestingly, the first domain of Cδ is highly homologous to Cμ1 demonstrating similarity of 96.6% and 93.5% at the DNA and protein levels, respectively [96]. A gene conversion model has been proposed from the comparisons of the μ and δ CH1 exon sequences in cows, where differences are congregated at the 3' end. This suggests that the δ gene was duplicated from the μ gene based on the structural similarity.

Cattle possess three subclasses of IgG (IgG1, IgG2, IgG3) [97, 104, 105] and these Igs are expressed in serum and milk [1] . Nucleotide sequences of allotypic variants of IgG2 (IgG2a and IgG2b) [104] and IgG3 (IgG3a and IgG3b) [105] in addition to IgG1 (IgG1a, IgG1b, IgG1c and IgG1d) [106, 107] have been described. The variation in BovCγ genes across species suggests that duplication of the BovCγ gene happened at different time points during evolution of the Ig heavy chain locus. For example, cattle have 3 γ genes [97] compared to 4 in humans. It has been demonstrated that the bovine γ1 gene is most likely the ancestral gene since there is an 87.1% similarity to ovine γ1 at the protein level which is significantly higher than the similarity between the γ2 of the two ruminant species (79.8%). This suggests that during evolution γ1 gene was duplicated to form the γ2 gene and further duplicated to generate the γ3 gene. This is supported by the fact that there is greater sequence homology of the γ3 gene with the γ1 gene (85.1%) as opposed to the γ2 gene (83.4%) [98]. A novel feature of cattle IgG1c, is the presence of a unique *Pro-Ala-Ser-Ser* combination at positions 189-192 and again at 205-208 within its Cγ1 domain [107]. This is of interest since this sequence resembles a fibronectin synergy site used in integrin-mediated cell adhesion and migration [108]. The IgG3b differs from IgG3a by 6 amino acids in the coding region and an 84 base pair insertion in the intron between the CH2 and CH3 exons [105].

The bovine epsilon (ε) gene has four exons (Cε1-4) with only 55% sequence similarity with those from humans but 87% with sheep ε-gene. Bovine IgE possesses characteristics similar to human IgE where the skin sensitizing ability is heat labile [109].

The bovine genome has a single Cα gene similar to swine and rodents. Analysis of 50 Swedish bovine genomic DNA samples, using genomic blots and five different restriction enzymes, failed to detect any evidence of polymorphism. Earlier studies, however, demonstrated IgA allotypic variants serologically [110], consistent with demonstration by RFLP of two allelic variants of bovine IgA [111]. This strengthens the argument that even though a single Cα gene exists, there is presence of allelic restriction polymorphism in some cattle breeds (e.g., Holstein) [97]. Cattle IgA has the closest similarity at amino acid sequence level to IgA of swine, another artiodactyl. The nucleotide sequence of three bovine Cα exons, separated by two introns, has been determined from a genomic phage clone [111]. Bovine IgA shares with rabbit IgA3 and IgA4, an additional N-linked glycosylation site at position 282.

Table 3. CDRH lengths, V_H gene families and mechanisms of CDR3H diversification across species

Species	V_H gene families (Clan)	Alternate post-recombination diversification mechanisms	Length (Codons)*			Mechanisms of CDR3H diversification			Reference
			CDR1H	CDR2H	CDR3H	N*	P*	D-D	
Human	7 (I, II &III)	Extensive germline sequence diversity, combinatorial diversity	7	19	2-26	+	+	+ (rare)	[73-75]
Dog	3 (I, II &III)	Extensive germline sequence diversity, combinatorial diversity	5	17	4-24	+	+	?	[76]
Mouse	15 (I, II &III)	Extensive germline sequence diversity, combinatorial diversity	5	17	2-19	+	+	+	[74, 77, 78]
Bat	5	Extensive Combinatorial diversity	5	8-12	12-39	?	?	?	[79]
Rabbit	1	Gene conversion, Ag independent SHM	5-6	13-19	4-19	+	+	?	[21, 80, 81]
Pig	1 (III)	Junctional flexibility	5	16-23	3-25	+	+	?	[1, 20, 72]
Sheep	1 (II)	Ag independent SHM	5-7	16-18	3-23	+	+	?	[49]
Cattle	1 (II)	Long CDR3H, CSNS insertions and Ag independent SHM	5	16	3-61	+	+	?	[56, 62, 63, 82-85]
Horse	3/7 subgroups (I, II&III)	Combinatorial diversity, loop-based enhanced CDR3H flexibility	5-7	13-27	9-26	+	+	+	[86, 87]
Camel	1 & 7 V_{HH}	V_{HH} homodimers	5	16	10-24	+	+	?	[88]
Chicken	1 (III)	Gene conversion	5	17	15-30	?	+	+	[19, 89]

*Numbered according to Kabat [17]; *N or *P nucleotide addition or junctional flexibility via N or P deletions; CSNS = Conserved short nucleotide sequence; D-D = D fusion; SHM = somatic hypermutations; V_{HH} antibodies devoid of light chains; V_{HH}H variable domain/gene of a heavy chain antibody devoid of light chains.

2.4. Light-chain Immunogenetics

2.4.1. Surrogate Light Chains

Unlike mice and humans, where three and two surrogate light chain are identified respectively, four surrogate light chains Vpreb1, Vpreb2, Vpreb3 and IgLL1 are identified in cattle (Ekman *et al.* in press). Since the expression of Vpreb2 and Vpreb3 differs from Vpreb1 and IgLL1 the biological function of Vpreb2 and Vpreb3 seems to be unrelated to B-cell development at the pre-B-cell stage.

2.4.2. The lambda (λ)-light Chain Is Mainly Expressed in Cattle Antibodies

Across species, significant differences exists with regard to expression of either κ (kappa) or λ (lambda) light chains (reviewed by [112]). Chickens exclusively express λ light chains [113] whereas rodents, such as mice, predominantly express κ chains (95%) [69, 114] with a minor role for λ light chains (5%) [115]. In humans, κ and λ light chains are expressed at 60% and 40% frequencies, respectively [17, 116]. A similar κ:λ ratio is also noted in pig antibodies [25]. It is, however, reported that κ light chains may be expressed in 20-25% of sheep antibodies [117-119]. Such a situation is not found in cattle and other ruminant species were λ light chain expression essentially predominates in the antibody repertoire. In camel antibodies, both λ and κ light chains have been noted to be expressed where some of the camel antibodies (IgG2 and IgG3 isotypes) exist as homodimers of V_H chains, devoid of light chains altogether (V_{HH}) [120]. Since little information is available on κ light chain genes in cattle as these are expressed in low frequencies, the most discussion in the following section relates to λ light chain genes.

2.4.3. Kappa (κ) Light Chain Genes

Although earlier reports suggested >98% expression of λ-light chains [1, 121], later reports mention a λ:κ ratio of 91:9 [122] and 4:1 in peripheral blood lymphocytes [123] in cattle. This implies that although there is limited information available on κ light chains they might have a relatively greater role then previously suspected. Kappa genes are found on chromosome 11 localized on a ca. 280kb genomic segment [124]. Twenty two V_κ genes (segments), 3 J_κ and 1 C_κ segments have been identified where recombination occurs probably only by deletion [124]. Not enough data is available to conclude that the low frequency of expressed κ-light chains is due to seemingly lower number of $BovV_\kappa$ genes as compared to $BovV_\lambda$ genes in cattle genome. But additional mechanisms seen in mice, e.g., endogenous counter selection [125], relevant to shaping of developing antibody repertoire may be involved. More research on the number of functional V_κ gene families and their expression would shed more light on the role of the kappa light chain in the antibody repertoire of cattle.

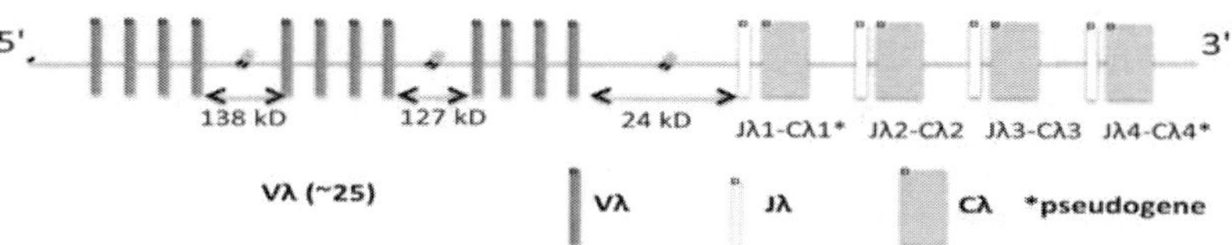

Figure 2. Organization of λ-light chain locus on chromosome 17 of cattle modified [127, 129].

2.4.4. Limited Germline Sequence Divergence Exists in λ-light Chain Genes

The bovine V_λ genes ($BovV_\lambda$) are classified into three V_λ gene families, $BovV_\lambda 1$, $BovV_\lambda 2$, and $BovV_\lambda 3$, based on nucleotide identity ≥80% [126]. The majority of $BovV_\lambda$ genes group into the $BovV_\lambda 1$ family that can also be classified on the bases of serine signatures. Such patterns of serine residues of $BovV_\lambda$ genes, similar to sheep and goat, differ from other mammals and thus provide a possible marker to track divergent evolution in V_λ genes [126]. The $BovV_\lambda 2$ and $BovV_\lambda 3$ gene families are small and comprise only few members. The $BovV_\lambda 1$ and $BovV_\lambda 2$ gene families are closest to sheep $V_\lambda 1$ (92.6%) and $V_\lambda 2$ (88.9%) gene families and also human $V_\lambda 1$ (74.8%) and $V_\lambda 2$ (79.3%) families, respectively. Similarly, $BovV_\lambda 3$ gene is closest to unclassified sheep $V_\lambda 6B$ gene (75%) and human $V_\lambda 3$ gene (LBR1104; 73.8%). Interestingly, the variable Serine content and distinct Serine distribution patterns in $BovV_\lambda$ domains closely match the phylogenetic tree indicating separation of $BovV_\lambda 1$, $BovV_\lambda 2$ and $BovV_\lambda 3$ gene families. Evidence exists for the presence of $BovV_\lambda$ pseudogenes (members of $BovV_\lambda 1$ and $V_\lambda 2$ gene family; [127]) that might contribute through gene conversion [128]. Lambda light chain genes are found on chromosome 17 and probably other yet unknown locations in the bovine genome [124]. Unlike mice, but similar to horse, four $BovJ_\lambda$-$BovC_\lambda$ units are identified on chromosome 17 (Figure 2) [129], where $J_\lambda 2$-$C_\lambda 2$ and $J_\lambda 3$-$C_\lambda 3$ are functional. Sequence analyses of the Hereford cow genome showed two copies of the $BovC_\lambda 2$ gene where the most 5' $C_\lambda 2$ proximal gene was lacking the $BovJ_\lambda$ gene to form $J_\lambda 1$-$C_\lambda 1$ cassette [127]. Such a discrepancy could be due to differences in the accuracy of sequencing or possible polymorphism at the λ-locus. $BovC_\lambda 1$ and $BovC_\lambda 4$ genes have been determined to be pseudogenes [129]. The $BovJ_\lambda 3$-$BovC_\lambda 3$ unit is preferentially used together with predominantly expressed $V_\lambda 1$ genes in the primary antibody repertoire [127, 129]. Interestingly, $V_\lambda 1d$, $V_\lambda 1e$ and $V_\lambda 1x$ preferentially pair with VDJ recombinations encoding exceptionally long CDR3H (up to 61 amino acids) [126]. Thus, restricted $V_\lambda 1$-$J_\lambda 3$-$C_{\lambda\lambda} 3$ recombinations encode most of the λ-light chain repertoire in cattle [127].

3. CONSTRUCTION OF BOVINE ANTIBODY REPERTOIRE

3.1. Mechanisms of Antibody Diversification

Given the limited sequence divergence and complexity, both at $BovV_H$ and $BovV_\lambda$ loci, only limited combinatorial diversity can be generated in the primary antibody repertoire of cattle. Although some evidence for gene conversion has been suggested for λ light chain variable region [53, 128], no such evidence is forthcoming for the variable heavy chain, though V_H pseudogenes exist [130]. The cattle heavy chain region employs two different strategies to diversify the developing antibody repertoire. First, somatic hypermutation contributes to the diversification of the developing nascent antibody repertoire early during B cell ontogeny without prior exposure to exogenous antigen. A similar strategy is also employed by another ruminant species, sheep, where somatic mutations diversify B cells developing in ileal PP without exposure to exogenous antigen [131]. By contrast, somatic hypermutations do not contribute to fetal antibody repertoire diversification in swine, another artiodactyl [20], though class switch recombination is seen. The CDR3H size in cattle antibodies is relative long as compared to other species rodent, pig, dog and horse) with an average length of 22.7±3.2 considering CDR3H loops ranging from 16 to 28 codons [86]. The CDR3H size further varies between IgM (21.7±1.8) and IgG (18.2±1.3) isotypes [130]. Interestingly, some of the cattle IgM antibodies have unusually long CDR3H size (>50 to 61 amino acids) that is not yet observed to occur in other mammalian species. These atypically long CDR3H with multiple cysteine residues [82] are likely to generate extensive configurational diversity via possible inter-CDR or intra-CDR3H disulphide bridging. As compared to IgM, higher diversity indicies are noted in the third framework region of IgG antibodies [130]. The antibodies expressing exceptionally long CDR3H, pair exclusively with V_λ light chains that have *Ser90* conserved in the CDR3L region [82]. The restricted V_H and V_λ pairing in antibodies with exceptionally long CDR3H suggests a minimal structural support role of lambda light chain in antigen binding with no direct contact with the target epitope [126]. Both N and/or P additions, apart from junctional flexibility, have been observed both in fetal and adult VDJ recombinations in cattle, in contrast to mice where such N or P insertions are few or absent in the neonatal VDJ recombinations. Most remarkable, however is the insertion of conserved short nucleotide sequences (CSNS; 13 to 18 'A' rich nucleotides) specifically at V_H-D_H junctions in adult VDJ recombinations that arise subsequent to antigen exposure in the periphery. Such CSNS insertions are absent in fetal VDJ rearrangements but contribute towards generation of CDR3H as long as 61 amino acids in adult VDJ recombinations. The mechanisms of such CSNS insertions specifically at V_H-D_H junction of $V_H D_H J_H C_\mu$ are yet to be delineated.

3.2. Development of Neonatal Variable Region Repertoire

The $V_H D_H J_H$ and $V_\lambda J_\lambda$ recombinations are seen in splenic B-cells at 125 days of gestation, including appearance of serum Ig by day 145 of fetal life (Table 2). Some of the splenic B-cells at this developmental stage show only $V_H D_H J_H$, but no $V_\lambda J_\lambda$ recombination. In some instances, λ light chains may be secreted alone due to non-productive VDJ rearrangement. Extensive CDR3H size heterogeneity (9-56 amino acids) is noted early during B cell ontogeny. The fetal VDJ recombinations with long CDR3H are encoded by a single germline $BovV_H$, gl.110.20, together with the longest $BovD_H$ gene, $BovD_H2$. In fact two $BovV_H$ genes (gl.110.20 and BF2B5 [56]) are preferentially expressed in fetal VDJ recombinations. Somatic hypermutation is evident in CDR1H and CDR2H of fetal VDJ recombinations (125 days old) without prior exposure to external antigens. Thus, somatic hypermutation provides the mechanism for diversifying developing nascent repertoire given the restricted germline sequence and combinatorial diversity. This is because of biased 'hot spot' triplets and nucleotide base use in CDR, which predispose them to mutation [130]. This is consistent with similar observations in sheep, where somatic hypermutation has been reported in the developing antibody repertoire in ileal PP without prior exposure to external antigen [131]. Unlike mice, both N and P additions, together with junctional flexibility have been observed in fetal VDJ recombination. Conserved $BovD_HQ52$ gene element is not expressed in fetal VDJ recombinations. This is contrary to preferential D_HQ52 gene usage seen in neonatal mice. In fact, D_H7 and D_H5 genes are predominantly expressed in fetal and adult B cells [92].

Table 4. Characteristic features of the Bovine immune system

1.	Limited germline sequence divergence of variable region heavy chains (V, D and J) and light chain (V and J) genes [132]
2.	Restricted potential combinatorial diversity in the development of primary antibody repertoire [62-64]. BovV$_H$ 11 functional genes, D$_H$ 10, J$_H$ 2, heavy variable region VxDxJ=11x10x2= 220 and V$_\lambda$ 17 genes J$_\lambda$ 2 genes [127] light chain variable region VxJ=17x2= 34 would generate combinatorial diversity of 220x34= 0.7x10^4 combinations.
3.	Antibodies expressing exceptionally long CDR3H, originating during B cell ontogeny, occurs at a frequency of 8-10% in IgM expressed on circulating B cells [56, 82].
4.	Restricted V$_\lambda$ and V$_H$ pairing occurs among IgM antibodies expressing exceptionally long CDR3H [126].
5.	Antigen independent somatic hypermutation contributes to antibody diversification early during B-cell ontogeny [130].
6.	Multiple cysteine residues in the CDR3H possibly permit inter- or intra- CDR3H disulphide bridging giving rise to possible configurational diversity of VDJ combining sites[82].
7.	Somatic hypermutation, significantly contributes to antibody diversification in the periphery during affinity maturation [130].
8.	Unlike other vertebrate species, insertion of conserved short nucleotide sequence (CSNS) specifically at V$_H$ D$_H$ junction provide molecular basis of atypical CDR3H length generation subsequent to antigen exposure in the periphery [92].
9.	The ileal Peyers' patches constitute the primary lymphoid organ where nascent immune repertoire develops [1].
10.	Lambda light chains provide a minimal role in antigen binding and provide a supporting platform in the context of antigen recognition [126].
11.	Bovine IgM is relatively less flexible because of fewer proline residues in the Cμ region that acts as a hinge [102].
12.	Apart from allotypic variants, bovine IgM variants also arise due to alternate cryptic splice donor sites [102].
13.	Genes for encoding IgD are present in the genome but IgD is not expressed [103].
14.	IgG1 protects mucosal surfaces in addition to of IgA [29, 42] in cattle.
15.	The Cγ1 domain of IgG1c allotype has characteristic *Pro-Ala-Ser-Ser* and, hence, it may have a role in cell adhesion and migration [107].

Analyses of BovJ$_H$ gene encoded FR4 region shows that bovine J$_H$1 gene (pB7S2), homolog of human J$_H$5, is predominantly expressed both in fetal and adult VDJ recombinations [62]. In addition to possible gene conversion [128], λ light chain diversification might occur via untemplated somatic hypermutations [53].

3.3. Development of Adult Variable Region Immunoglobulin Repertoire

As in fetus and neonates, exceptionally long CDR3H is encoded by a member of BovV$_H$1, the longest BovD$_H$2 segment and BovJ$_H$1 genes in the adult antibody repertoire, apart from junctional flexibility and/or N or P insertions. Nevertheless, 13-18 nucleotides are specifically inserted at V_H-D_H junctions that extend the CDR3H size, up to 61 amino acids, beyond the germline encoded potential. The unusually long CDR3H undergoes somatic mutation during affinity maturation as well upon antigen exposure in the periphery [130, 132]. While most BovV$_H$ and BovD$_H$ genes are expressed in adult VDJ recombinations, with the exception of BovD$_H$Q52, there is predominant expression of BovJ$_H$1 gene. In general, extensive somatic hypermutation in the CDRs, common to many species, occur during affinity maturation in the periphery. As would be expected, transition nucleotide substitutions predominate over transversions in adult VDJ recombinations [130], consistent with evolutionary conservation of somatic mutation machinery. What is not understood, however, is IgM isotype restricted expression of exceptionally long CDR3H in B cells that constitute an important proportion (8-10%) of circulating B cells. The possibility of exceptionally long CDR3H in other bovine antibody isotypes is not excluded. Nevertheless, IgM antibodies with an exceptionally long CDR3H provide protection against blood-borne infectious agents throughout the vasculature.

CONCLUSION

Significant advances in knowledge about the genetic elements and their organization in cattle, though some gaps exist, provide novel insights into the generation of antibody repertoire relevant to development of new generation of immunodiagnostics and therapeutics. While the molecular origin of unusually long CDR3H is now elucidated [93], the mechanism of specific addition of 'A' rich CSNS at the V_H-D_H junction needs to be elucidated. The restriction of exceptionally long CDR3H to IgM isotype [130] is yet to be defined. Despite a significant number of Vκ genes in cattle, it remains to be determined as to why λ-light chains are predominantly expressed in cattle antibodies. The ability of IgG1 isotype to protect mucosal surfaces in cattle needs to be examined in functional context. Certain unique characteristics of the bovine immune system (Table 4), have advanced our understanding of the origin of humoral immunity taking into consideration comparative functional immunogenetics across species. For example, exceptionally long CDR3H ($\leq$61 amino acids) in cattle antibodies provides new opportunities to engineer desired antibodies and new generation of vaccines, e.g., via antigenization or epitope grafting. A better understanding of the bovine immune system has an economic impact directly as a means to enhance production in beef and dairy cattle by preventing diseases and, also, as a potential economic target, e.g., production of specific antibodies in milk for pharmaceutical purposes. Cloning methods have permitted the generation of transgenic cattle that express human immunoglobulin [133], but their regulation in is not understood. Further, desired minimal antigen binding fragments against a target infectious agent have been developed for disease prevention and diagnosis in cattle, e.g., Bovine Herpes Virus-1 [83]. Engineered bovine Igs are also relevant to disease prevention and diagnosis in humans by exploiting bovine Ig for antigenization for the purpose of oral immunization relevant to enteric infectious diseases.

REFERENCES

[1]   Butler JE. Immunoglobulin diversity, B-cell and antibody repertoire development in large farm animals. *Rev Sci Tech.* 1998;17(1):43-70.

[2]   Flajnik MF, Du Pasquier L. Evolution of innate and adaptive immunity: can we draw a line? *Trends Immunol.* 2004;25(12):640-4.

[3]   Cooper MD, Alder MN. The evolution of adaptive immune systems. *Cell.* 2006;124(4):815-22.

[4]   Pancer Z, Cooper MD. The evolution of adaptive immunity. *Annu Rev Immunol.* 2006;24497-518.

[5]   Saha NR, Smith J, Amemiya CT. Evolution of adaptive immune recognition in jawless vertebrates. *Semin Immunol.* 2010;22(1):25-33.

[6]   Flajnik MF. Comparative analyses of immunoglobulin genes: surprises and portents. *Nat Rev Immunol.* 2002;2(9):688-98.

[7]   Du Pasquier L. Meeting the demand for innate and adaptive immunities during evolution. *Scand J Immunol.* 2005;62 Suppl 139-48.

[8]   Marchalonis JJ, Adelman MK, Schluter SF, Ramsland PA. The antibody repertoire in evolution: chance, selection, and continuity. *Dev Comp Immunol.* 2006;30(1-2):223-47.

[9]   Das S, Nozawa M, Klein J, Nei M. Evolutionary dynamics of the immunoglobulin heavy chain variable region genes in vertebrates. *Immunogenetics.* 2008;60(1):47-55.

[10]   Criscitiello MF, Flajnik MF. Four primordial immunoglobulin light chain isotypes, including lambda and kappa, identified in the most primitive living jawed vertebrates. *Eur J Immunol.* 2007;37(10):2683-94.

[11]   Das S, Nikolaidis N, Klein J, Nei M. Evolutionary redefinition of immunoglobulin light chain isotypes in tetrapods using molecular markers. *Proc Natl Acad Sci U S A.* 2008;105(43):16647-52.

[12]   Tonegawa S. Somatic generation of antibody diversity. *Nature.* 1983;302(5909):575-81.

[13]   Jones JM, Simkus C. The roles of the RAG1 and RAG2 "non-core" regions in V(D)J recombination and lymphocyte development. *Arch Immunol Ther Exp (Warsz).* 2009;57(2):105-16.

[14]   Kaushik A, Lim W. The primary antibody repertoire of normal, immunodeficient and autoimmune mice is characterized by differences in V gene expression. *Res Immunol.* 1996;147(1):9-26.

[15]   Neuberger MS, Scott J. Immunology. RNA editing AIDs antibody diversification? *Science.* 2000;289(5485):1705-6.

[16]   Hackney JA, Misaghi S, Senger K, Garris C, Sun Y, Lorenzo MN, et al. DNA targets of AID evolutionary link between antibody somatic hypermutation and class switch recombination. *Adv Immunol.* 2009;101163-89.

[17]   Kabat EA, Wu TT. Identical V region amino acid sequences and segments of sequences in antibodies of different specificities. Relative contributions of VH and VL genes, minigenes, and complementarity-determining regions to binding of antibody-combining sites. *J Immunol.* 1991;147(5):1709-19.

[18]   Pink JR, Vainio O, Rijnbeek AM. Clones of B lymphocytes in individual follicles of the bursa of Fabricius. *Eur J Immunol.* 1985;15(1):83-7.

[19] Reynaud CA, Anquez V, Dahan A, Weill JC. A single rearrangement event generates most of the chicken immunoglobulin light chain diversity. *Cell.* 1985;40(2):283-91.

[20] Butler JE, Weber P, Sinkora M, Sun J, Ford SJ, Christenson RK. Antibody repertoire development in fetal and neonatal piglets. II. Characterization of heavy chain complementarity-determining region 3 diversity in the developing fetus. *J Immunol.* 2000;165(12):6999-7010.

[21] Knight KL. Restricted VH gene usage and generation of antibody diversity in rabbit. *Annu Rev Immunol.* 1992;10593-616.

[22] Weinstein PD, Anderson AO, Mage RG. Rabbit IgH sequences in appendix germinal centers: VH diversification by gene conversion-like and hypermutation mechanisms. *Immunity.* 1994;1(8):647-59.

[23] Brandon MR, Watson DL, Lascelles AK. The mechanism of transfer of immunoglobulin into mammary secretion of cows. *Aust J Exp Biol Med Sci.* 1971;49(6):613-23.

[24] Schultz RD, Dunne HW, Heist CE. Transport, distribution and synthesis of bovine immunoglobulins. Ontogeny of the bovine immune response. *J Dairy Sci.* 1971;54(9):1321-2.

[25] Butler JE, Zhao Y, Sinkora M, Wertz N, Kacskovics I. Immunoglobulins, antibody repertoire and B cell development. *Dev Comp Immunol.* 2009;33(3):321-33.

[26] Butler JE, Kerli ME. Immunocytes and immunoglobulins in milk. In: al OPe, editor. *Mucosal Immunology.* 3 ed. New York: Academic Press, 2004. p. 1763-93.

[27] Farrell HM, Jr., Jimenez-Flores R, Bleck GT, Brown EM, Butler JE, Creamer LK, et al. Nomenclature of the proteins of cows' milk--sixth revision. *J Dairy Sci.* 2004;87(6):1641-74.

[28] Hurley W. Proteins. *Advanced dairy chemistry.* 3 ed. New York: Kluwer Academic, 2003. p. 421-47.

[29] Newby TJ, Bourne FJ. Relative resistance of bovine and porcine immunoglobulins to proteolysis. *Immunol Commun.* 1976;5(7-8):631-5.

[30] Leach JL, Sedmak DD, Osborne JM, Rahill B, Lairmore MD, Anderson CL. Isolation from human placenta of the IgG transporter, FcRn, and localization to the syncytiotrophoblast: implications for maternal-fetal antibody transport. *J Immunol.* 1996;157(8):3317-22.

[31] Kacskovics I. Fc receptors in livestock species. *Vet Immunol Immunopathol.* 2004;102(4):351-62.

[32] Cervenak J, Kacskovics I. The neonatal Fc receptor plays a crucial role in the metabolism of IgG in livestock animals. *Vet Immunol Immunopathol.* 2009;128(1-3):171-7.

[33] Kacskovics I, Kis Z, Mayer B, West AP, Jr., Tiangco NE, Tilahun M, et al. FcRn mediates elongated serum half-life of human IgG in cattle. *Int Immunol.* 2006;18(4):525-36.

[34] Brambell FW, Hemmings WA, Morris IG. A Theoretical Model of Gamma-Globulin Catabolism. *Nature.* 1964;2031352-4.

[35] Anderson CL, Chaudhury C, Kim J, Bronson CL, Wani MA, Mohanty S. Perspective--FcRn transports albumin: relevance to immunology and medicine. *Trends Immunol.* 2006;27(7):343-8.

[36] Mayer B, Zolnai A, Frenyo LV, Jancsik V, Szentirmay Z, Hammarstrom L, et al. Redistribution of the sheep neonatal Fc receptor in the mammary gland around the time of parturition in ewes and its localization in the small intestine of neonatal lambs. *Immunology.* 2002;107(3):288-96.

[37] Laegreid WW, Heaton MP, Keen JE, Grosse WM, Chitko-McKown CG, Smith TP, et al. Association of bovine neonatal Fc receptor alpha-chain gene (FCGRT) haplotypes with serum IgG concentration in newborn calves. *Mamm Genome.* 2002;13(12):704-10.

[38] Mayer B, Kis Z, Kajan G, Frenyo LV, Hammarstrom L, Kacskovics I. The neonatal Fc receptor (FcRn) is expressed in the bovine lung. *Vet Immunol Immunopathol.* 2004;98(1-2):85-9.

[39] Story CM, Mikulska JE, Simister NE. A major histocompatibility complex class I-like Fc receptor cloned from human placenta: possible role in transfer of immunoglobulin G from mother to fetus. *J Exp Med.* 1994;180(6):2377-81.

[40] Telemo E, Hanson LA. Antibodies in milk. *J Mammary Gland Biol Neoplasia.* 1996;1(3):243-9.

[41] Adamski FM, Demmer J. Immunological protection of the vulnerable marsupial pouch young: two periods of immune transfer during lactation in Trichosurus vulpecula (brushtail possum). *Dev Comp Immunol.* 2000;24(5):491-502.

[42] Butler J, Kerli ME. Immunocytes and immunoglobulins in milk. In: al OPe, editor. *Mucosal Immunology.* 3 ed. New York: Academic Press, 2004. p. 1763-93.

[43] Chhabra PC, Goel MC. Normal profile of immunoglobulins in sera and tracheal washings of chickens. *Res Vet Sci.* 1980;29(2):148-52.

[44] Gapper LW, Copestake DE, Otter DE, Indyk HE. Analysis of bovine immunoglobulin G in milk, colostrum and dietary supplements: a review. *Anal Bioanal Chem.* 2007;389(1):93-109.

[45] Butler JE. Why I agreed to do this. Dev Comp Immunol. 2006;301-17.

[46] Kim K, Keller MA, Heiner DC. Immunoglobulin G subclasses in human colostrum, milk and saliva. *Acta Paediatr.* 1992;81(2):113-8.

[47] Yasuda M, Fujino M, Nasu T, Murakami T. Histological studies on the ontogeny of bovine gut-associated lymphoid tissue: appearance of T cells and development of IgG+ and IgA+ cells in lymphoid follicles. *Dev Comp Immunol.* 2004;28(4):357-69.

[48] Alitheen NB, McClure S, McCullagh P. B-cell development: one problem, multiple solutions. *Immunol Cell Biol.* 2010;88(4):445-50.

[49] Yasuda M, Jenne CN, Kennedy LJ, Reynolds JD. The sheep and cattle Peyer's patch as a site of B-cell development. *Vet Res.* 2006;37(3):401-15.

[50] Butler JE, Maxwell, C.F., Pierce, C.S., Hylton, M.B., Asofsky, R., Kiddy, C.A. Studies on the relative synthesis and distribution of IgA and IgG1 in various tissues and body fluids of the cow. *J Immunol.* 1972;10938–46.

[51] Schultz RD, Dunne HW, Heist CE. Ontogeny of the bovine immune response. *Infect Immun.* 1973;7(6):981-91.

[52] David CW, Norrman J, Hammon HM, Davis WC, Blum JW. Cell proliferation, apoptosis, and B- and T-lymphocytes in Peyer's patches of the ileum, in thymus and in lymph nodes of preterm calves, and in full-term calves at birth and on day 5 of life. *J Dairy Sci.* 2003;86(10):3321-9.

[53]   Lucier MR, Thompson RE, Waire J, Lin AW, Osborne BA, Goldsby RA. Multiple sites of V lambda diversification in cattle. *J Immunol.* 1998;161(10):5438-44.

[54]   Schultz RD, Confer F, Dunne HW. Occurrence of blood cells and serum proteins in bovine fetuses and calves. *Can J Comp Med.* 1971;35(2):93-8.

[55]   Osburn BI, MacLachlan NJ, Terrell TG. Ontogeny of the immune system. *J Am Vet Med Assoc.* 1982;181(10):1049-52.

[56]   Saini SS, Kaushik A. Extensive CDR3H length heterogeneity exists in bovine foetal VDJ rearrangements. Scand J Immunol. 2002;55(2):140-8.

[57]   Ishino S, Kadota K, Matsubara Y, Agawa H, Matsui N. Immunohistochemical studies on ontogeny of bovine lymphoid tissues. *J Vet Med Sci.* 1991;53(5):877-82.

[58]   Meyer A, Parng CL, Hansal SA, Osborne BA, Goldsby RA. Immunoglobulin gene diversification in cattle. *Int Rev Immunol.* 1997;15(3-4):165-83.

[59]   Zhao Y, Jackson SM, Aitken R. The bovine antibody repertoire. *Dev Comp Immunol.* 2006;30(1-2):175-86.

[60]   Senogles DR, Muscoplat CC, Paul PS, Johnson DW. Ontogeny of circulating B lymphocytes in neonatal calves. *Res Vet Sci.* 1978;25(1):34-6.

[61]   Tobin-Janzen TC, Womack JE. Comparative mapping of IGHG1, IGHM, FES, and FOS in domestic cattle. *Immunogenetics.* 1992;36(3):157-65.

[62]   Saini SS, Hein WR, Kaushik A. A single predominantly expressed polymorphic immunoglobulin VH gene family, related to mammalian group, I, clan, II, is identified in cattle. *Mol Immunol.* 1997;34(8-9):641-51.

[63]   Berens SJ, Wylie DE, Lopez OJ. Use of a single VH family and long CDR3s in the variable region of cattle Ig heavy chains. *Int Immunol.* 1997;9(1):189-99.

[64]   Sinclair MC, Gilchrist J, Aitken R. Bovine IgG repertoire is dominated by a single diversified VH gene family. *J Immunol.* 1997;159(8):3883-9.

[65]   Zimin AV, Delcher AL, Florea L, Kelley DR, Schatz MC, Puiu D, et al. A whole-genome assembly of the domestic cow, Bos taurus. *Genome Biol.* 2009;10(4):R42.

[66]   Tomlinson IM, Cook GP, Carter NP, Elaswarapu R, Smith S, Walter G, et al. Human immunoglobulin VH and D segments on chromosomes 15q11.2 and 16p11.2. *Hum Mol Genet.* 1994;3(6):853-60.

[67]   Flajnik MF, Kasahara M. Origin and evolution of the adaptive immune system: genetic events and selective pressures. *Nat Rev Genet.* 2010;11(1):47-59.

[68]   Saini S, Teo K, Nangpal A, Mallard BA, Kaushik A. Homologues of murine Vh11 gene are conserved during evolution. *Exp Clin Immunogenet.* 1996;13(3-4):154-60.

[69]   Kofler R, Geley S, Kofler H, Helmberg A. Mouse variable-region gene families: complexity, polymorphism and use in non-autoimmune responses. *Immunol Rev.* 1992;1285-21.

[70]   Charlton KA, Moyle S, Porter AJ, Harris WJ. Analysis of the diversity of a sheep antibody repertoire as revealed from a bacteriophage display library. *J Immunol.* 2000;164(12):6221-9.

[71]   Dufour V, Malinge S, Nau F. The sheep Ig variable region repertoire consists of a single VH family. *J Immunol.* 1996;156(6):2163-70.

[72]   Sun J, Kacskovics I, Brown WR, Butler JE. Expressed swine VH genes belong to a small VH gene family homologous to human VHIII. *J Immunol.* 1994;153(12):5618-27.

[73]   Matsuda F, Ishii K, Bourvagnet P, Kuma K, Hayashida H, Miyata T, et al. The complete nucleotide sequence of the human immunoglobulin heavy chain variable region locus. *J Exp Med.* 1998;188(11):2151-62.

[74]   Wu TT, Johnson G, Kabat EA. Length distribution of CDRH3 in antibodies. *Proteins.* 1993;16(1):1-7.

[75]   Corbett SJ, Tomlinson IM, Sonnhammer EL, Buck D, Winter G. Sequence of the human immunoglobulin diversity (D) segment locus: a systematic analysis provides no evidence for the use of DIR segments, inverted D segments, "minor" D segments or D-D recombination. *J Mol Biol.* 1997;270(4):587-97.

[76]   Bao Y, Guo Y, Xiao S, Zhao Z. Molecular characterization of the VH repertoire in Canis familiaris. *Vet Immunol Immunopathol.* 2010;137(1-2):64-75.

[77]   Gangemi RM, Singh AK, Barrett KJ. Independently derived IgG anti-DNA autoantibodies from two lupus-prone mouse strains express a VH gene that is not present in most murine strains. *J Immunol.* 1993;151(9):4660-71.

[78]   Mainville CA, Sheehan KM, Klaman LD, Giorgetti CA, Press JL, Brodeur PH. Deletional mapping of fifteen mouse VH gene families reveals a common organization for three Igh haplotypes. *J Immunol.* 1996;156(3):1038-46.

[79]   Bratsch S, Wertz N, Chaloner K, Kunz TH, Butler JE. The little brown bat, M. lucifugus, displays a highly diverse V(H), D(H) and J(H) repertoire but little evidence of somatic hypermutation. *Dev Comp Immunol.* 2010.

[80]   Allegrucci M, Young-Cooper GO, Alexander CB, Newman BA, Mage RG. Preferrential rearrangement in normal rabbits of the 3' VHa allotype gene that is deleted in Alicia mutants; somatic hypermutation/ conversion may play a major role in generating the heterogeneity of rabbit heavy chain variable region sequences. *Eur J Immunol.* 1991;21(2):411-7.

[81]   Friedman ML, Tunyaplin C, Zhai SK, Knight KL. Neonatal VH, D, and JH gene usage in rabbit B lineage cells. *J Immunol.* 1994;152(2):632-41.

[82]   Saini SS, Allore B, Jacobs RM, Kaushik A. Exceptionally long CDR3H region with multiple cysteine residues in functional bovine IgM antibodies. *Eur J Immunol.* 1999;29(8):2420-6.

[83]   Koti M, Farrugia W, Nagy E, Ramsland PA, Kaushik AK. Construction of single-chain Fv with two possible CDR3H conformations but similar inter-molecular forces that neutralize bovine herpesvirus 1. *Mol Immunol.* 2010;47(5):953-60.

[84]   Armour KL, Tempest PR, Fawcett PH, Fernie ML, King SI, White P, et al. Sequences of heavy and light chain variable regions from four bovine immunoglobulins. *Mol Immunol.* 1994;31(17):1369-72.

[85]   Sinclair MC, Gilchrist J, Aitken R. Molecular characterization of bovine V lambda regions. *J Immunol.* 1995;155(6):3068-78.

[86]   Almagro JC, Martinez L, Smith SL, Alagon A, Estevez J, Paniagua J. Analysis of the horse V(H) repertoire and comparison with the human IGHV germline genes, and sheep, cattle and pig V(H) sequences. *Mol Immunol.* 2006;43(11):1836-45.

[87]   Sun Y, Wang C, Wang Y, Zhang T, Ren L, Hu X, et al. A comprehensive analysis of germline and expressed immunoglobulin repertoire in the horse. *Dev Comp Immunol.* 2010;34(9):1009-20.

[88] Conrath KE, Wernery U, Muyldermans S, Nguyen VK. Emergence and evolution of functional heavy-chain antibodies in Camelidae. *Dev Comp Immunol.* 2003;27(2):87-103.

[89] Reynaud CA, Anquez V, Weill JC. The chicken D locus and its contribution to the immunoglobulin heavy chain repertoire. *Eur J Immunol.* 1991;21(11):2661-70.

[90] Meek KD, Hasemann CA, Capra JD. Novel rearrangements at the immunoglobulin D locus. Inversions and fusions add to IgH somatic diversity. *J Exp Med.* 1989;170(1):39-57.

[91] Shojaei F, Saini SS, Kaushik AK. Unusually long germline DH genes contribute to large sized CDR3H in bovine antibodies. *Mol Immunol.* 2003;40(1):61-7.

[92]   M, Kataeva G, Kaushik AK. Organization of D(H)-gene locus is distinct in cattle. *Dev Biol (Basel).* 2008;132307-13.

[93] Koti M, Kataeva G, Kaushik AK. Novel atypical nucleotide insertions specifically at VH-DH junction generate exceptionally long CDR3H in cattle antibodies. *Mol Immunol.* 2010;47(11-12):2119-28.

[94] Merelli I, Guffanti A, Fabbri M, Cocito A, Furia L, Grazini U, et al. RSSsite: a reference database and prediction tool for the identification of cryptic Recombination Signal Sequences in human and murine genomes. *Nucleic Acids Res.* 2010;38(Web Server issue):W262-7.

[95] Hosseini A, Campbell G, Prorocic M, Aitken R. Duplicated copies of the bovine JH locus contribute to the Ig repertoire. *International immunology.* 2004;16(6):843-52.

[96] Zhao Y, Kacskovics I, Pan Q, Liberles DA, Geli J, Davis SK, et al. Artiodactyl IgD: the missing link. *J Immunol.* 2002;169(8):4408-16.

[97] Knight KL, Suter M, Becker RS. Genetic engineering of bovine Ig. Construction and characterization of hapten-binding bovine/murine chimeric IgE, IgA, IgG1, IgG2, and IgG3 molecules. *J Immunol.* 1988;140(10):3654-9.

[98] Zhao Y, Kacskovics I, Rabbani H, Hammarstrom L. Physical mapping of the bovine immunoglobulin heavy chain constant region gene locus. *J Biol Chem.* 2003;278(37):35024-32.

[99] Chowdhary BP, Fronicke L, Gustavsson I, Scherthan H. Comparative analysis of the cattle and human genomes: detection of ZOO-FISH and gene mapping-based chromosomal homologies. *Mamm Genome.* 1996;7(4):297-302.

[100] Gu F, Chowdhary BP, Andersson L, Harbitz I, Gustavsson I. Assignment of the bovine immunoglobulin gamma heavy chain (IGHG) gene to chromosome 21q24 by in situ hybridization. *Hereditas.* 1992;117(3):237-40.

[101] Mousavi M, Rabbani H, Pilstrom L, Hammarstrom L. Characterization of the gene for the membrane and secretory form of the IgM heavy-chain constant region gene (C mu) of the cow (Bos taurus). *Immunology.* 1998;93(4):581-8.

[102] Saini SS, Kaushik A. Origin of bovine IgM structural variants. *Mol Immunol.* 2001;38(5):389-96.

[103] Naessens J. Surface Ig on B lymphocytes from cattle and sheep. *Int Immunol.* 1997;9(3):349-54.

[104] Kacskovics I, Butler JE. The heterogeneity of bovine IgG2--VIII. The complete cDNA sequence of bovine IgG2a (A2) and an IgG1. *Mol Immunol.* 1996;33(2):189-95.

[105] Rabbani H, Brown WR, Butler JE, Hammarstrom L. Polymorphism of the IGHG3 gene in cattle. *Immunogenetics.* 1997;46(4):326-31.

[106] Symons DB, Clarkson CA, Beale D. Structure of bovine immunoglobulin constant region heavy chain gamma 1 and gamma 2 genes. *Mol Immunol.* 1989;26(9):841-50.

[107] Saini SS, Farrugia W, Muthusamy N, Ramsland PA, Kaushik AK. Structural evidence for a new IgG1 antibody sequence allele of cattle. *Scand J Immunol.* 2007;65(1):32-8.

[108] Ochsenhirt SE, Kokkoli E, McCarthy JB, Tirrell M. Effect of RGD secondary structure and the synergy site PHSRN on cell adhesion, spreading and specific integrin engagement. *Biomaterials.* 2006;27(20):3863-74.

[109] Hammer DK, Kickhofen B, Schmid T. Detection of homocytotropic antibody associated with a unique immunoglobulin class in the bovine species. *Eur J Immunol.* 1971;1(4):249-57.

[110] De Benedictis G, Capalbo P, Dragone A. Identification of an allotypic IgA in cattle serum. *Comp Immunol Microbiol Infect Dis.* 1984;7(1):35-42.

[111] Brown WR, Rabbani H, Butler JE, Hammarstrom L. Characterization of the bovine C alpha gene. *Immunology.* 1997;91(1):1-6.

[112] Saini SS KA. Immunoglobulin genes and their diversification in vertebrates. *Curr Trends in Immunol.* 2002;4161-76.

[113] Reynaud CA, Dahan A, Weill JC. Complete sequence of a chicken lambda light chain immunoglobulin derived from the nucleotide sequence of its mRNA. *Proc Natl Acad Sci U S A.* 1983;80(13):4099-103.

[114] Hood L, McKean D, Farnsworth V, Potter M. Mouse immunoglobulin chains. A survey of the amino-terminal sequences of kappa chains. *Biochemistry.* 1973;12(4):741-9.

[115] Sanchez P, Nadel B, Cazenave PA. V lambda-J lambda rearrangements are restricted within a V-J-C recombination unit in the mouse. *Eur J Immunol.* 1991;21(4):907-11.

[116] Blomberg BB, Glozak MA, Donohoe ME. Regulation of human lambda light chain gene expression. *Ann N Y Acad Sci.* 1995;76484-98.

[117] Hein WR, Dudler L. Diversity of Ig light chain variable region gene expression in fetal lambs. *Int Immunol.* 1998;10(9):1251-9.

[118] Griebel PJ, Kennedy L, Graham T, Davis WC, Reynolds JD. Characterization of B-cell phenotypic changes during ileal and jejunal Peyer's patch development in sheep. *Immunology.* 1992;77(4):564-70.

[119] Jenne CN, Kennedy LJ, Reynolds JD. Antibody repertoire development in the sheep. *Dev Comp Immunol.* 2006;30(1-2):165-74.

[120] Hamers-Casterman C, Atarhouch T, Muyldermans S, Robinson G, Hamers C, Songa EB, et al. Naturally occurring antibodies devoid of light chains. *Nature.* 1993;363(6428):446-8.

[121] Butler JE. Immunoglobulin gene organization and the mechanism of repertoire development. *Scand J Immunol.* 1997;45(5):455-62.

[122] Arun SS, Breuer W, Hermanns W. *Immunohistochemical examination of light-chain expression (lambda/kappa ratio) in canine, feline, equine, bovine and porcine plasma cells.* Zentralbl Veterinarmed A. 1996;43(9):573-6.

[123] Beyer J, Kollner B, Teifke JP, Starick E, Beier D, Reimann I, et al. Cattle infected with bovine leukaemia virus may not only develop persistent B-cell lymphocytosis but also persistent B-cell lymphopenia. *J Vet Med B Infect Dis Vet Public Health.* 2002;49(6):270-7.

[124] Ekman A, Niku M, Liljavirta J, Iivanainen A. Bos taurus genome sequence reveals the assortment of immunoglobulin and surrogate light chain genes in domestic cattle. *BMC Immunol.* 2009;10(1):22.

[125] Knott J, Bona C, Kaushik A. The primary antibody repertoire of kappa-deficient mice is characterized by non-stochastic Vlamda1 + V(H) gene family pairings and a higher degree of self-reactivity. *Scand J Immunol.* 1998;48(1):65-72.

[126] Saini SS, Farrugia W, Ramsland PA, Kaushik AK. Bovine IgM antibodies with exceptionally long complementarity-determining region 3 of the heavy chain share unique structural properties conferring restricted VH + Vlambda pairings. *Int Immunol.* 2003;15(7):845-53.

[127] Pasman Y, Saini SS, Smith E, Kaushik AK. Organization and genomic complexity of bovine lambda-light chain gene locus. *Vet Immunol Immunopathol.* 2010.

[128] Parng CL, Hansal S, Goldsby RA, Osborne BA. Gene conversion contributes to Ig light chain diversity in cattle. *J Immunol.* 1996;157(12):5478-86.

[129] Chen L, Li M, Li Q, Yang X, An X, Chen Y. Characterization of the bovine immunoglobulin lambda light chain constant IGLC genes. *Vet Immunol Immunopathol.* 2008;124(3-4):284-94.

[130] Kaushik AK, Kehrli ME, Jr., Kurtz A, Ng S, Koti M, Shojaei F, et al. Somatic hypermutations and isotype restricted exceptionally long CDR3H contribute to antibody diversification in cattle. *Vet Immunol Immunopathol.* 2009;127(1-2):106-13.

[131] Weill JC, Reynaud CA. Early B-cell development in chickens, sheep and rabbits. *Curr Opin Immunol.* 1992;4(2):177-80.

[132] Kaushik A, Shojaei F, Saini SS. Novel insight into antibody diversification from cattle. *Vet Immunol Immunopathol.* 2002;87(3-4):347-50.

[133] Kuroiwa Y, Kasinathan P, Choi YJ, Naeem R, Tomizuka K, Sullivan EJ, et al. Cloned transchromosomic calves producing human immunoglobulin. *Nat Biotechnol.* 2002;20(9):889-94.

In: Cattle: Domestication, Diseases and the Environment
Editor: George Liu
ISBN: 978-1-62417-820-7
© 2013 Nova Science Publishers, Inc.

Chapter 2

THE TRAPPIN GENE FAMILY: STRUCTURE, FUNCTION AND EVOLUTION

George E. Liu[1], and Derek M. Bickhart[1]*

[1]USDA-ARS, ANRI, Bovine Functional Genomics Laboratory, Beltsville, MD, US

ABSTRACT

Trappins are a family of small secretary host-defense peptides that have many functions. Most members exhibit antiprotease and antimicrobial activities, while others influence inflammation, immunity and the promotion of tissue repair. Considered to be important guardians of mucosal surfaces, trappins possess an N-terminal transglutaminase substrate (TGS) domain and a C-terminal whey acidic protein (WAP) four-disulphide core (WFDC) domain. The numbers and compositions of trappin genes vary among eutherian mammalian species. While there is a single trappin-2 gene in human and sheep, no trappin gene was found in mouse and rat. By contrast, multiple duplicated trappin paralogs were found in pig, cattle, guinea pig, armadillo and Afrotherian species (elephant, tenrec, and hyrax). Trappin duplication events appear to have occurred independently in these mammalian lineages over a long time period, suggesting their potential roles in species formation and animal domestication. Recent duplication and accelerated evolution of trappin genes in pig, cattle and armadillo demonstrate that mammalian genomes have the capability to form trappin multigenes to acquire antimicrobial activities for niche-specific pathogens.

Keywords: Trappin, elafin, structure, function, evolution

---

* Corresponding Author: GEL: Bovine Functional Genomics Laboratory, USDA-ARS, Building 200, Room 124B, BARC-East, Beltsville, MD 20705, USA. E-mail: George.Liu@ars.usda.gov, Voice Phone: +1-301-504-9843, Fax: +1-301-504-8414.

1. INTRODUCTION

One of the barriers between an organism and the external environment is the layer of mucosal fluids critical for maintaining interface integrity and protecting host from damage or infection. Mucosal fluids, including seminal fluid, cervical mucus, bronchial and nasal secretions and tears, are complicated in composition, containing many small peptides, ions and polysaccharides. Trappins are a family of small secretory host defense peptides found in mucosal fluids belonging to the WFDC (*Wh*ey Acidic Protein *Fo*ur-*Di*sulphide *Co*re)-type protein family. Although trappins were first considered to be simple, local protease inhibitors, we now realize their broad roles in orchestrating intracellular communication, host defense mechanisms and immune system modulations. In this chapter, we use human trappin-2/elafin as an example of the trappin family of genes, thereby discussing the family's gene and protein structures as well as their pleiotropic functions. We will then examine their roles in mammalian evolution and domestication and conclude with their therapeutic potentials in human and animal health.

2. STRUCTURE AND EXPRESSION

2.1. Trappin-2/elafin Protein Structure

As mentioned before, trappins belong to the four-disulphide core (4DSC) protein or WAP (Whey Acidic Protein) family. The name of 'trappin' stands for *TR*ansglutaminase substrate and w*AP* domain containing Prote*IN* (Zeeuwen et al., 1997; Furutani et al., 1998). This unifying nomenclature reflects their two domain structure and their tendency to "trap" inhibitors in extracellular matrix proteins. Human trappin-2, which is also known as elastase-specific inhibitor (ESI) or protease inhibitor 3 (PI3), is a well studied skin-derived antileukoproteinase (SKALP). The trappin-2 protein was first isolated from human lung sputum and skin tissues (Wiedow et al., 1990; Sallenave and Ryle, 1991). The human trappin-2 gene (*PI3*) encodes 117 amino acids in length, containing a 22-residue signal peptide, followed by an N-terminal TGS (transglutaminase substrate) or cementoin domain (38 amino acids) and a C-terminal inhibitory WAP domain (57 amino acids) (Figure 1). All known trappin genes consist of three exons: exon 1 typically encodes a signal peptide, exon 2 encodes most of the TGS and WAP domains, and exon 3 encodes the 3' untranslated region (Figure 1). After the signal peptide is cleaved during secretion, the mature human trappin-2 product is a 9.9 kDa, nonglycosylated, 95-residue cationic protein. Elafin is a ~6 kDa C-terminus product created after an additional cleavage of the trappin-2 protein (Schalkwijk et al., 1999). The N-terminal TGS or cementoin domain contains multiple GQDPVK motifs that act as a transglutaminase substrate, permitting cross-linking, or 'trapping', of the inhibitor to extracellular matrix proteins (Schalkwijk et al., 1999). The C-terminal WAP domain of the trappin family is structurally similar to other WAP proteins. For example, it is highly homologous to the second WAP domain of SLPI (secretory leucocyte protease inhibitor), which is also a WFDC-type protease inhibitor.

2.2. Expression and Regulation in Cells and Tissues

Trappin-2 is typically found in mucosal fluids and mucosal surfaces within the lungs, skin, gastrointestinal tract, genital tract and other organs (Table 1). Often, epithelial cells and inflammatory cells are the primary producers of trappin-2 (Williams et al., 2006; Sallenave, 2010).

Multiple studies have focused on the regulation of trappin-2 expression in healthy and inflamed states. Trappin-2/elafin mRNA expression can be increased to high concentrations (μM levels) by high concentrations of free neutrophil elastase (NE) in bronchial epithelial cells at inflammatory sites (Reid et al., 1999; van Wetering et al., 2000). Although normal bronchial epithelial cells, alveolar epithelial cells and keratinocytes produce little trappin-2 protein *in vitro*, IL-1β and TNFα can dramatically increase its production in these cell types (Sallenave et al., 1994; Tanaka et al., 2000). Several signal pathways are implicated in these responses, involving c-Jun, mitogen-activated protein kinase (MAPK) and nuclear factor-κB (NF-κB) (Pfundt et al., 2000; Pfundt et al., 2001; Bingle et al., 2001). These cytokines also appear to induce a higher level of trappin-2 expression than antileukoproteinase (SLPI) (Sallenave et al., 1994). This observation suggests that SLPI functions as a microbial defense peptide for normal cellular states and trappin-2/elafin provides acute protection during inflammatory conditions.

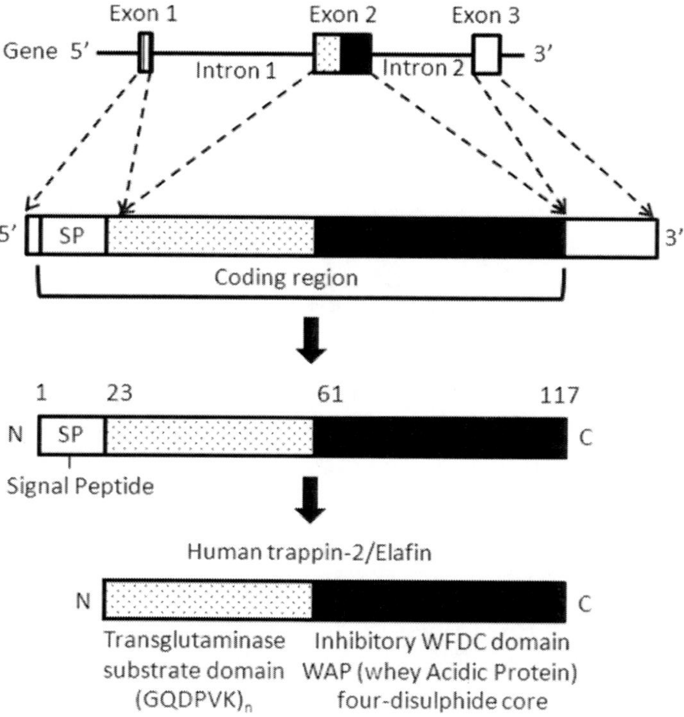

Figure 1. Structure of human trappin-2 gene. Structure of the gene and biosynthesis process of human trappin-2. Human trappin-2 gene encodes 117 amino acids in length, comprising a 22-residue signal peptide, followed by an N-terminal TGS (transglutaminase substrate) or cementoin domain and a C-terminal inhibitory WAP domain.

3. FUNCTION

In addition to its antiprotease function, trappin-2 has increasingly been shown to provide antimicrobial and immunomodulatory activities (Williams et al., 2006; Sallenave, 2010).

Table 1. Properties of trappin-2/elafin and SLPI

Protein	Trappin, Elafin	Secretory leukocyte pepridase inhibitor
Gene	PI3	SLPI
Molecular mass (pI)	10/6 kDa (9.0/8.5)	12 kDa (9.5)
Number of WAP domain(s)	1	2
Tissue expression	Skin, endometrim, large intestine, brochial secretions, seminal plasma	Seminalervical mucus, endometrium, bronchial secretions
Protease inhibitory spectrum	Neutrophil elastase and proteinase 3	Neutrophil elastase, cathepsin G, trypsin, chymotrypsin and mast cell chymase and tryptase.
Function	Innate immunity, antibacterial, antifungal, antiviral, anti-inflammatory, tissue repair	Innate immunity, antibacterial, antifungal, antiviral, anti-inflammatory, tissue repair
Antimicrobial properties	*E. coli, P. aeruginosa, S. aureus, K. pneumoniae, S. pneumoniae, H. influenzae, A. fumigatus and C. albicans*	*E. coli, P. aeruginosa, S. aureus, A. fumigatus and C. albicans*
LPS binding	Yes	Yes
Antiviral activity	HIV-1	HIV-1
Anti-inflammatory properties	Inhibition of NF-kB and AP-1 activation and proinflammatory cytokine production	Inhibition of NF-kB activation and pro-inflammatory cytokine production

3.1. Antiprotease Function

Trappin-2 inhibits NE, pancreatic elastase and proteinase-3, but does not inhibit cathepsin G, trypsin or chymotrypsin. By contrast, SLPI can inhibit cathepsin G but not proteinase 3 (Eisenberg et al., 1990; Henriksen et al., 2004). Compared to SLPI, trapping-2 has a distinct and more restricted spectrum of inhibitory specificities (Table 1). Trappin-2's antiprotease activity appears to be exclusive to its C-terminal WAP domain, with one leucine residue working as the active site responsible for inhibitory activity (Eisenberg et al., 1990). Although both trappin-2 and elafin have antiprotease activity, elafin has a reduced inhibitory effect.

3.2. Antimicrobial Activity

Antimicrobial peptides play a crucial role in human immunity. Important antimicrobial peptides include defensins, cathelicidins, lysozymes, and lactoferrins. Trappin-2/elafin and SLPI, belonging to the WAP domain containing class of antimicrobial peptides, are also important in inhibition of NE and killing of microbes.

Trappin-2 and elafin are broad-spectrum antimicrobial peptides, capable of inhibiting both Gram-positive and Gram-negative bacteria. Both trappin-2 and elafin have been shown to be effective against *Pseudomonas aeruginosa*, *Staphylococcus aureus*, *Streptococcus pneumonia* and *Escherichia coli* (Table 1). Their cationic charges could allow them to disrupt bacterial membranes in a similar mechanism employed by cationic antimicrobial proteins (Williams et al., 2006). Trappin-2/elafin antimicrobial activity was found to be attenuated by both high salt and heparin, further suggesting cationic charge is involved (Baranger et al., 2008). It was demonstrated that both the cementoin and WFDC domains of elafin/trappin-2 possess significant independent antibacterial activity (Simpson et al., 1999). As elafin contains only one WFDC domain, the precursor protein trappin-2 shows greater antibacterial activity than elafin (Simpson et al., 1999). Trappin-2 and elafin have also been shown to possess antifungal activity against *Aspergillus fumigatus*, a common airway pathogen, and *Candida albicans*, which is most commonly found on the epidermis (Tomee et al., 1997; Baranger et al., 2008).

Another important function of trappin-2 and elafin is their antiviral activity. Elevated trappin-2/elafin in the female genital tract is associated with protection against HIV infection (Iqbal et al., 2009). A better studied example is SLPI, in which two potential anti-HIV modes were reported: (1) SLPI blocks viral entry/fusion via binding to annexin II, a macrophage receptor for HIV(Ma et al., 2004); (2) SLPI interferes with HIV fusion with the T-cell by binding to scramblase 1, a membrane protein that interacts with CD4 and controls the movement of the plasma membrane (Py et al., 2009). Given the structural similarity between their WFDC domains, trappin-2/elafin is believed to interact similarly with key cell surface cofactors to prevent HIV invasion (Iqbal et al., 2009).

3.3. Anti-inflammatory Activity

Trappin-2 and elafin can inhibit the inflammatory response both *in vitro* and *in vivo* by preventing the activation of NF-κB (nuclear factor κB) in the presence of LPS (lipopolysaccharide) and LTA (lipoteichoic acid) (McMichael et al., 2005). Trappin-2/elafin achieves their anti-inflammatory activity via both extracellular and intracellular mechanisms (Henriksen et al., 2004). Outside of the cell, elafin can bind and neutralize LPS thereby preventing TLR (Toll-like receptor) activation (McMichael et al., 2005). Interaction of trappin-2 with LPS results in an augmentation of the LPS-induced TNFα response. Elafin also plays a role in the resolution of inflammation by inhibiting NE-mediated cleavage of CD14 (Williams et al., 2006). Within the cell, elafin prevents AP-1 (activator protein 1) and NF-κB activation by inhibiting LPS-induced phosphorylation of AP-1, c-Jun, and JNK (c-Jun Nterminal kinase) (Butler et al., 2006). Elafin can also inhibit the ubiquitin-proteasome degradation pathway, leading to an accumulation of ubiquitinated IRAK-1 (IL-1R-associated kinase 1) and IκB (inhibitor of NF-κB) α/β in LPS-activated cells (Butler et al., 2006).

In a mouse model of LPS-induced inflammation, recombinant human trappin-2 significantly inhibited MIP-2 (macrophage inflammatory protein-2) and KC (keratinocyte chemoattractant) levels, neutrophil influx and protease activity in bronchoalveolar lavage fluids (Vachon et al., 2002). Similarly, trappin-2 overexpression (using adenovirus constructs or in elafin-transgenic mice) led to lower serum-to-BAL ratios of proinflammatory cytokines such as TNFα, MIP-2 and monocyte chemoattractant protein 1 than found in wild-type mice (Sallenave et al., 2003). Trappin-2 overexpression also results in an increased influx of inflammatory cells in response to infection/inflammation (Sallenave et al., 2003). Since SLPI and trappin-2 respond differently to proinflammatory cytokines such as IL-1β and TNFα, they seem to have distinct functions instead of redundant roles.

3.4. Immunomodulatory Activity

Beyond their previously described functions, trappin-2/elafin can also modulate innate and adaptive immune responses. Sallenave et al. demonstrated that trappin-2 induces a type 1-biased inflammatory and immunological response (Th1; cellular and humoral) in the lungs and spleens of mice overexpressing the protein (Sallenave et al., 2003). The Th1 skewing effect of trappin-2 is likely to be mediated through the increase in numbers and/or activation status of lung APCs (antigen presenting cells). Along with the number increase of activated dendritic cells, increased levels of proinflammatory cytokines IL-12, TNFα and IFNγ (interferon γ) were observed in bronchoalveolar lavage fluids (Roghanian et al., 2006). Similar clinic observations can be found in farmer's lung and psoriasis patients, where increased levels of trappin-2 are associated with a type I immune response (Schalkwijk et al., 1993; Tremblay et al., 1996).

Cultures of human γ δ T-cells can produce trappin-2/elafin (both mRNA and protein) when induced by *Pseudomonas aeruginosa*. While most CD3+ T-cells express the α β TCR (T-cell receptor) in the peripheral blood, 2-5% of them express the γ δ TCR. In contrast to the peripheral blood, 20–30% of local T-cells in the small intestine are γ δ T-cells, suggesting γ δ T-cells are a major T-cell population in mucosal surfaces (Kabelitz et al., 2000; Hayday, 2000). γ δ T cells can also function as APCs and secret antimicrobial peptides like granulysin and LL37/cathelicidin (Agerberth et al., 2000; Dieli et al., 2001; Brandes et al., 2005). Therefore, γ δ T-cells are considered to link innate and adaptive immunity by sharing both the adaptive (e.g. TCR expression) and the innate immune system (e.g. Toll-like receptor expression and antigen-presenting capacity) (Hayday, 2000). Through the secretion of antimicrobial peptides like trappin-2/elafin, defensins and cathelicidins, γ δ T-cells contribute to the recruitment of neutrophils and the opsonization of pathogens on mucosal surfaces.

These results suggest that trappin-2/elafin may have dual immune functions depending on the environment. Trappin-2/elafin can down-regulate undesired systemic inflammatory responses while promoting immunostimulation, thereby priming the immune system.

4. EVOLUTION

4.1. Identification of Trappin and other Genes in Mammals

The numbers and compositions of trappin genes vary among mammalian species as indicated by cDNA cloning, PCR and sequence similarity search efforts. While there is a single trappin-2 gene in humans and sheep, no trappin gene was found in mouse and rat. A single trappin-2 was also found in 11 eutherian mammals, including chimpanzee, rhesus macaque, bushbaby, dog, cat, horse, cow, European shrew, European hedgehog, megabat, and microbat.

Additional trappin duplicates exist in pig, cattle, guinea pig, armadillo (5, 5, 2 and 5 additional copies, respectively) and Afrotherian species (1 additional copy for each species in elephant, tenrec, and hyrax).

Since no trappin gene was found in chicken, zebra finch, xenopus, fish, sea squirt, insects, and *C. elegans*, trappin-2 is likely the ancestral form of the trappin gene family. Other trappins are likely lineage-specific paralogs, with trappin-null species such as mouse and rat being the exception.

Pigs have at least six trappin genes: trappins 1, 2, 3, 7, 8, and 9. A short mobile element (SINE) is found in intron 2 of the trappin genes of the Suidae (Tamechika et al., 1996; Furutani et al., 1998). Cattle also have 6 known trappin genes: trappins 2, 4, 5, 6, 19 and 20 (Zeeuwen et al., 1997).

Bovine trappin-19 and trappin-20 are closely related to bovine trappin-2, suggesting that they are recently duplicated bovine specific paralogous genes. Afrotherian species have two trappin paralogs: trappins 2 and 18. Afrotherian trappin-18 is a unique paralog and analyses suggest that it is likely derived from an ancient duplication (Kato et al., 2010).

4.2. Origin of Trappin Genes

The two domain structure of trappins is likely derived from exon shuffling. The introns, exons and other non-coding regions near the first TGS domain of trappin genes have significant similarity with rapidly evolving seminal vesicle transcribed (REST) genes (Lundwall and Ulvsback, 1996).

The REST genes, as their name suggests, encode a group of seminal-vesicle TGS substrates. The second WAP domain of trappin-2 and the second WAP domain of SLPI are quite similar in their sequences and functions (antiproteolytic and antimicrobial activities), suggesting that the WAP domains of trappin and SLPI share a common ancestor.

This mosaic pattern of homology in trappin genes indicates that trappin genes likely originated from the shuffling of exons between ancestral TGS-like and WFDC-like genes (Figure 2).

As described below, trappin-2, SLPI and semenogelin genes (members of the REST gene family) are all localized together in the genome, providing strong support for this hypothesis.

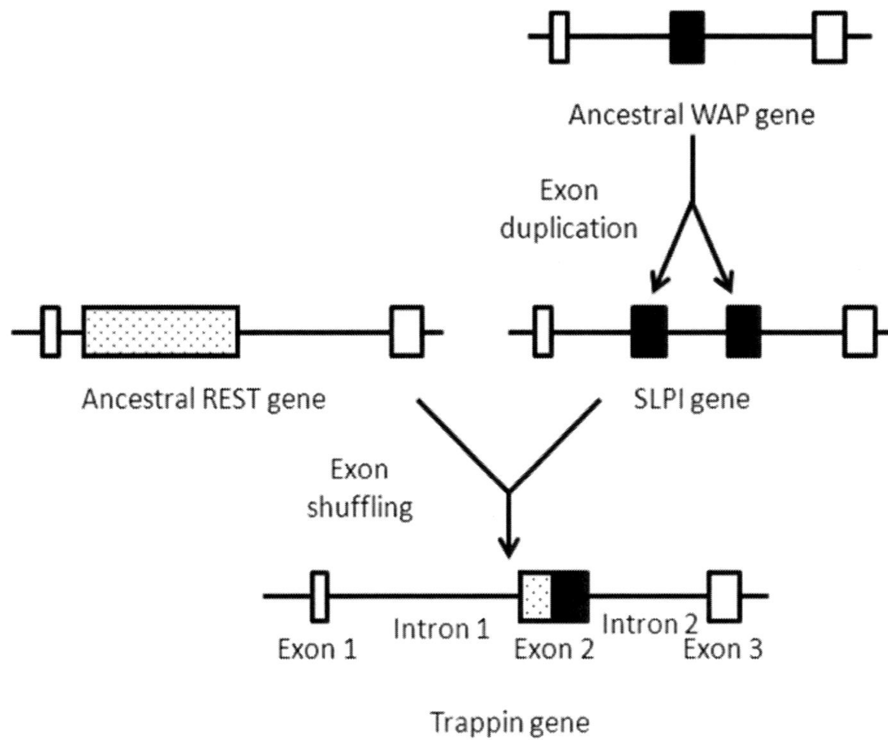

Figure 2. Evolution of trappin genes. Trappin genes may originate from an ancient TGS (transglutaminase substrate) gene and obtain a WAP domain possibly by exon shuffling.

4.3. Genomic Loci around Trappin Genes

Human Trappin-2 is encoded by the *PI3* gene which is located in the same chromosome region 20q12-13 as the other WFDC genes, such as the SLPI and semenogelin genes. The conserved synteny of WFDC loci has been observed in primates, rodents, pigs, dogs and cattle (Clauss et al., 2002; Hurle et al., 2007; Kato et al., 2010). Hurle et al. found that primate WFDC locus contains two tandem duplicons (WFDC12-to-ΨPI3 and PI3-to-ΨWFCD15d), and suggested that trappin-2 and WFDC12 have a common ancestral gene (Hurle et al., 2007). As expected, the trappin-2 gene was not found in the mouse WFDC locus. By contrast, WFDC12 and ΨWFDC15 were not found in the bovine WFDC locus. The bovine trappin genes (trappins 19, 20, 5 and 2) display a tandem pattern, suggesting that these genes could arise through recent local duplications (Figure 3).

4.4. Dates of Duplications

Using different phylogenetic software (BEAST or MEGA) and various reference points, Kato et al. estimated the time range of the trappin gene duplication in pig, cow, armadillo, guinea pig, and Afrotheria (elephant, hyrax, and tenrec) as 3.3-7.8, 8.8-12.6, 11.4-15.9, 35-79, and 161-244 Mya (million-years ago), respectively (Figure 4) (Kato et al., 2010). Pig and cattle trappin genes were predicted to be relatively young. For example, when the divergence time between sheep and cattle (18.3 Mya) was used as a reference point, the date of the duplication of pig and cattle trappin gene families were calculated as 7.8 and 9.7 Mya, respectively. Similarly, the date of the duplication of the armadillo trappins was calculated as 15.5 Mya. Conversely, the guinea pig trappin family was estimated to have originated 55.2 Mya, and the Afrotherian trappin subfamily was calculated to have originated 91.9 Mya (Figure 4).

4.5. Accelerated Evolution and Positive Selection

Normally most important genes are under purifying selection due to functional constrains. One of the striking features of the trappin genes is a surprisingly low degree of conservation of exon sequences compared to that of the intron sequences (Schalkwijk et al., 1999). The coding regions of trappin multigenes of almadillo, bovine, and pig have evolved much faster than the noncoding exons, introns, and the flanking regions, suggesting that these genes have undergone accelerated evolution. Based on their dN/dS ratios, significant positive Darwinian selection was observed in pig trappin-3 and trappin-9 (Furutani et al., 1998; Kato et al., 2010).

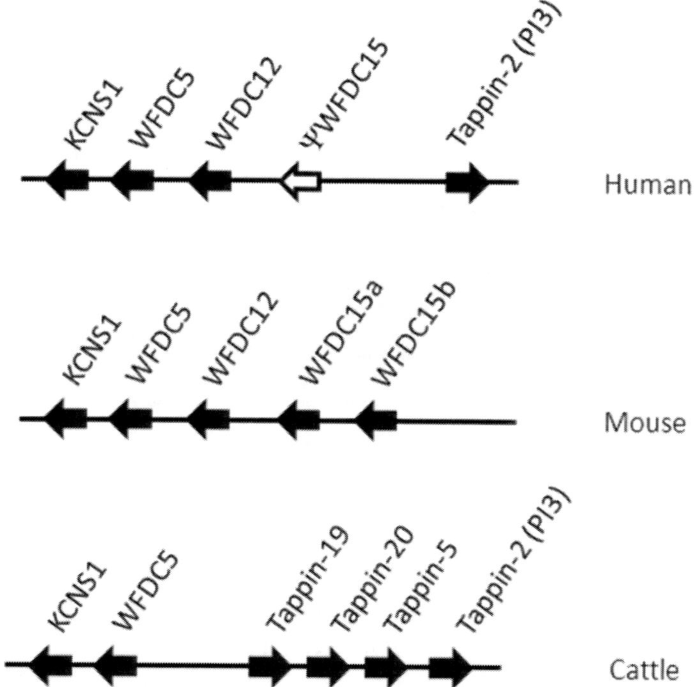

Figure 3. Conserved synteny around trappin(s) in the WFDC locus. Human WFDC locus contains a WFDC12 gene and its pseudogene (ΨWFDC15) while mouse WFDC locus contains no trappin-2 gene. Bovine WFDC locus does not have WFDC12 or ΨWFDC15. The bovine trappin genes (trappin-19, -20, -5 and -2) are arranged in a tandem duplication pattern.

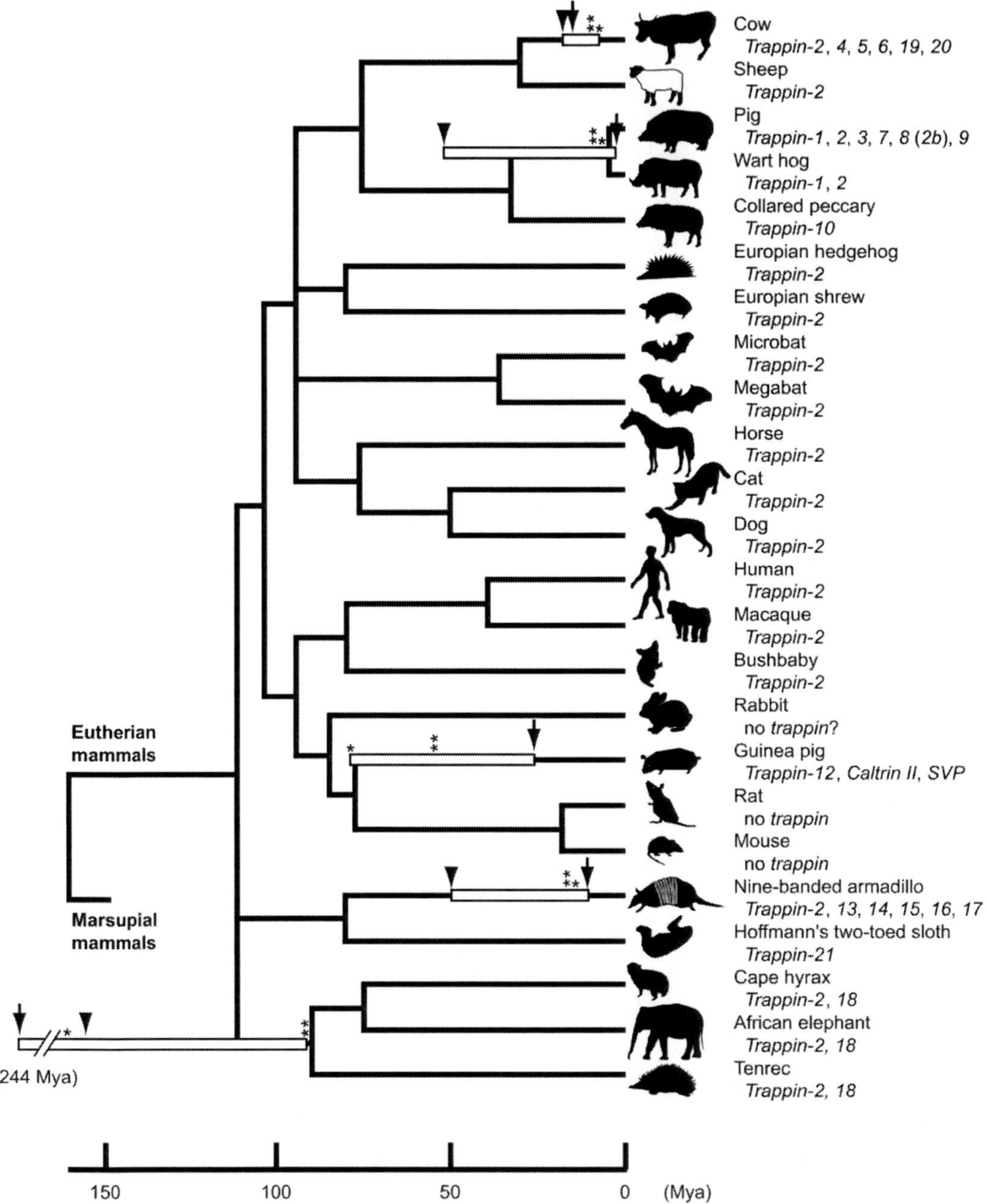

Figure 4. History of the evolution of trappin genes in mammals. Estimated time ranges of trappin gene duplications are indicated by open boxes on the generally accepted mammalian phylogeny. BEAST/Bayesian estimations of duplications using the nucleotide and the amino acid sequences of trappin genes are indicated by arrows and arrow heads, respectively (Drummond and Rambaut, 2007). The dates of duplication estimated by MEGA software (Tamura et al., 2007) using single reference point are indicated by asterisks. The dates of duplications individually estimated by MEGA software for each species are indicated by double asterisks. Mya, million years ago. Adapted from (Kato et al., 2010).

The findings of recently-duplicated, accelerated-evolved trappin multigenes in three individual species demonstrate that mammalian genomes have the potential to form trappin multigenes within a short period (several million years). As pointed out by Kato et al., selective pressures that formed the trappin multigenes may be relate to some niche-specific pathogens, and the variety of amino acid sequences in the WAP-domain may contribute to the acquisition of antimicrobial activities for a large spectrum of pathogens (Kato et al., 2010). Tissue distribution of trappin paralogs in pig and cow has been shown to vary among genes: porcine trappin-2 is expressed in the trachea and the large intestine, porcine trappin-1 in the small intestine, bovine trappin-2 in the epidermis and the tongue, bovine trappin-4 in the trachea and the tongue, and bovine trappin-5 in the trachea (Zeeuwen et al., 1997). Therefore, the aforementioned selective pressures might also affect the regulation of the tissue-specific expression of trappin genes.

5. THERAPEUTICS FUNCTIONS

As described previously, SLPI and trappin-2/elafin can protect the female genital tract against HIV. Muto et al. also reported that UVA light induces the expression of elafin in skin fibroblasts to protect against proteolytic damage (Muto et al., 2007). Trappin-2 is also highly protective against gut colitis inflammation (Sallenave, 2010). In clinic settings, reduced expressions of trappin-2/elafin contributed to inflammatory processes in Crohn's disease and ulcerative colitis (Schmid et al., 2007). These findings highlight important roles of these peptides in innate viral recognition and tissue protection. Therefore, understanding the mechanisms of these factors in mucosal fluids may significantly impact human health.

There is a potential to develop SLPI and trappin-2/elafin as novel therapeutics in animal models and clinical trials. For example, SLPI and elafin/trappin-2 can be used as inhaled drugs for treating chronic lung diseases such as CF (cystic fibrosis) and COPD (chronic obstructive pulmonary disease). In a phase II trials, elafin was tested in the treatment of a variety of human inflammatory diseases. These include elafin's therapeutic effects on post-operative inflammation and its reduction of post-operative morbidity after cancer, heart surgery and organ transplantation. However, host and bacterial proteases may reduce the benefits of these types of protein therapies. Future improvement of their resistances to protease degradation will be needed to provide effective treatment strategies.

ACKNOWLEDGMENTS

G.E.L. was supported by NRI/AFRI grants no. 2007-35205-17869 and 2011-67015-30183 from the USDA CSREES (now NIFA) and Project 1265-31000-098-00 from USDA-ARS. Mention of trade names or commercial products in this article is solely for the purpose of providing specific information and does not imply recommendation or endorsement by the US Department of Agriculture. The USDA is an equal opportunity provider and employer.

REFERENCES

Agerberth, B., J. Charo, J. Werr, B. Olsson, F. Idali, L. Lindbom, R. Kiessling, H. Jornvall, H. Wigzell, and G. H. Gudmundsson. 2000. The human antimicrobial and chemotactic peptides LL-37 and alpha-defensins are expressed by specific lymphocyte and monocyte populations. *Blood* 96:3086-3093.

Baranger, K., M. L. Zani, J. Chandenier, S. Dallet-Choisy, and T. Moreau. 2008. The antibacterial and antifungal properties of trappin-2 (pre-elafin) do not depend on its protease inhibitory function. *FEBS J* 275:2008-2020.

Bingle, L., T. D. Tetley, and C. D. Bingle. 2001. Cytokine-mediated induction of the human elafin gene in pulmonary epithelial cells is regulated by nuclear factor-kappaB. *Am. J Respir. Cell Mol. Biol.* 25:84-91.

Brandes, M., K. Willimann, and B. Moser. 2005. Professional antigen-presentation function by human gammadelta T Cells. *Science* 309:264-268.

Butler, M. W., I. Robertson, C. M. Greene, S. J. O'Neill, C. C. Taggart, and N. G. McElvaney. 2006. Elafin prevents lipopolysaccharide-induced AP-1 and NF-kappaB activation via an effect on the ubiquitin-proteasome pathway. *J Biol. Chem.* 281:34730-34735.

Clauss, A., H. Lilja, and A. Lundwall. 2002. A locus on human chromosome 20 contains several genes expressing protease inhibitor domains with homology to whey acidic protein. *Biochem. J* 368:233-242.

Dieli, F., M. Troye-Blomberg, J. Ivanyi, J. J. Fournie, A. M. Krensky, M. Bonneville, M. A. Peyrat, N. Caccamo, G. Sireci, and A. Salerno. 2001. Granulysin-dependent killing of intracellular and extracellular Mycobacterium tuberculosis by Vgamma9/Vdelta2 T lymphocytes. *J Infect. Dis.* 184:1082-1085.

Drummond, A. J. and A. Rambaut. 2007. BEAST: Bayesian evolutionary analysis by sampling trees. *BMC Evol. Biol.* 7:214.

Eisenberg, S. P., K. K. Hale, P. Heimdal, and R. C. Thompson. 1990. Location of the protease-inhibitory region of secretory leukocyte protease inhibitor. *J Biol. Chem.* 265:7976-7981.

Furutani, Y., A. Kato, H. Yasue, L. J. Alexander, C. W. Beattie, and S. Hirose. 1998. Evolution of the trappin multigene family in the Suidae. *J Biochem.* 124:491-502.

Hayday, A. C. 2000. [gamma][delta] cells: a right time and a right place for a conserved third way of protection. *Annu. Rev. Immunol.* 18:975-1026.

Henriksen, P. A., M. Hitt, Z. Xing, J. Wang, C. Haslett, R. A. Riemersma, D. J. Webb, Y. V. Kotelevtsev, and J. M. Sallenave. 2004. Adenoviral gene delivery of elafin and secretory leukocyte protease inhibitor attenuates NF-kappa B-dependent inflammatory responses of human endothelial cells and macrophages to atherogenic stimuli. *J Immunol.* 172:4535-4544.

Hurle, B., W. Swanson, and E. D. Green. 2007. Comparative sequence analyses reveal rapid and divergent evolutionary changes of the WFDC locus in the primate lineage. *Genome Res.* 17:276-286.

Iqbal, S. M., T. B. Ball, P. Levinson, L. Maranan, W. Jaoko, C. Wachihi, B. J. Pak, V. N. Podust, K. Broliden, T. Hirbod, R. Kaul, and F. A. Plummer. 2009. Elevated elafin/trappin-2 in the female genital tract is associated with protection against HIV acquisition. *AIDS* 23:1669-1677.

Kabelitz, D., A. Glatzel, and D. Wesch. 2000. Antigen recognition by human gammadelta T lymphocytes. *Int. Arch. Allergy Immunol.* 122:1-7.

Kato, A., A. P. Rooney, Y. Furutani, and S. Hirose. 2010. Evolution of trappin genes in mammals. *BMC Evol. Biol.* 10:31.

Lundwall, A. and M. Ulvsback. 1996. The gene of the protease inhibitor SKALP/elafin is a member of the REST gene family. *Biochem. Biophys. Res. Commun.* 221:323-327.

Ma, G., T. Greenwell-Wild, K. Lei, W. Jin, J. Swisher, N. Hardegen, C. T. Wild, and S. M. Wahl. 2004. Secretory leukocyte protease inhibitor binds to annexin II, a cofactor for macrophage HIV-1 infection. *J Exp. Med.* 200:1337-1346.

McMichael, J. W., A. Roghanian, L. Jiang, R. Ramage, and J. M. Sallenave. 2005. The antimicrobial antiproteinase elafin binds to lipopolysaccharide and modulates macrophage responses. *Am. J Respir. Cell Mol. Biol.* 32:443-452.

Muto, J., K. Kuroda, H. Wachi, S. Hirose, and S. Tajima. 2007. Accumulation of elafin in actinic elastosis of sun-damaged skin: elafin binds to elastin and prevents elastolytic degradation. *J Invest Dermatol.* 127:1358-1366.

Pfundt, R., I. Vlijmen-Willems, M. Bergers, M. Wingens, W. Cloin, and J. Schalkwijk. 2001. In situ demonstration of phosphorylated c-jun and p38 MAP kinase in epidermal keratinocytes following ultraviolet B irradiation of human skin. *J Pathol.* 193:248-255.

Pfundt, R., M. Wingens, M. Bergers, M. Zweers, M. Frenken, and J. Schalkwijk. 2000. TNF-alpha and serum induce SKALP/elafin gene expression in human keratinocytes by a p38 MAP kinase-dependent pathway. *Arch. Dermatol. Res.* 292:180-187.

Py, B., S. Basmaciogullari, J. Bouchet, M. Zarka, I. C. Moura, M. Benhamou, R. C. Monteiro, H. Hocini, R. Madrid, and S. Benichou. 2009. The phospholipid scramblases 1 and 4 are cellular receptors for the secretory leukocyte protease inhibitor and interact with CD4 at the plasma membrane. *PLoS One* 4:e5006.

Reid, P. T., M. E. Marsden, G. A. Cunningham, C. Haslett, and J. M. Sallenave. 1999. Human neutrophil elastase regulates the expression and secretion of elafin (elastase-specific inhibitor) in type II alveolar epithelial cells. *FEBS Lett.* 457:33-37.

Roghanian, A., S. E. Williams, T. A. Sheldrake, T. I. Brown, K. Oberheim, Z. Xing, S. E. Howie, and J. M. Sallenave. 2006. The antimicrobial/elastase inhibitor elafin regulates lung dendritic cells and adaptive immunity. *Am. J Respir. Cell Mol. Biol.* 34:634-642.

Sallenave, J. M. 2010. Secretory leukocyte protease inhibitor and elafin/trappin-2: versatile mucosal antimicrobials and regulators of immunity. *Am. J Respir. Cell Mol. Biol.* 42:635-643.

Sallenave, J. M., G. A. Cunningham, R. M. James, G. McLachlan, and C. Haslett. 2003. Regulation of pulmonary and systemic bacterial lipopolysaccharide responses in transgenic mice expressing human elafin. *Infect. Immun.* 71:3766-3774.

Sallenave, J. M. and A. P. Ryle. 1991. Purification and characterization of elastase-specific inhibitor. Sequence homology with mucus proteinase inhibitor. *Biol. Chem. Hoppe Seyler* 372:13-21.

Sallenave, J. M., J. Shulmann, J. Crossley, M. Jordana, and J. Gauldie. 1994. Regulation of secretory leukocyte proteinase inhibitor (SLPI) and elastase-specific inhibitor (ESI/elafin) in human airway epithelial cells by cytokines and neutrophilic enzymes. *Am. J Respir. Cell Mol. Biol.* 11:733-741.

Schalkwijk, J., I. M. van Vlijmen, J. A. Alkemade, and G. J. de Jongh. 1993. Immunohistochemical localization of SKALP/elafin in psoriatic epidermis. *J Invest Dermatol.* 100:390-393.

Schalkwijk, J., O. Wiedow, and S. Hirose. 1999. The trappin gene family: proteins defined by an N-terminal transglutaminase substrate domain and a C-terminal four-disulphide core. *Biochem. J* 340 (Pt 3):569-577.

Schmid, M., K. Fellermann, P. Fritz, O. Wiedow, E. F. Stange, and J. Wehkamp. 2007. Attenuated induction of epithelial and leukocyte serine antiproteases elafin and secretory leukocyte protease inhibitor in Crohn's disease. *J Leukoc. Biol.* 81:907-915.

Simpson, A. J., A. I. Maxwell, J. R. Govan, C. Haslett, and J. M. Sallenave. 1999. Elafin (elastase-specific inhibitor) has anti-microbial activity against gram-positive and gram-negative respiratory pathogens. *FEBS Lett.* 452:309-313.

Tamechika, I., M. Itakura, Y. Saruta, M. Furukawa, A. Kato, S. Tachibana, and S. Hirose. 1996. Accelerated evolution in inhibitor domains of porcine elafin family members. *J Biol. Chem.* 271:7012-7018.

Tamura, K., J. Dudley, M. Nei, and S. Kumar. 2007. MEGA4: Molecular Evolutionary Genetics Analysis (MEGA) software version 4.0. *Mol. Biol. Evol.* 24:1596-1599.

Tanaka, N., A. Fujioka, S. Tajima, A. Ishibashi, and S. Hirose. 2000. Elafin is induced in epidermis in skin disorders with dermal neutrophilic infiltration: interleukin-1 beta and tumour necrosis factor-alpha stimulate its secretion in vitro. *Br. J Dermatol.* 143:728-732.

Tomee, J. F., P. S. Hiemstra, R. Heinzel-Wieland, and H. F. Kauffman. 1997. Antileukoprotease: an endogenous protein in the innate mucosal defense against fungi. *J Infect. Dis.* 176:740-747.

Tremblay, G. M., J. M. Sallenave, E. Israel-Assayag, Y. Cormier, and J. Gauldie. 1996. Elafin/elastase-specific inhibitor in bronchoalveolar lavage of normal subjects and farmer's lung. *Am. J Respir. Crit Care Med.* 154:1092-1098.

Vachon, E., Y. Bourbonnais, C. D. Bingle, S. J. Rowe, M. F. Janelle, and G. M. Tremblay. 2002. Anti-inflammatory effect of pre-elafin in lipopolysaccharide-induced acute lung inflammation. *Biol. Chem.* 383:1249-1256.

van Wetering, S., A. C. van der Linden, M. A. van Sterkenburg, W. I. de Boer, A. L. Kuijpers, J. Schalkwijk, and P. S. Hiemstra. 2000. Regulation of SLPI and elafin release from bronchial epithelial cells by neutrophil defensins. *Am. J Physiol Lung Cell Mol. Physiol* 278:L51-L58.

Wiedow, O., J. M. Schroder, H. Gregory, J. A. Young, and E. Christophers. 1990. Elafin: an elastase-specific inhibitor of human skin. Purification, characterization, and complete amino acid sequence. *J. Biol. Chem.* 265:14791-14795.

Williams, S. E., T. I. Brown, A. Roghanian, and J. M. Sallenave. 2006. SLPI and elafin: one glove, many fingers. *Clin. Sci. (Lond)* 110:21-35.

Zeeuwen, P. L., W. Hendriks, W. W. de Jong, and J. Schalkwijk. 1997. Identification and sequence analysis of two new members of the SKALP/elafin and SPAI-2 gene family. Biochemical properties of the transglutaminase substrate motif and suggestions for a new nomenclature. *J Biol. Chem.* 272:20471-20478.

In: Cattle: Domestication, Diseases and the Environment
Editor: George Liu

ISBN: 978-1-62417-820-7
© 2013 Nova Science Publishers, Inc.

Chapter 3

BODY FAT AND PLASMA LEPTIN INVOLVEMENT IN THE VOLUNTARY FEED INTAKE OF CATTLE

***Renato S. A. Vega**[1,2], **Hong-Gu Lee**[2], **Hideto Kuwayama**[3] **and Hisashi Hidari**[3]*

[1] Animal Breeding & Physiology Division, Animal and Dairy Sciences, College of Agriculture, University of the Philippines Los Baños, Laguna, Philippines
[2] Department of Animal Sciences, College of Natural Resources and Life Sciences, Pusan National University, Samangjin-eup, Miryang City, Gyeongnam, S. Korea
[3] Metabolism and Physiology Laboratory, Department of Animal Production Science, Obihiro University of Agriculture and Veterinary Medicine, Obihiro-shi, Hokkaido, Japan

ABSTRACT

The involvement of adipose derived leptin in feed intake regulation remains elusive. Hence, the purpose of this chapter is to clarify the involvement of body fat measures and endogenous leptin in feed intake of cattle. In *study one*, 6 16-month old Holstein steers were offered *ad libitum* feed for seven months.

Feed intake, body weight and backfat thickness (BFT) between 6th to 7th and 12th to 13th rib were measured at selected monthly ages from day 1 to 8. On day 8, pre-prandial blood was sampled to measure leptin, insulin, glucose, NEFA, triglyceride and total cholesterol, then ultrasound BFT was taken. In *study two*, eight heads of finishing (n=4) and growing (n=4) steers were used for cross-over experimental design to know the effects of 2-hour interval of physiological dose intravenous insulin administration (6 mU per kg $BW^{0.75}$) on plasma leptin and TDN intake per kg $BW^{0.75}$ from 08:00 until 22:00 hours. Blood was sampled 15 minutes before and after insulin administration to measure plasma metabolites and hormones of growing and finishing Holstein steers.

In *study one*, the inter-relationship of BFT, plasma leptin and TDN intake for the period of seven months, revealed significant positive relationship between backfat thickness and plasma leptin. Negative relationship of TDN intake to plasma leptin

---

* E-mail: renevega10@yahoo.com.

(P≤0.004; r=0.49) and backfat thickness (P≤0.005; r=0.048) was also observed. The reduction of TDN intake from 16 to 23 months was 25%.

This inter-relationship between backfat thickness, plasma leptin and TDN intake implies strongly that 12th to 13th rib backfat, an indicator of adiposity reflects correlated elevation of plasma leptin and TDN intake reduction per kg $BW^{0.75}$ of finishing steers. In *study two*, no daytime plasma leptin variation was observed for growing and finishing steers. Plasma glucose was depressed in growing, while depression was observed only at certain period after insulin administration for finishing steers.

Plasma leptin was not elevated significantly in growing steers, whereas significant plasma leptin elevation was observed among finishing steers at 11:45 and 15:45. At this period of plasma leptin elevation, insulin administration caused 25% reduction in short-term TDN intake of finishing steers (P<0.07), whereas no short-term TDN reduction was observed in growing steers. Both growing and finishing steers did not show reduction in the 24 hour feed intake. Briefly, the over-all results revealed that leptin elevation is necessary for feed intake reduction; hence leptin is involved only in long-term feed intake regulation in cattle.

INTRODUCTION

There are several evidences in the involvement of fat tissues in regulating feed intake and body weight in experimental animals. Kennedy [1] reported the involvement of fat depot in rats, while Coleman [2] in his parabiotically joined obese-diabetic and normal mice resulted to loss in weight, hypoglycemia, and death of normal partner due to starvation. The injection of acid ethanol extract from rat adipose tissues resulted to feed inhibition of mice [3].

The cloning of obesity gene and the expression of 164kDa peptide protein called leptin [4] set a landmark in understanding obesity and regulation of feed intake in mouse. In lambs, central infusion of leptin in well-fed ewes caused reduction on feed intake, but not in food deprived ewes [5]. In sheep, there was no evidence of circadian rhythm of plasma leptin [6], suggesting that the short-term meal intake may not be regulated by plasma leptin. In large animals, evidence of the regulation of feed intake, body weight or body fat by leptin remain unclear. Plasma leptin was positively related to body fat content in male and female subjects [7], backfat thickness of sheep [8] and fat score of sheep [9]. Subcutaneous fat was related highly to plasma leptin in human [10] and pigs [11].

Clearly, leptin has become a good indicator of body fat, but whether it regulates feed intake and body fat remains unclear. There has been no better alternative in measuring body fat directly in living animals but through ultrasonic technique of backfat thickness (BFT). It was reported that the ultrasound technique accurately measures BFT in cattle [12, 13].

Considering this, we performed ultrasonic scanning for seven months cross-sectional study of finishing Holstein steers fed with *ad libitum* of high concentrate diet to monitor the changes in TDN intake per kg $BW^{0.75}$ at fattening period and determine its relationship to plasma leptin and BFT. Insulin modulates the adipocytes' *ob* gene mRNA and *ob* protein (leptin) in humans [14, 15] rats [16].

Conflicting results on plasma leptin by insulin infusion was clearly demonstrated, and it was found out that the effect of insulin on leptin is more of chronic (long-term) rather than an acute effect [15]. In rat in vitro, it was shown that the insulin-induced leptin production was caused by glucose transport and metabolism [17].

Likewise, the glucose infusion rate was positively related to changes in plasma leptin after nine hours of insulin infusion in human [18]. However, there has been no evidence that the endogenous increase in plasma leptin leads to feed intake reduction. Hence, the second study aims to know if the two-hour interval intravenous physiological insulin administration increase endogenous plasma leptin and consequently reduce TDN intake in growing and finishing steer.

MATERIALS AND METHODS

Study 1: Relationship of Backfat Thickness, Plasma Leptin and TDN Intake per Kg BW at Finishing Stage in Holstein Steers

Care and Management of Animals

Six castrated Holstein steers were housed in a pen with individual electronic head gates. For the period of one month (15th month-old), the steers underwent adaptation and all steers readily consumed 2.0 to 2.3 % concentrate feed per kilogram body weight and 1.8 kg roughage feed every day. This level of feeding was the basis of *ad libitum* feeding (more than 10% feed refusal) and feed intake was measured at selected ages (16, 17, 18, 19, 20-21, 22 and 23 months). Since feed data gathering was conducted every last week of the month, the 20th month covered the period from Oct 30 to Nov 5, a seven day data collection. The commercial concentrate and roughage feed composition are shown in Table 1. The feeds were given twice daily at 09:00 and 15:00 hours. At selected ages body weight was taken at 08:00 hours in the first day and the following day after the last day of feed data collection (day 8). Pre-prandial blood was sampled twice on day 8 through the jugular vein at 08:00 (am) and 14:00 (pm). Morning and afternoon plasma were pooled for blood analysis. All experimental animals were treated according to the Guidelines for Care and Use of Experimental Animals of Obihiro University.

Back Fat Thickness (BFT) Measurement

Ultrasound (Aloka SSD338, Japan) was used for BFT determination between the 6th to 7th and 12th to 13th rib every month. At similar location below the lumbar column (40 cm at 6th to 7th rib and 44 cm at 12th to 13th rib) of the left torso the probe was placed consistently throughout the measurement at selected ages in months. The skin hair was clipped and *Konnyaku*, a firm gelatinous pad was used to avoid deformation of skin surface when pressed, allowing visual accuracy of BFT. Mineral oil was liberally applied between the skin surface and *Konnyaku* and the probe to ensure proper contact and propagation of the sound waves. Real-time ultrasound images (5.0 MHz) on the monitor were recorded in videotape and photo-printed. The BFT was measured using micro-caliper with lowest calibration of 0.05 mm. The photo-printed BFT measurement was performed according to the guidelines of Brethour (13). The backfat measured at 6th to 7th and 12th to 13th rib were not significantly different (p>0.16), and obtained higher association with body weight (r^2=0.81 and r^2=0.80, respectively). Clearly, BFT at 12th to 13th rib represent general backfat thickness and an indicator of levels of body fatness in steers.

Table 1. Concentrate and roughage feed composition offered to finishing Holstein steers from 16 to 23 months of age

Ingredients	Percentage of diet as fed	
Concentrate Ingredients: Wheat	29.78	
Soybean meal	5.96	
Corn	39.70	
Wheat bran	23.82	
Feed supplement (Vitamin A, D, E[1] and Trace mineral premix[2])	0.74	
Feed Analysis (DM Basis);	Concentrate	Timothy hay
DM, %	88.21	90.8
TDN, %	73.44	53.8
CP,%	13.25	6.1
Ash,%	3.39	4.3

Note: [1]Each vitamin contains 1,000 IU.
[2]Trace mineral premix contained (ppm): Fe (66), Cu (7.46), Co (0.09), Zn (48), Mn (41), Se (0.2) and I (0.04).

Study 2: Effects of Serial Insulin Injection on Plasma Leptin and TDN Intake of Growing and Finishing Holstein Steers

Care and Management

Experiment was conducted to determine the effect of chronic insulin injection on plasma leptin and feed intake of finishing and growing Holstein steers. Castrated and individually penned four heads of growing (body weight = 271.5±3.4kg) and four heads of finishing steers (body weight = 706.9±28.1 kg) were conditioned to concentrate feed (1.6%kg BW) and *ad libitum* roughage 4 weeks prior to the experiment. The experimental animals were grouped for saline (n=2) and insulin (n=2) administration. Then after 1 week, the treatment administration was reversed, allowing all animals to undergo both saline and insulin injections. An indwelling catheter was implanted at the jugular vein, a day before conducting the trial for blood collection and insulin administration. Finishing and growing steers were given a concentrate mix feed of 1.6% per kg BW per day. *Ad libitum* water and roughage were provided daily. The roughage was composed mainly of timothy hay. The roughage composition offered were 90.2% DM, 52.9% TDN and 6.2% CP (DM basis). Both were given concentrate diets containing 88.21% DM, 81.59% TDN and 14.72 %CP (DM basis). Concentrate and roughage feeds were offered twice daily in the morning, at about 08:00 and in the afternoon at 16:00. Feeds were withdrawn and measured before blood collection at 07:45, 11:45, 15:45; 19:45 and 23:45 and were offered again after 30 minutes to determine the TDN intake. Animal procedures were carefully done in conformity with the Guidelines for the Care and Use of Experimental Animals of Obihiro University which were derived from the *Declaration of Helsinki and Guiding Principles in the Care and Use of Animals.*

Insulin Administration and Blood Collection

Growing and finishing steers' experiments were performed with jugular injection of 0.9% saline (n=4) and 6mU insulin (n=4). The bovine pancreas insulin was acquired from SIGMA Chem. Co. (St Louis, MO) and was administered at 6 mU per kg BW dissolved in 5 ml 0.9% NaCl as vehicle. The 5 ml saline and insulin solutions were administered every two hours interval from 08:00 to 22:00 having eight doses in a day. Blood was sampled at 07:45, 08:15, 11:45, 15:45; 19:45 and 23:45. Samples were placed in a heparinized tube then into the ice bucket. The aliquot plasma were collected and stored at -40 °C until analysis. Since significant plasma leptin was observed at least four hours after sequential insulin infusion (1-5 mU per kg BW per min) in human [37], plasma leptin levels were measured every four hours interval, i.e. 07:45, 11:45, 15:45; 19:45 and 23:45 hours.

Blood Assay

Plasma samples were analyzed for nonsterified fatty acids (NEFA) and glucose utilizing NEFA C kit and Glucose C-II kit, respectively (Wako Chemicals, Tokyo, Japan). Plasma was also assayed for bovine insulin utilizing ELISA kit (Mercodia AB, Sweden) and modified multi-species leptin radioimmunoassay (RIA) kit (Linco, St. Charles, MO, USA). The leptin kit utilized guinea pig anti-human leptin, and the human leptin standard was replaced by bovine leptin (rbleptin) standard. Serial dilutions of bovine plasma showed parallelism, sensitivity of 4.9 ng/ml, cross reactivity (11.22%) and 97.8% recovery of 41.9 ng/ml rbleptin in bovine plasma [19].

Statistical Analysis

In study 1. Linear regression analysis was used to determine the relationship between dependent (TDN intake, plasma leptin, and plasma insulin) and independent variables (backfact thickness at 6th to 7th and 12th to 13th rib). Correlation analysis was also used for the determination of association of TDN intake to plasma leptin and insulin as well as between plasma insulin and leptin. The declared significant level was set at 5% ($p \leq 0.05$) and 10% ($p \leq 0.01$) level. While in study 2. The cross-over experimental design utilized mixed model analysis to compare the differences between saline and physiological insulin administration, between growing and finishing steers, daytime variation and 1 week cross-over transition.

RESULTS AND DISCUSSION

Study 1: Relationship of Backfat Thickness, Plasma Leptin and TDN Intake per Kg BW at Finishing Stage in Holstein Steers

The age-related changes in plasma leptin revealed significant increase at fattening period, suggesting parallel increase with body fat [19-21], hence this study was performed to substantiate the suggested parallel increase of plasma leptin and backfat and to include plasma leptin relationship with monthly TDN intake of steers offered constantly with high concentrate and roughage feed from 16 to 23 months of finishing period. High grain-fed condition at fattening period was performed to facilitate maximum body fat accumulation. In the experiment of Loerch (22), 85% concentrate plus 15% corn silage diet obtained significantly higher ADG, DM intake and feed/gain ratio compared to groups fed with 100% concentrate diet. Likewise, Kreikemier et al[23] reported that the optimum level of roughage necessary to obtain best animal performance was within 5 to 10% in high concentrate diet. In this study, the volume of roughage consumed declined from 13% to 5% of the diet (data not shown), which may still be optimum to cause the necessary physical stimulation of ruminal epithelial surface, allowing maximum animal performance.

Average Daily Gain (ADG)

The mean monthly ADG of Holstein steers across the finishing ages are shown in Figure 1. The decreasing ADG with monthly age cannot be attributed solely to reduction in TDN intake because the proportion of TDN intake and ADG was perceived higher at late fattening period, indicating increased energy requirement per kg weight gain observed in the considered ages in months. Insulin central effect on feed intake remain controversial [24], hence its involvement in TDN intake reduction with monthly ages was considered part of adipose metabolism.

Plasma leptin involvement in TDN intake cannot be concluded in the relationship study, because this experiment considered positive and negative relation of various variables associated with plasma leptin at fattening period.

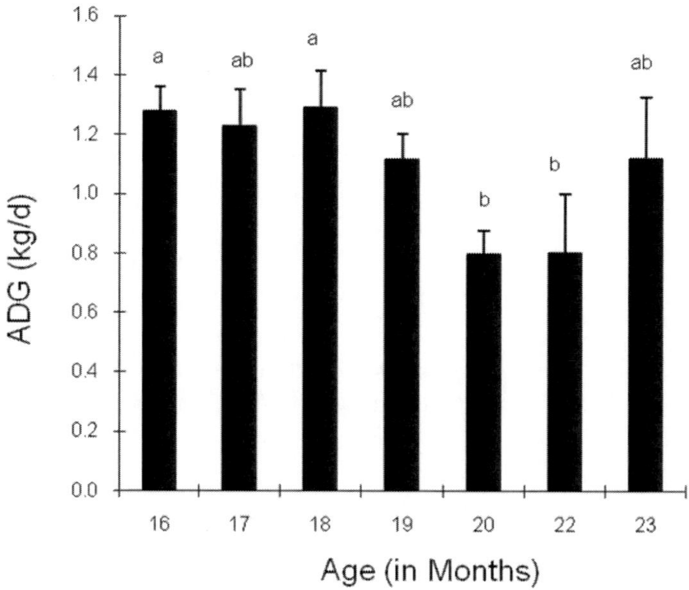

Figure 1. Means+SEM of average daily gain (kg/d) of Holstein steers across the finishing ages (months).

Research at micro-level such as leptin treatment or induction or elevation of endogenous leptin needs to be conducted to specifically clarify their role in the age-related TDN intake reduction of finishing steers offered with high grain diet.

Backfat Thickness

The BFT we observed from 490 to 704 kg bodyweight, ranges from 3 to 15 mm (see Figure 2), which shows similar results in two different species of steers reported by Wells and Preston [25] at about the same fattening period. Brethour [13] reported the accuracy and repeatability of ultrasound in measuring BFT in numerous cattle, and Houghton and Turlington [12] affirmed its accuracy in other livestock. Compared to actual measure of BFT the ultrasonic measures were 8% or about 1.2 mm underestimated [13]. Ultrasound can be used to track changes in absolute BFT in live animals [12, 13]. A little modification was included in the methodology of this study, *Konnyaku*, a firm gelatinous pad that can minimize error by absorbing pressure put upon the skin surface during ultrasound measurement was used. In film prints, the area covered by *Konnyaku* display a faded dark area distinctly recognizable before the skin line. Ten different commercially available materials were tested and 20 mm thickness showed excellent visual results. Backfat may not have similar thickness in other portions, but our measurements at 6th to 7th and 12th to 13th ribs were comparable, indicating that either of the two BFT measure can represent general backfat thickness.

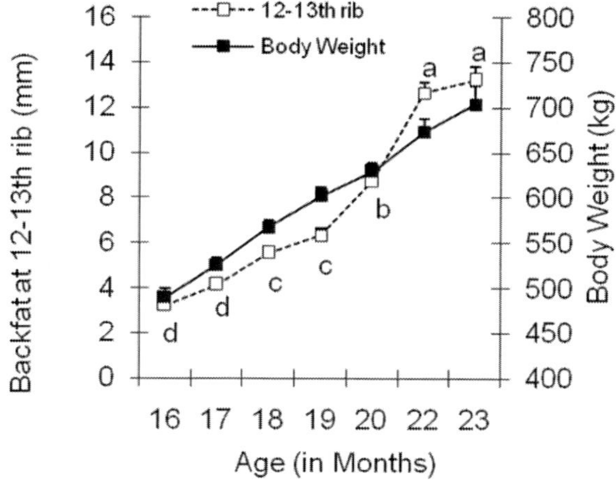

Figure 2. Means+SEM of backfat thickness at 12 to 13th rib and body weight of Holstein steers across the finishing ages (months). Open and solid squares represent backfat at 12 to 13th rib and body weight, respectively across the monthly ages of blood collection.

In humans, subcutaneous adipose tissue showed greater secretion of plasma leptin compared to omental adipose tissue [26, 27], and plasma leptin showed significant relationship with subcutaneous adiposity at umbilicus level but not with visceral fat area [10]. In sheep, backfat thickness to liveweight ratio showed significant linear relationship with plasma leptin [8]. The significant linear relationship between BFT and plasma leptin we observed in steer upholds the previous notion that the linear increase in plasma leptin at fattening period is associated to body fatness. The BFT at 6th to 7th and 12th to 13th rib generally showed significant bimonthly accumulation. However, plasma leptin concentration rose more steeply than BFT from 16 to 18 months, then it leveled-off from 18 to 22 months and attained the highest concentration at the last month.

The BFT did not perfectly reflect the changes in plasma leptin, which can be explained by one or combinations of the following hypothesis: (1) backfat accumulation differs significantly with other portions of fat depots, (2) different portions of fat depots differ in degree of plasma leptin secretion, and (3) leptin secretion and removal from plasma vary with monthly ages. Although significant association between plasma leptin and two BFT measurements was observed, BFT accumulation does not perfectly account for plasma leptin concentration in highly grain-fed Holstein steers.

TDN Intake per kg BW$^{0.75}$

The elevation of plasma leptin from 19 to 22 months compared to 16 months coincided with lower TDN intake/kg BW (see Figure 2 and Figure 3). Although BFT accumulation did not slow down within this period, there is a possibility that viscera could have attenuation during reduced ADG at later finishing period. Some authors reported that internal organs of the body are sensitive to changes in nutrition, possibly because they are metabolically active than muscle and fats [28, 29]. The reduction in TDN intake per kg BW across ages in this study can be influenced by adipose plasma leptin elevation. In sheep, increase in plasma leptin due to nutrition also increased cerebrospinal leptin concentration[8], and the central infusion of leptin in ewe and male sheep resulted to decrease in voluntary feed intake [5, 30]. However, in undernourished ewe lamb there was no reduction in feed intake [5]. The TDN intake declined from 1.6 to 1.2% per kg BW in this study.

Most likely if the offered TDN was maintained at moderate level, i.e. 1.2% per kg BW$^{0.75}$ across the monthly ages, plasma leptin may be increased without age-related decline in TDN intake. In the experiment of Blache (8), high and medium diet obtained significant backfat thickness differences, but plasma leptin concentration were not statistically different.

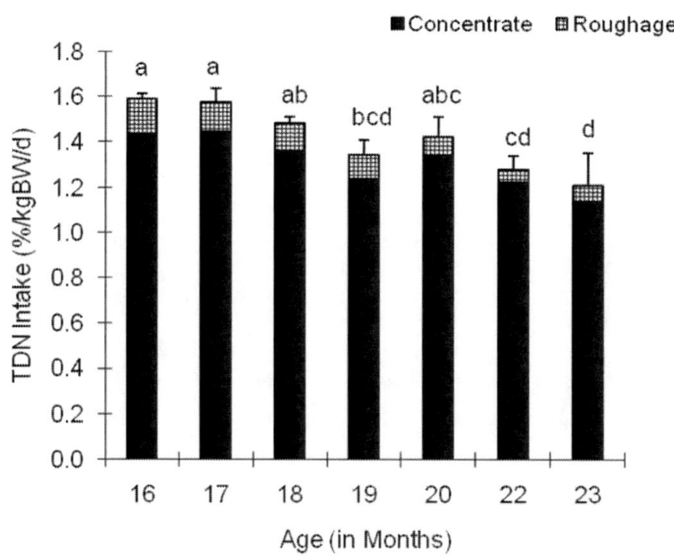

Figure 3. Means+SEM of TDN intake/kg BW of Holstein steers across the finishing ages (months).

Focusing on central leptin action on feed intake, there is possibility that in ruminants, condition of moderate feeding may increase plasma leptin and body fat, but it may not have significant effect on TDN intake per kg BW at the same period. Thus, it is suggested that high TDN intake or high concentrate diet in beef steers at finishing period shows involvement of backfat thickness and plasma leptin in age-related reduction of TDN intake per kg BW.

Metabolite Concentration

Blood metabolites manifested its availability or utilization and may indicate animal's nutritional condition. Extremely high plasma glucose from 16 to 20 months confirmed high grain-fed consumption and the drop to normal levels during the last two months implied glucose utilization necessary for acclimatization because of cold season. Likewise the significantly higher preprandial plasma NEFA obtained may reflect the actual body lipid loss because of coldness.

Birkelo et al [31] reported that acute cold stress was responsible for poorer feedlot performance during winter. In this study, the level of plasma cholesterol was higher, while plasma NEFA and triglyceride were lower than those reported in similar breed by Matsuzaki et al [32]. The lower NEFA concentration in our experiment can be explained by higher level of concentrate consumption (2.3% vs 1.0% per kg $BW^{0.75}$), showing lesser breakdown of long chain fatty acids in highly grain-fed steers.

The plasma total cholesterol and triglyceride increased with fattening age, but failed to show significant differences ($P<0.08$). The elevation in plasma cholesterol with monthly ages from 16 to 23 months was not statistically significant and can be explained by narrow range of ages in months.

Hormone Concentrations

The *in vitro* experiment demonstrated the insulin increased leptin secretion from adipocyte or tissues of rat [16, 33, 34], mouse [35, 36] and human [27]. The *in vivo* study in human showed a chronic effect of insulin on leptin production [15], and hyperinsulinemia increased plasma leptin concentration after 4 hours [37], but leptin increase induced by insulin was recorded lower in obese insulin-resistant men [18].

It was demonstrated that decreased insulin binding was related to obesity and caused by a decreased number of insulin receptor site per cell in rats [38] and bovine [39].

The results indicate that the effect of insulin on leptin production decreases with insulin resistance and increasing adiposity, as highlighted by Saad [18]. Therefore the significant linear relationship of plasma insulin to BFT and to plasma leptin at fattening period supports: (1) the concept of relative insulin resistance with increasing adiposity [38, 39, 18] and age [40]; and (2) the involvement of endogenous insulin in plasma leptin secretion from adipocyte.

Plasma leptin's follow through on plasma insulin level across the monthly ages may represent adipose metabolism (see Figure 4). Although the age-related increase in backfat thickness did not perfectly mimic plasma leptin and insulin level, it obtained significant relationship with both hormones. Furthermore, the persistence of plasma leptin mimic on plasma insulin level may be explained by the blunting of relative tissue insulin resistance with adiposity and age through progressive increase in endogenous insulin.

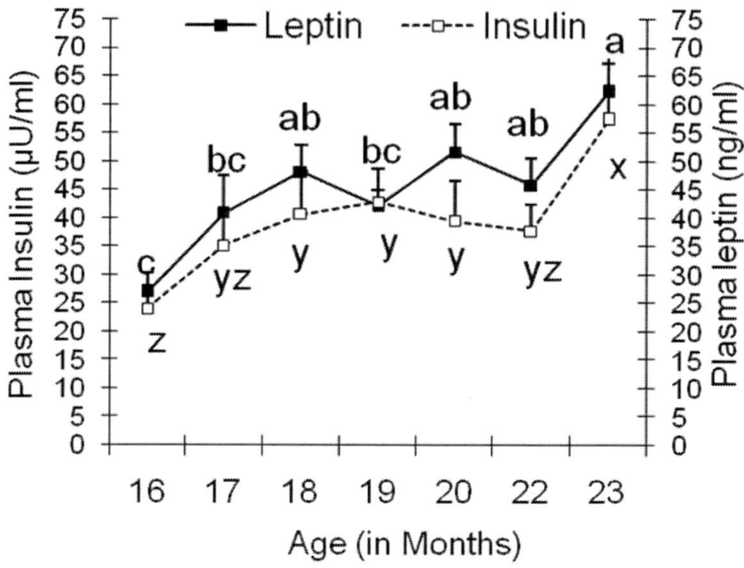

Figure 4. Means+SEM of plasma leptin and insulin across the monthly ages of castrated Holstein steers. Means having different alphabets across the monthly ages show significant differences at P<0.01.

Correlation Coefficient of TDN and Other Parameters

The elevation of plasma leptin closely mimicked the elevation of plasma insulin, which resulted to a highly significant association between the two hormones (Figure 4). Since plasma leptin and insulin are recognized to cause feed intake inhibition in sheep [5, 41, 42], we determined the correlation of TDN to plasma leptin and insulin. The age-related reduction of TDN intake was negatively associated to plasma leptin (r^2=0.24, P<0.004) and plasma insulin (r^2=0.17; P<0.02) as shown in Table 2.

Table 2. Correlation coefficients (r^2) with corresponding level of significance (P value) of castrated Holstein steers between variables from 16 to 23 monthly ages

Variables	Plasma Insulin	TDN Intake	BFT 6th -7th	BFT 12th-13th
Plasma Leptin				
r^2	0.29	0.24	0.25	0.20
slope	0.44	-0.0077	2.15	1.73
P value	0.0013	0.0042	0.0034	0.0096
Plasma Insulin				
r^2		0.17	0.13	0.10
slope		-0.005	1.62	1.27
P value		0.0173	0.0406	0.0761
TDN Intake				
r^2			0.14	0.23
slope			-0.025	-0.029
P value			0.0321	0.0052

Note: [a] BFT means backfat thickness (mm).

The inter-relationships and correlation coefficients (r^2), slope and statistical values (P) of TDN, plasma leptin and insulin against backfat thickness (6th to 7th and 12th to 13th rib) are shown in Table 2. The data reveals significant positive relationship of plasma leptin to BFT at 6th to 7th and 12th to 13th rib. Plasma insulin shows positive but weaker relationship with BFT compared to plasma leptin. This can be attributed to insulin reduced NEFA/FFA having reduced hepatic – oxidation or continues production of liver ATP that is also considered involved in feed intake reduction in ruminants [43]. The potential future application of leptin in cattle is the association of polymorphism of the leptin gene with blood leptin levels, feed intake, and carcass measures [44], unraveling the thrifty genotype among breeds of cattle. This polymorphism study is expected to lead to the selection of cattle for good marbling characteristics, meat production, reproductive performance, and milk production.

Study 2: Effects of Series of Insulin Injection on Plasma Leptin and TDN Intake of Growing and Finishing Holstein Steers

Effect on Blood NEFA and Glucose

Figure 5 shows the baseline (07:45) plasma NEFA concentrations after insulin injections of growing (square) and finishing (triangle) steers. The mixed model analysis resulted to significant cross-over (P<0.0356), and daytime (P<0.0001) variations while treatment and growth stages were not significant at P>0.05. The daytime plasma NEFA level was highest at midnight and early in the morning for both steers. Although plasma NEFA did not show significant responses after insulin injection (P>0.05), it tends to show depression after insulin treatment in both steers. Significant effect of cross-over experimental procedure was also observed (P<0.05) indicating carry-over effect of insulin injection on plasma NEFA within and few days after 7 days cross-over interval.

Figure 6 demonstrates the significant depression of plasma glucose (P<0.01) after insulin injection of growing (square) and finishing (triangle) steers. The mixed model analysis resulted to plasma glucose having significantly higher level (P<0.01) in growing compared to finishing steers, and continuous glucose depression after insulin treatment in growing, while in finishing non-significant differences was observed at 08:15 and 19:15 hours of the day.

Plasma NEFA concentration obtained significant daytime variation, which may not be associated to direct influence of plasma leptin. Blood NEFA seemed depressed by insulin injection in growing and finishing steers. Plasma glucose was significantly depressed in insulin treated growing and finishing steers, showing continuous daytime depression in growing and finishing steers. The data shows possible glucose and NEFA uptake of the adipose tissues. At finishing stage, it is notable that animals accumulated more body fat relative to bones and lean tissues.

Generally, in ruminants FFA rather than glucose is involved in the metabolic activity. However, with insulin administration this mechanism is altered favoring glucose utilization more than the FFA. Insulin induced plasma leptin elevation may be associated to glucose utilization during lipogenesis.

Regulation of leptin secretion and production by glucose metabolism has been demonstrated with the inclusion of inhibitors of glucose transport and phosphorylation in rat adipocyte [17].

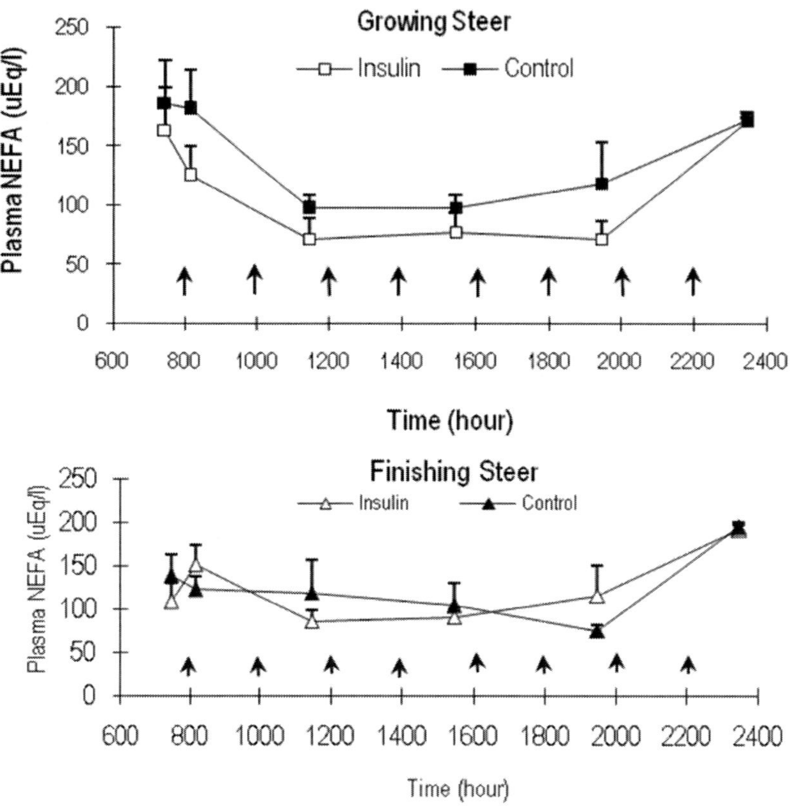

Figure 5. Plasma NEFA concentrations of control (closed symbols) and insulin treated (open symbols) growing (square) and finishing (triangle) steers. Arrows show the time of insulin injection.

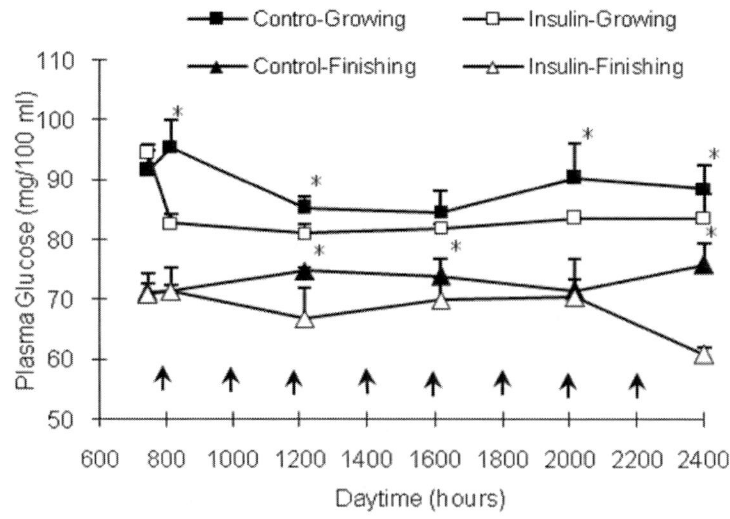

Figure 6. Plasma glucose of control (closed symbols) and insulin (open symbols) treatment of growing (square) and finishing (triangle) Holstein steers. Arrows show the time of insulin.

Insulin infusion with glucose metabolism caused chronic effect on plasma leptin elevation [15]. Also, in several studies on insulin causing leptin increase, glucose infusion has always been observed indicating involvement of both [14, 18, 37, 45].

The result of this study also reflects that insulin injection caused glucose depression and consequently plasma leptin elevation in finishing steers. Failure of plasma leptin elevation in growing steers could be very well understood because of proportionally higher lean growth relative to adipose tissues at this stage of growth and development. The absence of statistical difference has been due to significant effect of cross-over experimental procedure, implying carry-over influence of insulin on plasma leptin. The result of this study supports the results among subjects and experimental animals that the chronic insulin injection (6 mU per kg BW) causes tissue glucose utilization, thereby inducing plasma leptin elevation only in finishing steers.

Effect on Plasma Leptin

The changes in daytime plasma leptin in growing and finishing steers were also investigated. In human [15, 46] and mouse [47] diurnal leptin variation was reported. However, no significant plasma leptin variation was observed in both steers from 07:45 to 23:45 hours. In sheep, leptin concentration was not affected by feeding time and it did not vary within the day [30]. The reason for differences between monogastric and ruminants' plasma leptin behavior could be attributed to their physiological digestion and release of nutrients in the blood.

Ruminants' digestion undergoes fermentation and gradual nutrient release relative to monogastric animals. Plasma leptin concentration revealed that finishing steers had significantly higher concentration than the growing steers reflecting their differences in body weight and adiposity. The same was observed in the variation of plasma leptin in relation to body fat measures in cattle [48, 49] and in sheep [8].

Figure 7 shows the effect of serial injection of insulin on plasma leptin concentrations of growing and finishing steers. The mixed model analysis shows that plasma leptin concentrations of growing and finishing steers did not significantly differ within the day from 7:45 to 23:45.

There was no significant effect (P>0.05) of insulin injection in both steers. However, greater elevation in plasma leptin was observed in finishing compared to growing steers, which can be reflective of their degree of body fat accumulations. Finishing steers seemed to have tendency for greater plasma leptin elevation after four hours insulin injection, but its higher baseline concentration and significant cross-over effect (P<0.0004) may have caused the loss in significant effect on leptin level.

The significant effect of cross-over experimental procedure observed in plasma leptin of both steers implies that the seven days cross-over interval is not sufficient to bring the animal to normal baseline condition. The effect of insulin injection has longer effect on plasma leptin.

The significantly higher plasma leptin concentration of finishing over growing steers can be attributed to more body fat accumulation or deposition with age as presented in this paper and reported previously [19, 49]. The unelevated plasma leptin in 7-month growing steers can be supported by previous experiments showing significantly higher elevation of plasma leptin of cattle breeds only after the animal starts to deposit significant body fat [50].

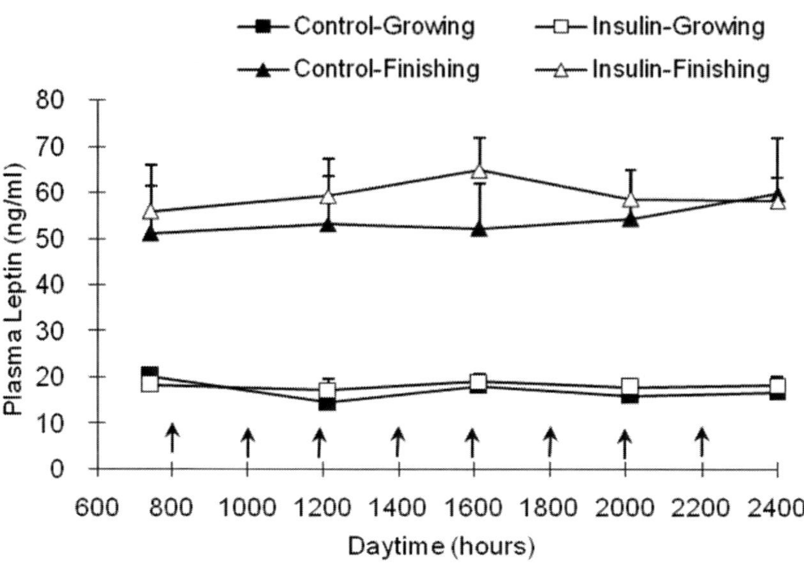

Figure 7. Plasma leptin of control (closed symbols) and insulin (open symbols) treatment of growing (square) and finishing (triangle) Holstein steers. Arrows show the time of insulin injection.

Effect on TDN Intake per kg BW$^{0.75}$

The feed intake response to insulin is complicated, low concentrations such as 6 mU per kg BW intravenous or 2 to 6mU per kg BW per min infusion for 15 minutes resulted to reduction in intake, whereas intermediate insulin dose level resulted to none while high doses resulted to stimulation of feed intake based on literature reviewed [51, 52]. Insulin-induced reduction on feed intake was observed only for a short-period (60 minutes) of 6mU per kg BW intravenous injection in sheep during meal intake [41]. In sheep 24 hours physiological dose of insulin injection (6mU per kg BW) during meal initiation (8x/day) caused significant depression in 24 hour feed intake [42]. Based on overwhelming positive effects of insulin-induced feed reduction in sheep [41, 42, 53], this research attempted to duplicate the result in cattle with the aim to understand the possible participation of plasma leptin in the short-term TDN intake. The insulin injection performed by Deetz and Wangsness [42] was done during meal initiation while this experiment administered it in every two hours injection interval from 08:00 to 22:00 for a period of 1 day to raise leptin level during the day. Likewise, 7-month old growing and 27-month old finishing Holstein steers were utilized with the possible consideration on the different responses of growing and finishing steers.

The TDN intake presented in Figure 8 and Figure 9 was the short-term (12:15 to 19:45) and 24 hours measurements, respectively. There was no significant effect of insulin injection on both short-term and 24 hour TDN intake of growing and finishing steers. However finishing steers experienced -25% and -8% decrease in short-term and 24 hours TDN intake, respectively. Furthermore finishing steers obtained significantly higher short-term (P<01) and 24 hours (P<0.05) TDN intake compared to growing steers.

The greater feed intake reduction (-25%) imply that sustained plasma leptin elevation above the baseline level caused by exogenous insulin administration is necessary to cause significant reduction in TDN intake at fattening or finishing stage. It has been shown that elevation of plasma leptin associated to backfat thickness is significantly related with reduction in TDN intake with age at finishing stage of Holstein steers as reported previously [49]. Serial injection of insulin administration in finishing steer revealed significant reduction on plasma glucose, tendency to elevate plasma leptin resulting to 25% and 8% reduction in short-term (12:15 to 19:45) and 24 hours TDN intake, respectively.

Further the significantly higher plasma leptin and significantly lower short-term TDN intake of finishing compared to growing steers, supports the action of adipose derived leptin on feed intake regulation. In growing steers serial injection of insulin resulted to depression of plasma glucose, failure to elevate plasma leptin and insignificant effect on short-term and 24 hour TDN intake.

The lower level of plasma leptin and greater TDN intake of growing steers is physiologically important for the development and growth of other tissues like bones, organs and lean tissues. Elevation of plasma and cerebrospinal fluid leptin concentration was observed in sheep with increased level of nutrition[30].

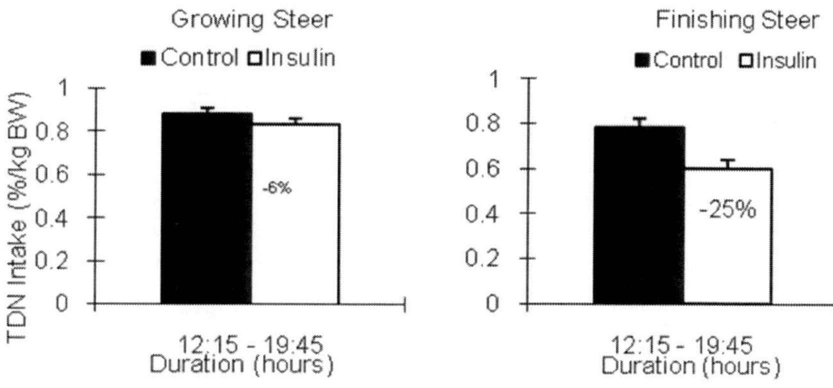

Figure 8. Short-term (12:15 to 19:45) Total Digestible Nutrients Intake (%/kg BW) of control (closed symbols) and insulin (open symbols) treatment of growing (left side) and finishing (right side) Holstein steers.

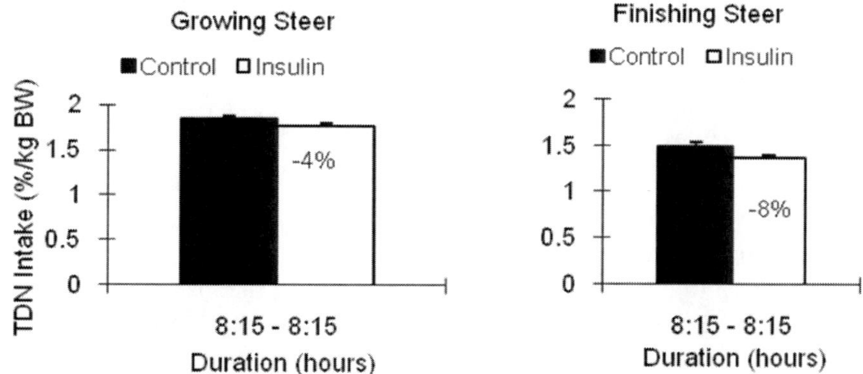

Figure 9. Twenty four hours Total Digestible Nutrients Intake (%/kg BW) of control (closed symbols) and insulin (open symbols) treatment of growing (left side) and finishing (right side) Holstein steers.

Likewise, central (i.c.v.) infusion of leptin revealed decrease in voluntary feed intake in male sheep[8] and in well-fed ewe lamb[5]. The greater magnitude of short-term TDN reduction (-25%) and the greater tendency to elevate plasma leptin of finishing steers suggest that leptin is involved in the insulin-induced feed reduction in finishing steers. The effect on short-term TDN reduction cannot solely be attributed to insulin but to the possible involvement of elevated plasma leptin in finishing steers. Moreover, significantly higher and sustained elevation of plasma leptin are the conditions necessary to cause greater feed intake reduction as shown by the responses of growing and finishing steers.

SUMMARY AND CONCLUSION

There is significant positive relationship of plasma leptin to measures of body fat (BFT at 6th to 7th and 12th to 13th rib) in cattle. Compared to plasma leptin, insulin shows weaker positive relationship with BFT. This can be attributed to dual influence on feed intake regulation of insulin together with free fatty acid in the hepatic – oxidation, i.e. effect of continues production of liver ATP involved in feed intake reduction in ruminants [43]. There was no significant variation in plasma leptin from morning to midnight implying absence of meal regulation of plasma leptin in ruminants. Chronic insulin injection caused slight depression in plasma NEFA and significant depression in glucose concentration. Higher plasma leptin elevation simultaneous to greater short-term TDN intake reduction was obtained in finishing steers compared to growing steers. The results of these studies revealed and support that plasma leptin elevation is involved, by causing reduction of 24% in TDN intake of high concentrate fed finishing steers.

The report of leptin gene polymorphism in cattle associated to blood leptin levels, feed intake and carcass measures [44] provide future application especially in identifying the thrifty genotype among breeds of cattle, important in animal selection.

REFERENCES

[1]	Kennedy GC. The role of depot fat in the hypothalamic control of food intake in rat. *Proc. Nutr. Soc.* 1953; 140B: 578-92.

[2]	Coleman DL, Hummel KP. Effect of parabiosis of normal with genetically diabetic mice. *Am. J. Physiol.* 1969; 215(5): 1928-34.

[3]	Goodner GC, Goodner CJ. Demosntration of acid-ethanol extracts of rat adipose tissue containing an inhibitor of feed intake in mouse. *Journal of Laboratory Clinical Medicine* 1996; 128(3):247 – 50.

[4]	Zang Y, Proenca R, Maffei M, Barone M, Leopold L, Friedman JM. Positional cloning of the mouse *obese* gene and its human homologue. *Nature* 1994;372:425-32.

[5]	Morrison CD, Daniel JA, Holmberg BJ, Djiane J, Raver N, Gertler A, Keisler DH. Central infusion of leptin in well-fed and undernourished ewe Lambs: effects on feed intake and serum concentration of growth hormone and luteinizing hormone. *Journal of Endocrinology* 2001;168: 317-24.

[6]   Marie MP, Findlay PA, Thomas L, Adam CL. Daily pattern of plasma leptin in sheep: effects of photoperiod and food intake. *J. Endocrinol.* 2001; 170:277 – 86.

[7]   Moller N., O'brien P, Nair KS. Disruption of the relationship of fat content and leptin levels with aging in humans. *J. Clin. Endocrinol.* 2001: 83:931-934.

[8]   Blache D, Celi P, Blackberry MA, Dynes DA, Martin GB. Decrease in voluntary feed intake and pulsatile luteinizing hormone secretion after intracerebroventricular infusion of recombinant bovine leptin in mature male sheep. *Reprod Fertil. Dev.* 2000; 12: 373-81.

[9]   Erhardt RA, Slepetis RM. Siegel-Willott J, Van Amburgh ME, Bell AW, Boisclair YR. Development of specific radioimmunoassay to measure physiological dose changes of circulating leptin in cattle and sheep. *J. Endocrinol.* 2000; 166:519-28.

[10] Takahashi M, Funahashi T, Shimomura I, Miyaoka K, Matsuzawa Y. Plasma leptin levels and body fat distribution. *Hormone Metabolic Research* 1996;28:751-52.

[11] Robert C, Palin M, Coulombe N, Roberge C, Silversides FG, Benkel BF, McKay RM, Pelletier G. Backfat thickness in pigs is positively associated with leptin mRNA levels. Can. J. Anim. Sci. 1998;78:473-82.

[12] Houghton PL, Turlington LM. Application of ultrasound for feeding and finishing animals: a review. *J. Anim. Sci.* 1992; 70:930-41.

[13] Brethour J.The repeatability and accuracy of ultrasound in measuring backfat of cattle. *J. Anim. Sci.* 1992;70:1039-1044.

[14] Boden G, Xinhua C, Kolaczynski J, Polansky M. Effect of prolonged hyperinsulinemia in normal human subjects. *J. Clin. Invest.* 1997;100:1107-13.

[15] Kolacynski JW, Nyce MR, Considine RV, Boden G, Nolan JJ, Henry R, Mudaliar SR, Olefsky J, Caro JF. Acute and chronic effect of insulin on leptin production in human. *Diabetes* 1996; 45:699-701.

[16] Mueller WM, Gregoire FM, Stanhope KL, Mobbs CV, Mizuno TM, Warden CH, Stern JS, Havel PJ. Evidence that glucose metabolism regulates leptin secretion form cultured rat adipocytes. *Endocrinology* 1998;139:551-58.

[17] Barr V, Malide D, Zarnowski MJ, Taylor SI, Cushman SW. Insulin stimulates both leptin secretion and production by rat white adipose tissue. *Endocrinology* 1997; 138:4463 – 72.

[18] Saad MF, Khan A, Sharma A, Michael R, Riad-Gabriel MG, Boyadjian R, Jinagouda SD, Steil GM, Kamdar V. Physiological insulinemia acutely modulates plasma leptin. *Diabetes* 1998;47:544-49.

[19] Vega RA, Lee HG, Kuwayama H, Matsunaga N, Hidari H. Age-related changes in plasma leptin from early growing to late finishing stages of castrated Holstein steers: Utilizing multi-species leptin RIA. *Asian-Australasian Journal of Animal Science* 2002;15 (5): 725-31.

[20] Vega RA, Kuwayama H, Hidari H. Effect of series of insulin injection on plasma leptin and TDN intake of growing and finishing Holstein steers. In: Lapitan RM, Oliveros MCR, Canaria TL, editors. *Proceedings of the 44th Scientific Seminar and Annual Convention*; 2007 Oct 18-19. Malate, Manila, Philippines. 2007: P.63.

[21] Vega RSA, Lee HG, Hidari H, Kuwayama H. Changes in plasma hormones and metabolites during compensatory growth of Holstein steers. *Philippine Journal of Veterinary Medicine and Animal Science* 2009;35(1):1-14.

[22] Loerch SC. Efficacy of plastic pot scrubbers as a replacement for roughage in high - concentrate cattle diets. *J. Anim. Sci.* 1991; 69:2321-28.

[23] Kreikemier KK, Harmon DL, Brandt RT Jr, Nagaraja TG, Cochran RC. Steem-rolled wheat diets for finishing cattle: effects of dietary roughage and feed intake on the finishing steer performance and ruminal metabolism. *J. Anim. Sci.* 1990; 68:2130-141.

[24] Ikeda H, West DB, Pustek JJ, Figlewicz DP, Greenwood MRC, Porte D Jr, Woods SC. Intraventricular insulin reduces food intake and body weight of lean but not obese Zucker rats. *Appetite* 1986; 7:381-86.

[25] Well RS, Preston RL. Effects of repeated urea dilution measurement on feedlot performance and consistency of estimated body composition in steers of different breed types. *J. Anim. Sci.* 1998;76:2799-804

[26] Hube F, Lietz U, Igel M, Jensen PB, Tornqvist H, Joost H-G, Hauner H. Difference in leptin mRNA levels between omental and subcutaneous abdominal adipose tissue from obese humans. *Hormone Metabolic Research* 1996;28:690-693.

[27] Russel CD, Pettersen RN, Rao SP, Ricci MR, Prasad A, Zang Y, Brolin RE, Fried SK. Leptin expression in adipose tissue from obese humans: depot specific regulation by insulin and dexamethasone. *Am. J. Physiol.* 1998;275:E507-E515.

[28] Hornick JL, Van Eanaeme C, Gerard O, Dufrasne I, Istasse L. Mechanism of reduced and compensatory growth. *Domest. Anim. Endocrinol.* 2000; 19:121-32.

[29] Koong LJ, Ferrel CL, Nienaber JA. Assessment of interrelationships among levels of feed intake and production, organ size and fasting heat production in growing animals. *J. Nutr.* 1985; 115:1383-390.

[30] Blache D, Tellam RL, Chagas LM, Blackberry MA, Vercoe PE, Martin GB. Level of nutrition affects leptin concentrations in plasma and cerebrospinal fluid in sheep. *J. Endocrinol.* 2000; 165;625-37.

[31] Birkelo CP, Johnson DE, Petteplace HP. Maintenance requirement of beef cattle as affected by season on different planes of nutrition. *J. Anim. Sci.* 1991; 69:1214 – 22.

[32] Matsuzaki M, Takizawa S, Ogawa M. Plasma insulin metabolite concentration and carcass characteristics of Japanese Black, Japanese Brown and Holstein steers. *J. Anim. Sci.* 1997; 75:3287-93.

[33] Hardie LJ, Guilhot N, Trayhurn P. Regulation of leptin production in cultured mature white adipocytes. *Hormone Metabolic Research* 1996;28:685-89.

[34] Siegrist-Kaiser CA, Pauli V, Judge-Aubrey CE, Boss O, Pernin A, Chin WW, Custin I, Rohner-Jeanrenaud F, Burger AG, Zapf J, Meier CA. Direct effects of leptin of brown aipose tissue. *J. Clin. Invest.* 1997;100 (11):2858-64.

[35] Rentsch J, Chiesi M. Regulation of *ob* gene mRNA in cultured adipocytes. *Federation of European Biochemical Societies Letters* 1996;379:55-59.

[36] Leroy P, Dessolin S, Villageois P, Moon BC, Friedman JM, Ailhaud G, Dani C. Expression of *ob gene* in adipose cells. *J. Biol. Chem.* 1996;271(5):2365-68.

[37] Ultrainen T, Malmstrom R, Makimattila S, Yki-Jarvinen H. Supraphysiological hyperinsulinemia increases plasma leptin concentrations after 4 h in normal subjects. *Diabetes* 1996; 45:1364-66.

[38] Olefsky JM, Reaven GM. Effects of age and obesity on insulin binding of isolated adipocytes. *Endocrinol.* 1975;96:1486-98.

[39] Vernon RG, Finley E, Taylor E, Flint DJ. Insulin binding and action on bovine adipocytes. *Endocrinol.* 1985; 116:1195-99.

[40] Rowe JW, Minaker KL, Pallota JA. Characterization of insulin resistance of aging. J. Clin. Invest. 1983;71:1581-87.

[41] Deetz LE, Wangsness PJ. Effect of intrajugular administration of insulin on feed intake, plasma glucose and plasma insulin. *J. Nutr.* 1980; 110:1976-1982.

[42] Deetz LE, Wangsness PJ. Influence of intrajugular administration of insulin, glucagon and propionate on voluntary feed intake of sheep. *J. Anim Sci.* 1981; 53:427-433.

[43] Allen MS, Bradford BJ, Oba M. The hepatic oxidation theory of the control of feed intake and its application to ruminants. *J .Anim. Sci.* 2009; 87:3317-3334.

[44] Nkrumah JD, Li C, Yu J, Hansen C, Keisler DH, Moore SS.. Polymorphism in the bovine leptin promoter associated to with serum leptin concentration, growth, feed intake, feeding behavior and measures of carcass merit. *J. Anim. Sci.* 2005;83:20-28.

[45] Koopsman S, Frolich J, Gribnau EH, Westendorp RGJ, Defrozo RA. Effect of hyperinsulinemia on plasma leptin concentration and food intake in rats. *Am. J. Physiol,* 1998; 274 : E998-1001.

[46] Sinha MK, Ohannesian JP, Heiman ML, Kriauciunas A, Stephens TW, Magosin S, Marco C, Caro JF. Nocturnal rise of leptin in lean, obese and non-insulin dependent diabetes mellitus subjects. *J. Clin. Invest.* 1996;97:1344-47.

[47] Ahima R, Prabakaran D, Mantzoros C, Qu D, Lowell B, Flier EM, Flier J. Role of leptin in neuroendocrine response to fasting. *Nature* 1996;382: 250-252.

[48] Delavaud C, Bocquier F, Chilliard Y, Keisler DH, Gertler A, Kann G. Plasma leptin determination in ruminants: effect of nutritional status and body fatness on plasma leptin concentration assessed by specific RIA in sheep. *J. Endocrinol.* 2000; 165; 519-26.

[49] Vega RA, Hidari H, Kuwayama H, Suzuki M, Manalo DD. The relationships of plasma leptin, backfat thickness and TDN intake across finishing stage of Holstein steers. *Asian-Asutralasian Journal of Animal Science* 2004;17(3): 330 – 36.

[50] Vega RA, Hidari H, Matsunaga N, Kuwayama H, Manalo DD, Lee HG, Hata H. Plasma leptin and performance of purebred and backcrossed Hereford throughout grazing and feedlot fattening. *Asian-Australasian Journal of Animal Science* 2004;17(7);954 – 59.

[51] Dulphy PJ, Faverdin P. L'ingestionalimentaire chez les ruminants: modalite'setphe'nome 'nesassocies. *Reprod. Nutr. Dev.* 1987;27:129-55.

[52] Grovum WL 1995. Mechanisms explaining the effects of short chain fatty acids on feed intake in ruminants – osmotic pressure, insulin and glucagon. In: Ruminant Phyisol: Digestion, Metabolism, Growth and Reproduction: *Proceedings of the 18th International Symposium on Ruminant. Physiol.,* 1995. P.173-97.

[53] Terashima Y, Achmadi J, Kurose Y. The physiological role of insulin in feed intake control exposed to a hot environment. *Journal of Reproduction and Development* 1996;42: 103-5.

In: Cattle: Domestication, Diseases and the Environment
Editor: George Liu
ISBN: 978-1-62417-820-7
© 2013 Nova Science Publishers, Inc.

Chapter 4

EPIGENETICS AND ENVIRONMENTAL IMPACTS IN CATTLE

Cong-jun Li[*] and Robert W. Li
[1]USDA-ARS, ANRI, Bovine Functional Genomics Laboratory,
Beltsville, MD, US

ABSTRACT

This chapter reviews the major advances in the field of epigenetics as well as the environmental impacts of cattle. Many findings from our own research endeavors related to the topic are also introduced. The phenotypic characterization of an animal can be changed through epigenetic mechanisms such as histone posttranslational modification, microRNA (miRNA), and other mechanisms. The interaction between genetics and epigenetics provides transcription regulation in cattle development and growth. The multiple layers of regulatory control of gene expression provide a multitude of paths by which cells can control their responses to external stimuli or environmental stresses. The number of research efforts to discover general molecular mechanisms fundamental to epigenetic phenomena has recently exploded.

Keywords: Cattle, environmental stress, epigenetics, gene regulation, nutrogenomics

INTRODUCTION

Epigenomics is the study of the phenomenon of changes in the regulation of gene expression and phenotype that do not depend on changes of gene sequences and establishes links between gene expression and phenotype. Epigenomics is genomics that goes beyond DNA sequences [1]. While epigenomics refers to the study of global changes across the entire genome, epigenetics is the study of single genes or groups of genes. In other words, the study

[*] Bovine Functional Genomics Laboratory, USDA-ARS, Building 200, Room 208, BARC-East, Beltsville, MD 20705, USA. E-mail: congjun.li@ars.usda.gov, Voice Phone: +1-301-504-7216, Fax: +1-301-504-8414.

of epigenomics/epigenetics explores heritable, reversible modifications of DNA and chromatin that do not change primary nucleotide sequences and is not a set of chemical modifications encoded within DNA, which orchestrate how and when genes are expressed [1]. Epigenomics illustrates the changes in the regulation of gene activities that act without, or independently from, changes in gene sequences. *TIME* magazine listed epigenetics as number two in the top ten discoveries in 2009.

Many life phenomena can be covered in the fields of epigenomics and epigenetics. Several different types of epigenetic mechanisms are involved in the regulation of gene expression in many biological processes. These mechanisms, such as DNA methylation and histone post- translational modifications, have been recognized for a long time and they are intricately interconnected with each other. Some of these processes, such as the formation of miRNA, have only recently been discovered. Genomic imprinting, gene silencing, X chromosome inactivation, position effects, reprogramming, and the progress of carcinogenesis are all known epigenetic processes.

By definition, in addition to DNA methylation and histone post-translational modifications, RNA splicing, RNA editing, miRNA, and prions also can be included as the epigenetic mechanisms for gene regulation. These regulatory mechanisms for modulation of gene function are multifaceted and complex. There are two intrinsic significant courses from epigenetic regulation of gene expression. First, this type of regulation determines up- or down-regulation and the scope of gene responses to the activation of different signaling pathways. Second, epigenetic mechanisms contribute to stable, cell-type-specific patterns of gene activities (silencing or activation) [2], a key property of living systems of robustness, e.g. the ability to maintain phenotypic stability in the face of diverse perturbations arising from environmental changes [3].

As this field continues to expend, it is becoming increasingly evident that a host of genomic interrelationships with aspects of the external environment, such as temperature or nutrient availability, exist.

For years, scientists have understood that biological fate is not completely controlled by DNA sequence and that genome sequences play only a partial role in determining an individual's biological characterization (phenotype). Cells, either free-living or part of a multi-cellular organism, must be able to rapidly respond to changes in their external environment, such as temperature or nutrient availability, to exploit and survive in changing conditions.

The function of DNA is not as fixed as previously thought. The interaction between genes and the environment plays a crucial role in determining human and animal resistance to various types of stress. Different environmental and nutritional factors are known to result in changes in phenotype in many organisms, described as phenotypic plasticity. The recognition that nutrient availability has the capacity to modulate the molecular mechanisms underlying an organism's physiological functions has prompted a revolution in the field of animal and human nutrition [4].

In this chapter, the discussion will be concentrated on environmental stress and nutrient and epigenetic interactions (nutrigenomics). Nutrigenomics is the intriguing topic of nutrition and epigenetics, concentrating especially on nutrient-epigenetic regulation in bovine cells.

NUTRIENTS AND EPIGENETICS IN BOVINE CELLS

Research in epigenomics, especially nutrigenomics, is still in its infancy in farm animals. One definitive example of the nutrient-epigenetic-phenotype relationship can be shown through the examination of volatile fatty acids (VFAs, i.e., acetate, propionate, and butyrate), also referred to as short-chain fatty acids (SCFAs), and the regulation of gene expression induced by SCFAs. SCFAs are formed during microbial fermentation of dietary fiber in the gastrointestinal tract of mammalian species and are then directly absorbed at the site of production. These compounds contribute up to 70% of the energy requirements of ruminant species [5]. Rates of SCFA production and absorption in ruminants, which have been calculated to be about 5 mol/kg of dry matter intake, are much greater than in humans and other animals. The major SCFAs in either the rumen or large intestine are acetate, propionate, and butyrate and they are produced in ratios varying from ~75:15:10 to 40:40:20. The concentrations of SCFAs in the rumen are highly variable and the total amount present usually fluctuates between 60 and 150 m*M*. In sheep, butyrate concentrations in the digestive tract and blood are usually between 0.5 and 13 mM [5]. Acetate and propionate have relatively higher concentrations as they have a prominent position in providing energy for ruminant metabolism. Butyrate is low in relative concentration but appears to be involved in metabolic processes beyond its role as a nutrient with high effectiveness as an inhibitor of histone deacetylases (HDACs). Butyrate involvement has been determined in cell differentiation, proliferation, motility, and, in particular, in induction of cell cycle arrest and apoptosis [6,7,8,9]. These biological effects on the cell cycle and apoptosis have undergone intensive investigation, with the aim of developing butyrate as a therapeutic agent for cancer treatment. All the evidence indicates that, in cattle, SCFAs are common and important nutrients. Therefore, understanding their biological importance, beyond their use as a simple energy supply, will aid in understanding critical control points in the cell cycle. This knowledge could lead to improvements in the efficiency of production of food animals.

The therapeutic potential of butyrate for cancer has been intensively studied [10]. The cell cycle regulatory effects of butyrate at the cellular and molecular levels in normal bovine cells also have been studied [9,11,12]. The principal biochemical change in cells treated with butyrate and other histone deacetylase (HDAC) inhibitors is the global hyperacetylation of histones [9,13,14]. The links of histone post-translational modifications and chromatin structure to cell cycle progression, DNA replication, and overall chromosome stability have become very clear [15]. However, the molecular basis for these effects on the cell cycle is still poorly defined. The modulation of genome expression as a consequence of chromatin structural changes is likely a mechanism with a major role in determining tissue responses. Data from *in vitro* experiments on bovine cells (MDBK) show that, as a direct result of the hyperacetylation of histones induced by butyrate treatment at physiological concentrations (2.5 to 10 m*M*), cultured bovine cells are arrested in the early G1 phase and DNA synthesis is eliminated, as assayed by BrdU incorporation and flow cytometric analyses [9]. At a relatively high concentration (10 mM), butyrate also induces apoptosis in an established bovine MDBK cell line [9]. In primary cultures of isolated ruminal epithelial cells, DNA replication is also inhibited by butyrate treatment [16]. In addition, butyrate may also alter histone methylation as a histone deacetylase inhibitor [17], suggesting an interplay between histone acetylation and methylation. Figure 1 shows that when bovine cells (MDBK) were treated with 10 m*M* butyrate for 24 hours, cell morphology became distorted [18]. Cells with large vacuoles or ragged membranes, lacking distinct intracellular organelles and increasing spaces between cells were readily visible and recurrent. Flow cytometry analysis of cell population profiles for DNA content and BrdU labeling also confirmed that the cells were arrested at the G1 and G1/S boundary. The incorporation of BrdU labeling suggested that DNA synthesis was blocked by butyrate treatment. Western blotting also confirmed that butyrate induced a hyper-acetylation of Histone 3.

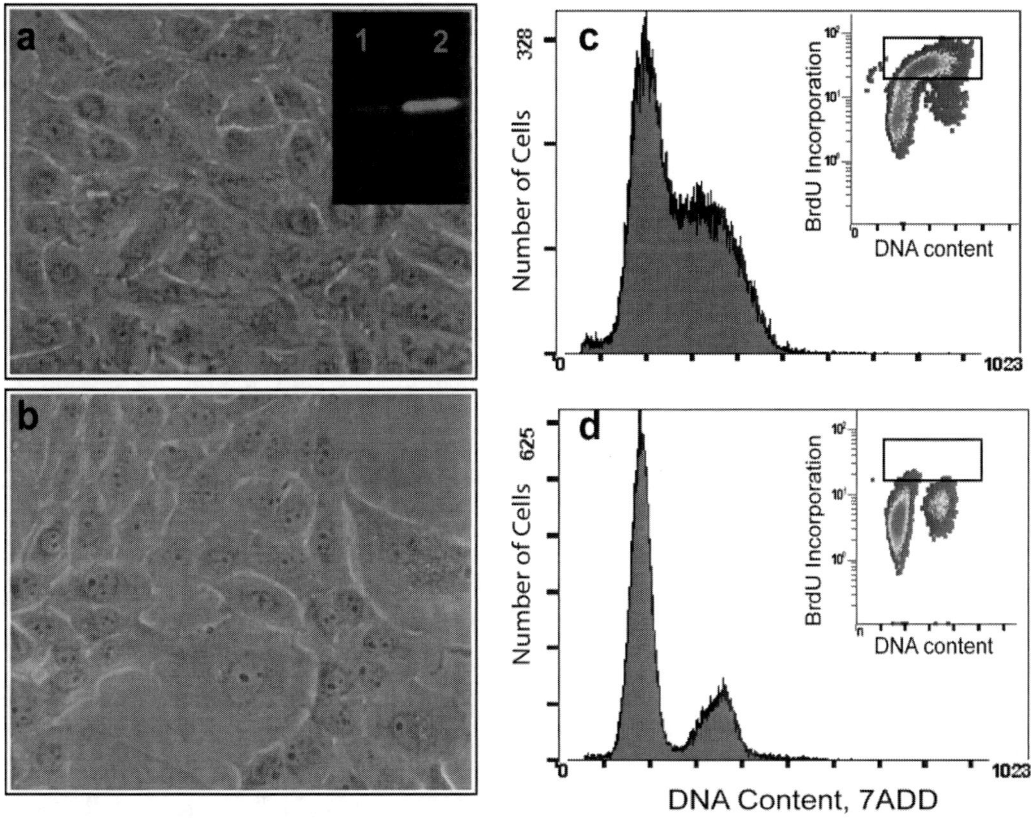

Figure 1. (Reproduced from [18]). Butyrate induces significant biological effects in cultured MDBK cells. a): normal cells; b): cells treated with 10mM butyrate for 24 hrs, showing morphological changes including large vacuoles, ragged membranes, lack of distinct intracellular organelles, and increasing spaces between cells. Insert in a) comparison of histone H3 acetylation of normal cells (1) and histone acetylation in butyrate-treated cells (2). c and d: Cell population profiles determined by flow cytometry. c); normal cells and d) cells treated with butyrate. Inserts: BrdU labeling show butyrate blocked the DNA synthesis after 24 hr treatment. Cells were first pulse labeled with BrdU for 30 min. Collected cells were first stained with diluted fluorescent (Fluorescent isothiocyanate, FITC) anti-BrdU antibody and then stained with DNA marker (7-ADD). The fluorescent signal generated by FITC was acquired in a logarithmic mode, and fluorescent signal from the DNA-content marker 7-ADD was normally acquired in the linear signal amplification mode. Cells were separated into three clusters by double staining analysis. Butyrate treatment eliminates cells in S phase (in rectangle box).

HISTONE ACETYLATION AND GENE REGULATION UNDERLYING THE MECHANISMS OF SHORT-CHAIN FATTY ACID EFFECTS ON CELLULAR FUNCTIONS

To understand the genetic basis of butyrate effects, a high-density oligonucleotide microarray was first employed to investigate the global gene expression profiles of bovine cells in response to sodium butyrate administration. These oligonucleotides represent approximately 45,383 unique cattle sequences. This investigation of global gene expression profiles of bovine kidney epithelial cells, regulated by sodium butyrate using a high-density oligonucleotide microarray [11,19], determined that as much as 8% of genes are regulated by butyrate. 450 genes were found to be significantly regulated by sodium butyrate at a very stringent false discovery rate (FDR) = 0% [11,19]. The single largest category of genes regulated by butyrate was represented by genes related to cell cycle control. Butyrate repressed the vast majority of these genes including cyclins, cyclin-dependent kinases, histone deacetylases, helicases, and chromosomal structure proteins. Extensive repression of cyclin-dependent kinases, as well as cell cycle related genes, such as *CDC2/CDK1, CDC20, CDC25A, CCNG1, CCNB1, CCNB2, CCNA2, CCNG1,* and *PCNA*, may be closely associated with the cell growth arrest induced by butyrate. This repression is also consistent with the growing body of evidence suggesting that disruption of the coordination between regulation of DNA synthesis and cyclin-dependent kinase activity is an important feature of apoptosis. Using microarray techniques, down regulation of *MCM2, MCM3, MCM4, MCM5, MCM6 (MCM*: minichromosome maintenance proteins, which are essential DNA replication initiation factors), and *ORC1* (Origin Recognition Complex subunit 1) genes, was found in response to butyrate treatment for the first time. All of the products of these genes are the critical elements for initiation of DNA replication as they are the essential components of the pre-replication complex. The functional category and pathway analyses of the microarray data revealed that four canonical pathways (Cell cycles: G2/M DNA damage checkpoint, pyrimidine metabolism, G1/S checkpoint regulation, and purine metabolism) were significantly perturbed. Moreover, the biologically relevant networks and pathways of these genes were also identified. They included genes such as *IGF2, TGFB1, TP53, E2F4,* and *CDC2*, which were established as central to these networks. The profound changes in gene expression elucidate the pleiotropic effects of histone acetylation induced by butyrate in bovine cells. A majority of these genes were repressed by butyrate and were associated with cell cycle control. It was also found that butyrate can greatly enhance the derivation of human pluripotent stem cells by promoting epigenetic remodeling and the expression of pluripotency-associated genes [20].

The development of next-generation sequencing (NGS) has provided novel tools for expression profiling and genome analysis [21,22,23]. A study using next-generation sequencing technology provided a more complete characterization of the RNA transcripts of MDBK cells [18]. The study was focused on the comparison between a control group of cells (without butyrate treatment) and cells treated with 10 m*M* butyrate for 24 hours. The samples were deep-sequenced, with an average of more than 67 million reads per sample, and the results were used to estimate the differences induced by butyrate treatment. The NGS results showed very reliable and detailed profiling of the changes in gene expression induced by butyrate in a normal bovine cell line.

IPA (Ingenuity Pathways Analysis, Ingenuity® Systems [www.ingenuity. com]) analysis revealed that butyrate exerts a very broad range of effects on many biological pathways through its action on HDACs in the MDBK cell line. NGS results, with a comparative transcriptomic profiling approach, extended far beyond the findings reported using microarray technologies [19,24]. The phenomenal number of genes fell within a broad range of functional categories, providing a very detailed molecular basis for the butyrate-induced biological effects. Figure 2 shows the major biological functions perturbed by butyrate-treatment and detected by transcriptomic characterization using deep RNA-sequencing (RNA-seq).

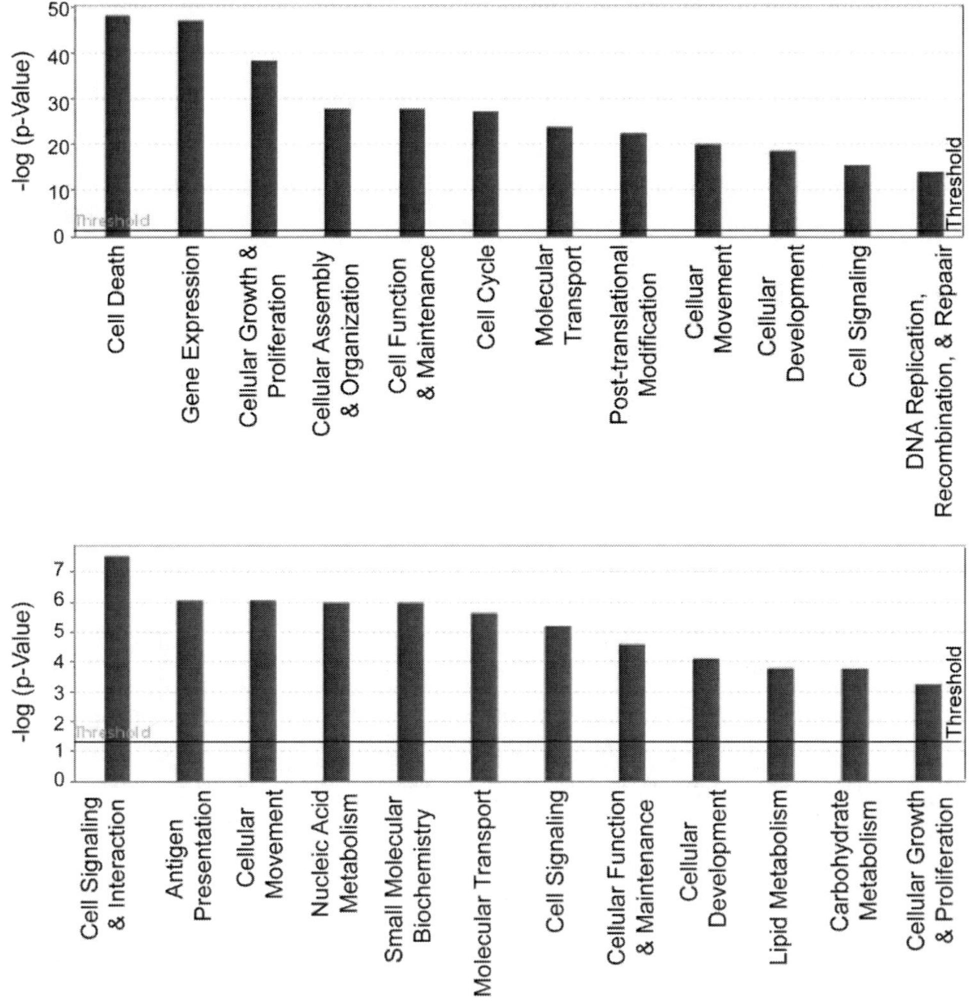

Figure 2. Global functional analysis. Datasets were analyzed by the Ingenuity Pathways Analysis software (Ingenuity® Systems, www.ingenuity.com). The significance value associated with a function in Global Analysis is a measure for how likely it is that genes from the dataset file under investigation participate in that function. The significance is expressed as a p-value, which is calculated using the right-tailed Fisher's Exact Test. Upper panel: Functional analysis of total genes perturbed by butyrate treatment; Lower panel: Functional analysis of genes uniquely expressed in butyrate treated cells.

The stable propagation of genetic information requires that the entire genome of an organism be faithfully replicated only once in each cell cycle. In eukaryotes, this replication is initiated at hundreds to thousands of replication origins distributed over the genome, each of which must be prohibited from re-initiating DNA replication within a single cell cycle [25]. Initiation of DNA replication is a two-step process. First, initiation proteins are assembled onto the replication origin in a stepwise fashion to develop a pre-replication complex. Second, the initiation complex is activated by protein kinases, resulting in the establishment of replication forks. This process is tightly regulated, such that initiation at a given replication origin occurs only once per cell cycle. In addition, initiation is down-regulated in response to agents that damage DNA or block DNA replication.

In eukaryotic cells, cell cycle checkpoint regulation assures the fidelity of cell division. The G1 (first gap phase)/S cell cycle checkpoint controls the passage of eukaryotic cells from the G1 into the S phase. Mitogen-dependent progression through the G1 of the cell-division cycle is accurately regulated to ensure that normal cell division is synchronous with cell growth and that the initiation of DNA synthesis (the S phase) is timed precisely to avoid inappropriate DNA amplification. The G1/S checkpoint control is vital for normal cell division and involves the key components that include cell cycle kinases, CDK4/6-cyclin D and CDK2-cyclin E, and the transcription complex composed of the retinoblastoma protein (Rb) and transcription factor E2F. The activation of E2F is necessary for the G1-S transition. In the present report, CDK4/6 and cyclins E and E2F were significantly down-regulated by butyrate-induced histone acetylation. In contrast, p21, a cell cycle inhibitor protein, was significantly up-regulated. All of these perturbations of gene expression in the G1/S cell cycle checkpoint pathways are consistent with the observed biological effects of butyrate, which induces cell cycle arrest at the G1/S boundary [9].

The first clear evidence that a six-subunit "origin recognition complex's" (ORC) activity in mammalian cells is regulated by cell cycle-dependent changes in the affinity of the largest subunit (Orc1) for chromatin has been reported [25,26]. Evidence has since confirmed these findings and extended them to show that mammalian Orc1 is selectively ubiquitinated and phosphorylated during the S-to-M–phase transition, while ORC subunits 2 to 5, which constitute a stable core complex, remain tightly bound to chromatin throughout cell division [27]. In addition, a second mechanism prevents the assembly of a functional ORC until the completion of mitosis: the selective association of Orc1 with Cdk1 (Cdc2)/cyclin A during the G2/M phase of cell division. This association accounted for the appearance in M-phase cells with hyperphosphorylated Orc1 that was subsequently dephosphorylated during the M-to-G1 transition [28]. The rebinding of Orc1 to chromatin follows the same time course as the degradation of cyclin B, suggesting that the exit from mitosis triggers Orc1 binding to chromatin. In fact, the inhibition of Cdk activity in metaphase cells resulted in the rapid binding of Orc1 to chromatin, and NGS profiling shows that all six subunits of ORC are down-regulated by butyrate-induced histone acetylation, adding yet another layer of regulation of ORC activities via the modified expression of those genes. In our previous microarray profiling [19], some of the components of this pathway were found to be perturbed by butyrate-induced gene regulation; however, *ORC1* was the only one of the six ORC complex genes that was detected to be a down-regulated gene. In the present report, *ORC1* is still the most significantly down-regulated gene, but the other ORC components (*ORC2* to *ORC6*) are all also identified as down-regulated. This result certainly indicates the superb sensitivity of deep RNA sequencing (Figure 3).

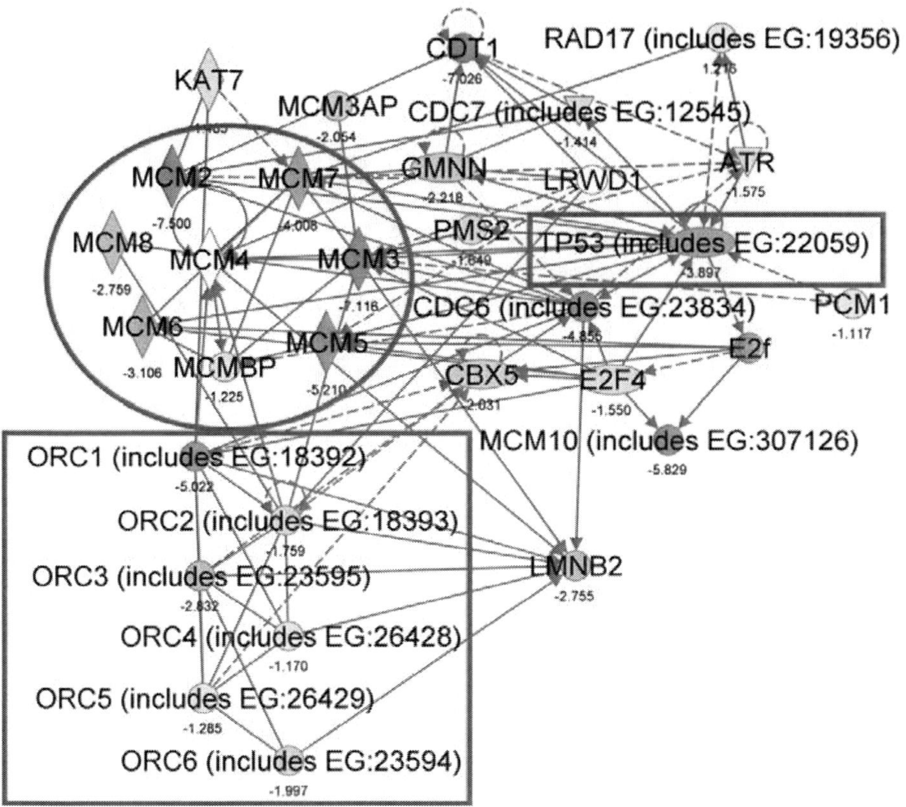

Figure 3. The biologically relevant gene network - genes related to DNA replication: The integrated network in cells treated with butyrate for 24 h. Data set was analyzed by the Ingenuity Pathways Analysis software (Ingenuity® Systems, www.ingenuity.com). All notes (genes) in this network are down-regulated. Notes and edges are displayed with various shapes and labels that present the functional class of genes and the nature of the relationship between the notes, respectively. Circle and two squares highlight the MCM (Mini Chromosome Maintenance complex); ORC (Origin Recognition Complex) and TP53.

It was very interesting that reports indicated that *ORC1* also effects transcriptional silencing in *Saccharomyces cerevisiae* and heterochromatin function in Drosophila [29,30] by mediation of chromatin acetylation. And these functions of ORC are conserved in mammals as well. A novel protein has been identified: *HBO1* (histone acetyltransferase binding to ORC), which interacts with human *ORC1* protein, the largest subunit of *ORC*. *HBO1* exists as part of a multi-subunit complex that possesses histone H3 and H4 acetyltransferase activities. *HBO1* is a member of the MYST domain family that includes *S. cerevisiae* Sas2p, a protein involved in control of transcriptional silencing that also has been genetically linked to ORC function. Thus the interaction between ORC and a MYST domain acetyltransferase is widely conserved. It was suggested that ORC-mediated acetylation of chromatin play roles in control of both DNA replication and gene expression [31].

We also found significant up-regulation of both *BTG1* and *BTG2*. The BTG family member-2 (*BTG2*) has antiproliferative activity, and the expression of *BTG2* in cycling cells induces the accumulation of hypophosphorylated, growth-inhibitory forms of retinoblastoma protein (Rb) and leads to G1 arrest through the impairment of DNA synthesis. These up-regulated antiproliferation activities are strengthened by the extensive repression of cyclin-dependent kinase and cell cycle-related genes that are clearly associated with the cell growth arrest induced by butyrate.

Tumor protein p53 (*TP53*, a nuclear protein), with transcription factor E2F4 and many other transcription factors, were deregulated by butyrate treatment in the present study. TP53 plays an essential role in the regulation of the cell cycle, specifically in the transition from G0 to G1. It is found in very low levels in normal cells; however, in a variety of transformed cell lines, it is expressed in high amounts and is believed to contribute to transformation and malignancy. p53 is a DNA-binding protein that contains DNA-binding, oligomerization, and transcription activation domains. p53 is postulated to bind as a tetramer to a p53-binding site and activate the expression of downstream genes that inhibit growth and/or invasion, thereby functioning as a tumor suppressor. p53 has been extensively studied for its function and involvement in butyrate-induced biological effects [32,33,34]. Butyrate efficiently suppresses the growth of WT p53-containing cells. It leads to a major G2/M arrest of cells in the presence of p53, while cells without wild-type p53 accumulate mainly in the G1 phase of the cell cycle. Apoptosis induction by butyrate is also greatly reduced in the absence of p53, suggesting that a p53 pathway mediates, in part, growth suppression by butyrate and that p53 status may be an important determinant of chemosensitivity to butyrate [35]. Our data also indicate that the *TP53* genes may have different responses and different roles to play in normal and transformed cells. In our dataset, 518 genes were potential targets for *TP53* regulation. Among these 518 genes, 238 genes showed expression directions consistent with the activation of *TP53*. However, one remaining question is why the expression of *TP53* was down-regulated, even as its function was more active [36].

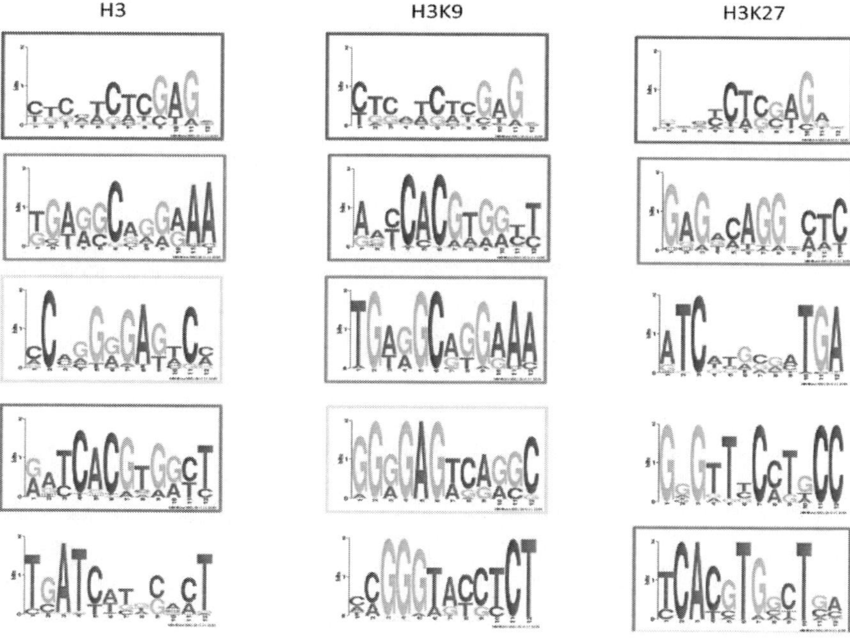

Figure 4. Characterization of histone H3, acetyl-H3K9 and acetyl-H3K27 binding motifs. Squares indicate the existing consensus with H3, acetyl-H3K9 and acetyl-H3K27

As an extremely regulated gene, two major factors may contribute to this complexity of *TP53*. First, the expression of *TP53* is subject to multiple regulations at transcriptional, post-transcriptional, and translational levels, with very complex expression patterns of alternative splicing, alternative promoter usage, and alternative translation. Secondly, the regulation of p53 function is extremely complex and occurs at many levels. Post-translational modifications of p53 (phosphorylation, methylation, acetylation, etc.) alter the functions of p53 (recognition of DNA sequences, interactions with transcription factors at promoters of target genes, etc.) [37]. Indeed, deep RNA-seq and IPA analysis revealed significant changes in the expression of genes related to the molecular function of protein post-translational modification. There are 333 genes related to the phosphorylation of proteins, 80 genes related to the tyrosine phosphorylation of proteins, and 106 genes related to the activation of protein kinase, which is up-regulated by butyrate. The possibility exists that the modification of p53 is affected by butyrate, directly or indirectly. Clearly, more studies are still required to understand the exact roles that *TP53* plays in butyrate-induced biological effects [18].

SHORT-CHAIN FATTY ACIDS, HISTONE ACETYLATION, HISTONE METHYLATION, DNA METHYLATION AND MICRORNA EXPRESSION

Butyrate is able to inhibit all class I HDACs. It also seems to affect many other epigenetic-related enzymes by regulating the expression of genes. The missing link is why this inhibition of enzymatic activities, in turn, regulates their own expression at the mRNA level. A vastly complicated depiction of the expression of HDACs induced by butyrate treatment was found by deep RNA sequencing. Whereas the expression of HCACs 7, 8, and 9 are down-regulated, HDACs 5 and 11 are up-regulated, and HDACs 1, 2, 4, and 6 are unchanged. HDAC inhibitors that affect the expression of the HDACs themselves have been observed in mouse neural cells [38]. In that report, both TSA and butyrate indeed elevated the expression of *HADC1, HDAC3, HDAC5,* and *HDAC6*, whereas the mRNA levels for *HDAC2* and *HDAC7* did not change. The mRNA levels of *HDAC8* and *HDAC10* were not detectable in these cells. The mechanism and biological relevance of HDAC inhibitors in the regulation of the expression of HDACs is not clear, but may possibly indicate the existence of an auto-regulatory feedback loop for the expression of several HDACs after their activities are inhibited [18].

As mentioned above, butyrate can also decrease histone methylation [17], suggesting an interplay between histone acetylation and histone methylation. An emerging possibility is that histone modifications can influence one another. In other words, there may be "crosstalk among histone modification" [39]. Consistently, *KDM5B*, a specific histone demethylase (H3-trimethyl-K4), was significantly up-regulated by butyrate treatment in bovine cells. However, *JSRID2*, which is directly related to histone methylation and responsible for maintaining the methylation level on histone H3 lysine 27 trimethylation (H3K27me3) [40], was also significantly up-regulated. *JARID2* possesses an *in vitro* methyl-protective activity, stabilizing Polycom Repressive Complex 2 (*PRC2*)-catalyzed H3K27me3 by protecting it from the activity of H3K27 demethylases [41]. These data may indicate that different histone marks (modifications) are differentially regulated and that in turn, differentially regulated histone marks regulate different biological functions [42].

On the other side, a reversal of DNA methylation by butyrate has also recently been reported to occur by the regulation of DNA (cytosine-5-)-methyltransferase 1 (*DNMT1*) through *ERK* signaling [43]. It was found that three DNA methyltransferases (DNMTs), *DNMT1, DNMT3A,* and *DNMT3B,* were significantly down-regulated by the butyrate treatment. While *DNMT1* functions in the establishment and regulation of tissue-specific patterns of methylated cytosine residues, *DNMT3A* and *DNMT3B* function in the *de novo* methylation of DNA [44,45]. These DNMTs are regulated by several mechanisms in terms of their expression and catalytic activity. However, deep RNA sequencing data directly indicated that histone modification has a role in the regulation of the expression of DNMTs, thereby affecting the level of DNA methylation [18].

miRNAs are a class of highly conserved, small non-coding RNAs (~22 nucleotides) that regulate gene expression post-transcriptionally [46]. miRNAs bind to complementary sequences in the 3'-untranslated regions (3' UTRs) of target messenger RNA transcripts (mRNAs), usually resulting in gene silencing [47]. miRNAs are encoded by specific genes in the genome, which are transcribed as primary transcripts called primary miRNAs. Biogenesis of miRNA has been extensively studied and excellent reviews are also available [48,49]. While Histone modification and miRNA are the two different epigenetic pathways for regulation of gene expression, in recent years, some evidence has suggested that these two pathways may cross-talk and interfere with each other [50]. Butyrate-induced histone acetylation may regulate miRNA expression, and in turn, miRNAs may interfere with butyrate-induced modulation of gene expression and cellular functions.

miRNA was first discovered from *C. elegans* in 1991 and was demonstrated as a novel mechanism for gene regulation. *lin-4* is a heterochronic gene in *C. elegans* that is required for proper cell fate specification in larval development. Genetic evidence indicated that the *lin-4* gene product negatively regulated the heterochronic lin-14 targeting the 3'UTR [51,52]. During the first 10 years after microRNA discovery, only a handful of publications appeared each year on the subject. Little was known about the mechanism of how miRNAs function lead to the translational repression of target mRNA. During the first 7 years, this novel mechanism was largely ignored and assumed to be a worm-specific anomaly. However, *let-7* was cloned from C. elegans [53,54] and was also found to be conserved in Drosophila and in humans [53]. Since then, the level of microRNA research has increased to become a microRNA revolution.

MicorRNAs are regulated by a variety of stimuli such as gene amplification, gene deletion, cellular stress, and inflammation, as well as by epigenetic mechanisms. The mechanism of miRNA silencing mRNA is based on the interaction between miRNAs and mRNAs. These interactions include competition for the nuclear cap-binding protein complex (which is an RNA-binding protein complex that binds to the 5' cap inside the nucleus), deadenylation and mRNA degradation, mRNA sequestration, and ribosome drop off. Many different miRNAs exist and each can target many mRNAs, which can be involved in various cellular processes such as cell division, cell death, DNA repair, differentiation, and epigenetic mechanisms. Therefore, the expression of miRNA can have a profound effect in regulating gene expression. Under certain cellular conditions, miRNA can also increase translation of target genes. For example, upon cell cycle arrest, miR-369-3 targets TNF-□ and leads to its translational activation [55,56].

SCFAs induced-transcriptional reprogramming is achieved through various and complex mechanisms not fully understood, including histone deacetylation, transcription factor or regulator (including *HDAC1*) deacetylation followed by chromatin remodeling, and positive or negative outcome regarding transcription initiation. While only a low percentage of protein-coding genes are affected by the action of HDAC inhibitors, it was found that about 40% of noncoding microRNAs are up-regulated or down-regulated. Moreover, a whole new world of long noncoding RNAs is emerging, revealing a new class of potential targets for HDAC inhibition. HDAC inhibitors might also regulate transcription elongation and have been shown to impinge on alternative splicing [57]. In bovine cells, miRNA microarray profiling of miRNAs and statistical tests, as well as clustering analysis, show that butyrate induces profound changes in miRNA expression in bovine cells. A total of 143 miRNA transcripts were differentially expressed and signal intensity was > 32. After eliminating the transcripts that had low signals (signal < 500), 35 transcripts remained that were significantly (p < 0.05) differentially expressed. Among these, expression of 11 transcripts was very significant (p < 0.01) [14]. These observations reflect cross-talk between miRNA and histone acetylation. Deep RNA-seq also reveals a significant amount of information regarding non-coding RNA (ncRNA) [18]. There are 24 ncRNAs that are differentially expressed due to the butyrate treatment. Those ncRNAs belong to different types of ncRNAs, including snoRNA (small nucleolar RNA), snRNA (splicesomal RNA), and some miscRNAs. Particularly, the expression of 10 snoRNAs (5 down-regulated and 5 up-regulated) was found to be disrupted by the butyrate treatment. snoRNAs are intermediate-sized ncRNAs (60-300 bp). They are components of small nucleolar ribonucleoproteins (snoRNPs), which are complexes that are responsible for the modification and processing of ribosomal RNA [58]. More importantly, a large proportion of snoRNAs have been found to be further processed into smaller molecules, such as miRNAs [59].

Very interestingly, a recent report also identified the important growth regulatory role for colonic epithelial miRNAs in mediating the effects of the microbe-derived short chain fatty acid butyrate on host gene expression [60]. In that report, it was found that in HCT-116 cells, butyrate suppressed many of the same miRNAs increased in human colon cancers. One of these miRNAs, miR-106b, was found to target p21. Butyrate and miR-106b treatment of a p21 3′UTR luciferase reporter construct in HCT116 cells indicates that butyrate-stimulated p21 expression is translationally inhibited in part by miR-106b. This partial inhibition by miR-106b confirms previous reports that butyrate also regulates p21 expression via a miRNA independent mechanism, through its inhibition of HDAC.

Understanding the regulatory mechanisms controlling miRNA expression is crucial because miRNA can have extensive effects through regulation of a variety of genes that are essential for cell functions and that are involved in all of the most crucial cellular processes. MicroRNA and epigenetic regulation present a very complicated interplay because miRNA can regulate the expression of components of the epigenetic machinery, by targeting molecules involved in methylation or acetylation of histone [61]. In bovine cells, butyrate-induced epigenetic modulation of gene expression resulted in profound changes in miRNA expression; in turn, miRNA modulate epigenetic regulation induced by butyrate by regulating expression of the genes targeted by differentially expressed miRNA. Functional network analysis indicated that differentially expressed miRNAs target some important gene networks. All of these findings indicate that a complicated interaction between the two different regulation machineries that use miRNA and histone acetylation results in a highly integrated regulation mechanism.

It is worth mentioning that histone deacetylase inhibitors (HDACi) are an emerging class of novel anti-cancer drugs that cause growth arrest, differentiation and apoptosis of tumor cells. The short chain fatty acids like butyrate are among the first class of HDACi to be identified [62]. Since then, a great effort has been devoted to develop HDAC inhibitors as antineoplastic drugs and some HDAC inhibitors are showing encouraging efficacy in cancer patients [63,64]. There are also many other beneficial effects of HDACi, such as their therapeutic implications in the innate immune system [65], in the generation of the anti-tumour immune response [66], modulation of antigen-presenting cells by HDAC inhibitors [67], as well as their anti-parasite activities [68], which have been studied intensively [69].

THE EXPRESSION OF GENES IN RESPONSE TO ENVIRONMENTAL STRESS

Cells exposed to different kinds of environmental stress rapidly alter gene transcription, resulting in the immediate down regulation of housekeeping genes, while drastically increasing crucial stress-responsive transcription [70]. Those changes are often referred to as a "cell stress response" [71,72]. Since a majority of the world's human and domestic animal population lies in regions where seasonal stressors adversely influence productivity and result in economic losses, there is renewed interest in identifying specific genes, which could improve resistance to stressors without adversely affecting productivity [73]. Certainly, these cell stress responses are also of great interest to basic biology and to biomedicine. It has been know for a long time that thermal stresses (both cold and heat) trigger a complex program of gene expression and biochemical adaptive responses [72,74,75]. Many of such responses that result in global transcriptional changes are highly conservative across the spectrum of living organisms, from bacteria to humans. Most stress responses follow a common two-pronged approach: a specific and immediate response, which allows the cell to survive immediate damage, while also preparing for more severe or long-term stress. The heat shock response, characterized by increased expression of heat shock proteins (Hsps) is induced by exposure of cells and tissues to extreme conditions that cause acute or chronic stress. Hsps function as molecular chaperones in regulating cellular homeostasis and promoting survival. If the stress is too severe, a signal that leads to apoptosis (programmed cell death) is activated, thereby providing a finely tuned balance between survival and death.

In addition to extracellular stimuli, several non-stressful conditions induce Hsps during normal cellular growth and development [76]. Heat shock transcription factors (HSFs) are transcription factors that regulate Hsps expression through interaction with a specific DNA sequence in the promoter, the heat shock element [77]. The importance of HSFs as regulators of the heat shock response is reflected by their high cross-species conservation in evolution [76]. The secondary stress response results in transcriptional changes that enable the cell to adapt to environmental stress and possibly enable the normal cell cycle to continue [70]. In domestic animals, a recent study utilizing microarrays to evaluate environmental stress tolerance at the cellular level in cattle [73] revealed that thermal stress triggers a dramatic and complex program of altered gene expression in bovine mammary epithelial cells (BMEC).

The patterns of altered gene expression are similar to patterns reported in other cells types exposed to heat stress [77]. The transcription profile indicated that genes involved in cell structure, metabolism, biosynthesis and intracellular transport are generally down-regulated, while genes involved in cellular repair, protein repair and degradation, and apoptosis after loss of thermo-tolerance are generally up-regulated when the Heat-shock protein (HSP)-70 gene expressed [73].

DIVERSE REGULATION MECHANISMS—THE ROLE OF EPIGENETIC REGULATIONS

Stress-induced transcription is very complex and involves diverse regulation mechanisms. It is becoming increasingly apparent that genetic information and environmental influences are not independent of each other and that information acquired from the environment provides instructions for how the genetic material is used [78]. The rapid activation of gene expression in response to stress is largely shown through the regulation of RNA polymerase II dependent transcription. In order to allow large amounts of genetic materials to fit into the relatively small nucleus, chromatin is organized into various levels of condensation. The first level of compaction is a histone octamer comprising 2 copies each of the core histones H2A, H2B, H3 and H4, which wraps around of DNA and forms nucleosomes. Every core histone has an amino-terminal tail and histone H2A also has a significant carboxyl-terminus. The core histone tails play a significant function in the further compaction of chromatin and the core histone tail domains are key regulators of eukaryotic chromatin structure and function [79,80]. Covalent and non-covalent modifications of histone proteins and DNA, as well as the mechanisms of such modification in changing overall chromatin structure, have been researched intensively in recent years as major epigenetic mechanisms that regulated the gene expression [81,82]. From a collection of diverse phenomena, epigenetics has evolved to a defined and far-reaching field of study [83].

Since the discovery of thermosensitive neurons in the preoptic anterior hypothalamus (POAH) [84], the primary importance of these neurons in thermoregulation has been established [85]. The thermal control set point is regulated by thermosensitive neurons of POAH and completes its development during a postnatal critical sensory period. However, until recently, it has been recognized that external stimuli, such as an increase in environmental temperature, influence the neuronal protein repertoire and, ultimately, cell properties via activation or silencing of gene transcription. Both activation and silencing of gene transcription are regulated by chromatin remodeling or histone modification. Chromatin remodeling is a dynamic means of altering chromatin structure so that transcription machinery can access previously condensed DNA. Much of chromatin remodeling occurs through interactions between chromatin remodeling/modifying complexes and histones. Histone modification is another mechanism used by cells to control access DNA in chromatin. Histone-modifying complexes alter the state of chromatin through covalent modification of histones [86].

The best such examples in farm animals are studies of chicks. It has been demonstrated in chicks that there is an increase in global histone H3 lysine 9 (H3K9) acetylation as well as H3K9 dimethylation in the chicks' POAH during heat conditioning at the critical period of sensory development. In contrast to the global profile of H3K9 modifications, acetylation and dimethylation patterns of H3K9 at the promoter of the catalytic subunit of eukaryotic translation initiation factor 2B (*Eif2b5*) were opposite to each other. During heat conditioning, there was an increase in H3K9 acetylation at the Eif2b5 promoter, simultaneously with decrease in H3K9 dimethylation. These alterations coincided with Eif2b5 mRNA induction. Exposure to excessive heat during the critical period resulted in long-term effect on both H3K9 tagging at the Eif2b5 promoter and Eif2b5 mRNA expression [87]. These data are the clearest indication that dynamic H3K9 post-translational modifications regulate the gene expression at translational level during the thermal control establishment. Findings of induction of global histone H3 lysine 27 (H3K27) dimethylation, with no changes in its trimethylation levels, in the frontal hypothalamus, as well as at the promoter of the brain-derived neurotrophic factor (BDNF) gene during thermal-control establishment also highlight the specific epigenetic role of chromatin modifications in thermal-control establishment [88].

Heat-shock transcription factor 1 (*HSF1*) also has a major regulatory function in a large-scale remodeling of the cell epigenome. In addition to its well-known transcriptional activities, *HSF1* mediates a genome-wide and massive histone deacetylation [89]. The heat-shock-dependent histone deacetylation is triggered by *HSF1,* and is specifically associated with and uses *HDAC1* and *HDAC2*. This heat-shock response indicates a potent and unique model to understand the link between gene activity and chromatin remodeling [89].

Increasing evidence suggests that Hsp90 has a role in modifying the chromatin conformation of many genes [90]. The data from Drosophila studies revealed that *HSP90* affecting chromatin remodeling might be the mechanism underline transgenerational inheritance of epigenetic information acquired from environmental stimuli [91]. Hsp90 is required for optimal activity of the histone H3 lysine-4 methyltransferase *SMYD3* in mammals. Hsp90 has been shown to increase the activity of the histone H3 lysine-4 methyltransferase *SMYD3*, which activates the chromatin of target genes [92,93]. Further evidence for chromatin-remodeling functions is that Hsp90 acts as a capacitor for morphological evolution by masking epigenetic variation. Release of the capacitor function of Hsp90, such as by environmental stress or by drugs that inhibit the ATP-binding activity of Hsp90, exposes previously hidden morphological phenotypes in the next generation and for several generations thereafter [94,95].

Steroid hormones also participate in the stress response. Epigenetic regulation of expression of genes involved in steroid hormone provides an additional layer of gene regulation, even though epigenetic regulation of key steroidogenic enzymes does not look like a predominant regulatory pathway [96]. Steroide hormones wield their action in target cells through steroid nuclear receptors belong to the NR3A and NR3C families. Those nuclear receptors include estrogen receptor, androgen receptor, glucocorticoid receptor, mineralocorticoid receptor, etc. DNA methylation and other epigenetic modifications play important roles in regulating and dictating the expression of the nuclear factors, and also have secondary impacts on the expression of these steroidogenic enzymes [96]. Epigenetic modification to either steroid hormone biosynthesis or steroid receptor functions is likely to modify their associated signaling.

Living organisms are constantly exposed to various stresses. It has been suggested that stress elicits a transgenerational modification of the genome. This heritable, transgenerational modification is not associated with a corresponding change in DNA sequence [97]. The mechanism of inheritance of stress-induced epigenetic change is unknown. A recent study shows that dATF-2 is involved in heterochromatin formation and that stress-induced activation of dATF-2 disrupts heterochromatin. The effect of stress-induced heterochromatin disruption can be inherited by subsequent generations. Heat shock or osmotic stress induced phosphorylation of dATF-2 and resulted in its release from heterochromatin. This heterochromatic disruption was an epigenetic event that was transmitted to the next generation. When embryos were exposed to heat stress over multiple generations, the defective chromatin state was maintained over multiple successive generations, though it gradually returned to the normal state. The results suggest a mechanism by which the effects of stress are inherited epigenetically via the regulation of a tight chromatin structure [98].

GENOME-WIDE ChIP-SEQ MAPPING AND ANALYSIS REVEAL BUTYRATE-INDUCED CHROMATIN MODIFICATION

The HDAC inhibition activity of butyrate makes it a great inducer of the hyperacetylation of histone in cells. Discovering how the epigenomic landscape is modified by butyrate-induced histone acetylation is a critical step in the path to understanding how this nutrient-affecting specific transcriptome changes at the mechanistic level. Utilizing next-generation sequencing technology, combined with ChIP (Chromatin Immunoprecipitation) technology, and histone modification (acetylation) induced by butyrate, the large-scale mapping of the epigenomic landscape of normal histone H3 and acetylated histone H3K9 and H3K27 has recently been completed [99]. To determine the location of histone H3, acetyl-H3K9 and acetyl-H3K27 binding sites within the bovine genome, the H3, acetyl-H3K9 and acetyl-H3K27 enriched binding regions in the proximal promoter within 5 Kb upstream or at the 5'untranslated region (UTR) from the transcriptional start site (TSS), exon, intron and intergenic regions (defined as regions 25 Kb upstream or 10 Kb downstream from the TSS) were analyzed. The analysis indicated that the distribution of histone H3, acetyl-H3K9, and acetyl-H3K27 correlated with transcription activity induced by butyrate. Analysis of the consensus sequences bound to H3, acetyl-H3K9, and acetyl-H3K27 reveals several consensus sequences (motifs) from each of the ChIP-seq data sets (Figure 4). Sequence motifs are short, recurring patterns in DNA that are presumed to have a biological function [100]. The motifs usually indicate sequence-specific binding sites for proteins such as nucleases and transcription factors, and in our case, one important chromatin component, histone H3. Computational analysis of the ChIP-seq data makes it possible to derive genome-wide binding patterns for the histone H3 core, acetyl-H3K9, and acetyl-H3K27.

Those results reveal that butyrate-induced acetylation of H3K9 and H3K27 changes the sequence-based binding preference of histone H3. The differences in the binding motifs for acetyl-H3K9 and acetyl-H3K27 indicate that histone modification (acetylation) at various lysine sites changes the histone H3 binding preferences either independently or cooperatively [99]. In either situation, it is evident that butyrate-induced acetylation of histone plays a role in changing chromatin structure and in defining genetic regulatory networks and interpreting the regulatory program of individual genes.

In addition to the variation of the binding preferences of acetylated histone H3 as the results of acetylation, it is very interesting that a high degree of conservation in histone binding is also evidently presented. This may present a key property of living systems of robustness, e.g. the ability to maintain phenotypic stability in the face of diverse perturbations arising from environmental changes [3]. Recent progress on understanding of epigenetics at the molecular level is remarkable, however, epigenetics is closely related to robustness, as both lie between genotypes and phenotypes [101]. Developing a better understanding of robustness and epigenetics on a molecular level is certainly an imperative task. The mapping of epigenomic landscape modified by butyrate-induced histone acetylation was a crucial starting-point for an in-depth evaluation of the mechanisms involved in bovine rumen epithelial epigenomic regulation.

THE BACTERIAL COMMUNITY COMPOSITION OF THE BOVINE RUMEN, RUMINAL FUNCTIONS AND ENVIRONMENTAL IMPACTS

The rumen is a complex microbial ecosystem and plays a critical role in sustainable agriculture throughout human civilization. Microorganisms in the rumen, such as bacteria, archaea, protozoa, and fungi, perform essential fermentation, including the conversion of plant fiber to small molecules, such as volatile fatty acids (VFA) and vitamins, used for the production of meat, milk, and wool for human consumption, thereby influencing the host's nutrition. In addition, rumen microorganisms modulate the host's immunity and enhance the host's resistance to invading pathogens [102]. Furthermore, certain bacteria detoxify naturally-occurring compounds in the diet that are harmful to the host [103]. Microorganisms in the rumen are highly responsive to changes in diet, host genetics, and physiology, as well as geographical and environmental factors.

In the rumen, hydrogen is produced during the anaerobic fermentation of nutrients. This hydrogen can be used during the synthesis of volatile fatty acids (VFAs) and microbial proteins. Ruminal methanogens reduces carbon dioxide to methane (CH_4) and eliminate the excess hydrogen from NADH. Methane production in the ruminants is an energetically-wasteful process (2-15% of ingested gross energy), since the portion of animal's feed that is converted to methane is eructed as gas. Furthermore, emission of methane, a greenhouse gas, into the environment contributes to global warming by trapping outgoing terrestrial infrared radiation [104].

It is clear that the capacity of the rumen microbiota to produce volatile fatty acids (VFAs) has important implications in animal's well-being and productivity, as well as environmental impacts. We investigated temporal changes of the rumen microbiota in response to butyrate infusion using pyrosequencing of the 16S rRNA gene [105]. Twenty one phyla were identified in the rumen microbiota of dairy cows. The rumen microbiota harbored 54.5 ± 6.1 genera (mean $\pm$ SD) and 127.3 ± 4.4 operational taxonomic units (OTUs), respectively. However, the core microbiome comprised of 26 genera and 82 OTUs. Butyrate infusion altered molar percentages of 3 major VFAs. Butyrate perturbation had a profound impact on the rumen microbial composition. A 72 h-infusion led to a significant change in the numbers of sequence reads derived from 4 phyla, including 2 of the most abundant phyla, Bacteroidetes and Firmicutes. As many as 19 genera and 43 OTUs were significantly impacted by butyrate infusion. Elevated butyrate levels in the rumen seemingly had a stimulating effect on butyrate-producing bacteria populations. The resilience of the rumen microbial ecosystem was evident as the abundance of the microorganisms returned to their pre-disturbed status after infusion withdrawal.

Our findings provide insight into perturbation dynamics of the rumen microbial ecosystem and should guide efforts in formulating optimal uses of probiotic bacteria to treat human diseases. A solid understanding of major components of rumen microbial ecosystems and their interactions is a prerequisite to successful ruminal manipulation, such as increasing efficiency of fiber digestion and reducing ruminal methanogenesis.

SUMMARY AND PERSPECTIVE

The phenotypic characterization of an animal can be changed through modification of epigenetic mechanisms, such as histone posttranslational modification, miRNA, and other mechanisms.

The multiple layers of regulatory control of the gene expression provide a multitude of paths through which cells can control their responses to external stimuli. An explosion of research efforts in recent years has begun to uncover common molecular mechanisms underlying epigenetic phenomena.

The relationship between genetics and epigenetics endow us with information about transcription regulation in cattle development and growth. With the rapid development of biotechnologies, epigenomic approaches will help us to characterize genome-wide epigenetic markers that are targets for dietary regulation.

The discovery and characterization of these novel epigenetic markers and epigenetic mechanisms will facilitate an understanding of how dietary factors modulate these epigenetic regulatory mechanisms. This area will provide a great research opportunity and a better understanding of the role of dietary components in changing epigenetic patterns and certainly will have important impacts on functional genomic research in bovines and in the farm animal industry.

On the other hand, rumen fermentation is a poorly understood process controlled by the interacting rumen microbiota constituents. Understanding of microbial interactions and dynamics in the rumen microbial ecosystem should provide a scientific basis for successful manipulation of ruminal fermentation for optimal outcomes, such as increasing efficiency of fiber digestion and reducing ruminal methanogenesis.

In the meantime, we have to realize that epigenetics and epigenomics are much more complicated and more dynamic than previously thought. Epigenomics research and the development of maps of the epigenomic markers in farm animals are increasingly required for the standardization of platforms and procedures.

Quick and efficient detection of epigenomic markers and better understanding of the factors that induce changes in these markers require a great effort. Substantial international collaboration is essential to accomplish this goal.

The fast development in this field has attracted strong interests to exploit epigenetic phenomena. We are convinced that the near future will bring many new developments in this field and that the epigenetic landscape will take shape in the field of animal science.

ACKNOWLEDGMENT

Mention of trade names or commercial products in this article is solely for the purpose of providing specific information and does not imply recommendation or endorsement by the US Department of Agriculture. The USDA is an equal opportunity provider and employer.

REFERENCES

[1] Katsnelson A (2010) Genomics goes beyond DNA sequence. *Nature* 465: 145.

[2] Tarakhovsky A (2010) Tools and landscapes of epigenetics. *Nature immunology* 11: 565-568.

[3] Stelling J, Sauer U, Szallasi Z, Doyle FJ, 3rd, Doyle J (2004) Robustness of cellular functions. *Cell* 118: 675-685.

[4] Mutch DM, Wahli W, Williamson G (2005) Nutrigenomics and nutrigenetics: the emerging faces of nutrition. *FASEB journal : official publication of the Federation of American Societies for Experimental Biology* 19: 1602-1616.

[5] Bergman EN (1990) Energy contributions of volatile fatty acids from the gastrointestinal tract in various species. *Physiol Rev* 70: 567-590.

[6] Chen JS, Faller DV, Spanjaard RA (2003) Short-chain fatty acid inhibitors of histone deacetylases: promising anticancer therapeutics? *Curr Cancer Drug Targets* 3: 219-236.

[7] Gassull MA, Cabre E (2001) Nutrition in inflammatory bowel disease. *Curr Opin Clin Nutr Metab Care* 4: 561-569.

[8] Scheppach W, Bartram HP, Richter F (1995) Role of short-chain fatty acids in the prevention of colorectal cancer. *Eur J Cancer* 31A: 1077-1080.

[9] Li CJ, Elsasser TH (2005) Butyrate-induced apoptosis and cell cycle arrest in bovine kidney epithelial cells: involvement of caspase and proteasome pathways. *J Anim Sci* 83: 89-97.

[10] Myzak MC, Dashwood RH (2006) Histone deacetylases as targets for dietary cancer preventive agents: lessons learned with butyrate, diallyl disulfide, and sulforaphane. *Curr Drug Targets* 7: 443-452.

[11] Li RW, Li CJ (2006) Butyrate induces profound changes in gene expression related to multiple signal pathways in bovine kidney epithelial cells. B*MC Genomics* 7: 234.

[12] Li RW, Li CJ (2007) Effects of butyrate on the expression of insulin-like growth factor binding proteins in bovine kindery epithelial cells. *The Open Veterinary Science Journal* 2007: 14-19.

[13] Riggs MG, Whittaker RG, Neumann JR, Ingram VM (1977) n-Butyrate causes histone modification in HeLa and Friend erythroleukaemia cells. *Nature* 268: 462-464.

[14] Li CJ, Li WR, Elsasser TH (2010) MicroRNA (miRNA) expression in regulated by butyrate-induced epigenetic modulation of gene expression in bovine cells. *Genetics & Epigentics* 2010: 23-32.

[15] Wolffe AP, Guschin D (2000) Review: chromatin structural features and targets that regulate transcription. *J Struct Biol* 129: 102-122.

[16] Baldwin RL (1999) The proliferative actions of insulin, insulin-like growth factor-I, epidermal growth factor, butyrate and propionate on ruminal epithelial cells in vitro. *Small Ruminant Research* 32: 261-268.

[17] Marinova Z, Leng Y, Leeds P, Chuang DM (2011) Histone deacetylase inhibition alters histone methylation associated with heat shock protein 70 promoter modifications in astrocytes and neurons. *Neuropharmacology* 60: 1109-1115.

[18] Wu S, Li RW, Li W, Li CJ (2012) Transcriptome characterization by RNA-seq unravels the mechanisms of butyrate-induced epigenomic regulation in bovine cells. *PLoS One* 2012;7(5):e36940.

[19] Li CJ, Li RW, Wang YH, Elsasser TH (2007) Pathway analysis identifies perturbation of genetic networks induced by butyrate in a bovine kidney epithelial cell line. *Funct Integr Genomics* 7: 193-205.

[20] Mali P, Chou BK, Yen J, Ye Z, Zou J, et al. (2010) Butyrate greatly enhances derivation of human induced pluripotent stem cells by promoting epigenetic remodeling and the expression of pluripotency-associated genes. *Stem cells* 28: 713-720.

[21] Kahvejian A, Quackenbush J, Thompson JF (2008) What would you do if you could sequence everything? Nature biotechnology 26: 1125-1133.

[22] Shendure J, Ji H (2008) Next-generation DNA sequencing. *Nature biotechnology* 26: 1135-1145.

[23] Ozsolak F, Milos PM (2011) RNA sequencing: advances, challenges and opportunities. *Nature reviews Genetics* 12: 87-98.

[24] Tabuchi Y, Takasaki I, Doi T, Ishii Y, Sakai H, et al. (2006) Genetic networks responsive to sodium butyrate in colonic epithelial cells. *FEBS letters* 580: 3035-3041.

[25] Li CJ, Bogan JA, Natale DA, DePamphilis ML (2000) Selective activation of pre-replication complexes in vitro at specific sites in mammalian nuclei. *J Cell Sci* 113 (Pt 5): 887-898.

[26] Li CJ, DePamphilis ML (2002) Mammalian Orc1 protein is selectively released from chromatin and ubiquitinated during the S-to-M transition in the cell division cycle. *Mol Cell Biol* 22: 105-116.

[27] DePamphilis ML (2003) The 'ORC cycle': a novel pathway for regulating eukaryotic DNA replication. *Gene* 310: 1-15.

[28] Li CJ, Vassilev A, DePamphilis ML (2004) Role for Cdk1 (Cdc2)/cyclin A in preventing the mammalian origin recognition complex's largest subunit (Orc1) from binding to chromatin during mitosis. *Mol Cell Biol* 24: 5875-5886.

[29] Bell SP, Kobayashi R, Stillman B (1993) Yeast origin recognition complex functions in transcription silencing and DNA replication. *Science* 262: 1844-1849.

[30] Fox CA, Rine J (1996) Influences of the cell cycle on silencing. *Current opinion in cell biology* 8: 354-357.

[31] Iizuka M, Stillman B (1999) Histone acetyltransferase HBO1 interacts with the ORC1 subunit of the human initiator protein. *The Journal of biological chemistry* 274: 23027-23034.

[32] Watson AJ (2006) An overview of apoptosis and the prevention of colorectal cancer. *Crit Rev Oncol Hematol* 57: 107-121.

[33] Jung JW, Cho SD, Ahn NS, Yang SR, Park JS, et al. (2005) Ras/MAP kinase pathways are involved in Ras specific apoptosis induced by sodium butyrate. *Cancer Lett* 225: 199-206.

[34] Shi SL, Wang YY, Liang Y, Li QF (2006) Effects of tachyplesin and n-sodium butyrate on proliferation and gene expression of human gastric adenocarcinoma cell line BGC-823. *World J Gastroenterol* 12: 1694-1698.

[35] Joseph J, Wajapeyee N, Somasundaram K (2005) Role of p53 status in chemosensitivity determination of cancer cells against histone deacetylase inhibitor sodium butyrate. *Int J Cancer* 115: 11-18.

[36] Shin JH, Li RW, Gao Y, Baldwin Rt, Li CJ (2012) Genome-wide ChIP-seq mapping and analysis reveal butyrate-induced acetylation of H3K9 and H3K27 correlated with transcription activity in bovine cells. *Functional & integrative genomics.*

[37] Hollstein M, Hainaut P (2010) Massively regulated genes: the example of TP53. *The Journal of pathology* 220: 164-173.

[38] Ajamian F, Salminen A, Reeben M (2004) Selective regulation of class I and class II histone deacetylases expression by inhibitors of histone deacetylases in cultured mouse neural cells. *Neuroscience letters* 365: 64-68.

[39] Berger SP (2007) Old laws stop drugs being used in valuable new ways. *Nature* 449: 972.

[40] Pasini D, Cloos PA, Walfridsson J, Olsson L, Bukowski JP, et al. (2010) JARID2 regulates binding of the Polycomb repressive complex 2 to target genes in ES cells. *Nature* 464: 306-310.

[41] Jones A, Wang H (2010) Polycomb repressive complex 2 in embryonic stem cells: an overview. *Protein & cell* 1: 1056-1062.

[42] Xu C, Bian C, Yang W, Galka M, Ouyang H, et al. (2010) Binding of different histone marks differentially regulates the activity and specificity of polycomb repressive complex 2 (PRC2). *Proceedings of the National Academy of Sciences of the United States of America* 107: 19266-19271.

[43] Sarkar S, Abujamra AL, Loew JE, Forman LW, Perrine SP, et al. (2011) Histone deacetylase inhibitors reverse CpG methylation by regulating DNMT1 through ERK signaling. *Anticancer research* 31: 2723-2732.

[44] Kinney SR, Pradhan S (2011) Regulation of expression and activity of DNA (cytosine-5) methyltransferases in mammalian cells. *Progress in molecular biology and translational science* 101: 311-333.

[45] Jurkowska RZ, Jurkowski TP, Jeltsch A (2011) Structure and function of mammalian DNA methyltransferases. *Chembiochem : a European journal of chemical biology* 12: 206-222.

[46] Bartel DP (2009) MicroRNAs: target recognition and regulatory functions. *Cell* 136: 215-233.

[47] Bartel DP (2004) MicroRNAs: genomics, biogenesis, mechanism, and function. *Cell* 116: 281-297.

[48] Esquela-Kerscher A, Slack FJ (2006) Oncomirs - microRNAs with a role in cancer. *Nat Rev Cancer* 6: 259-269.

[49] Winter J, Jung S, Keller S, Gregory RI, Diederichs S (2009) Many roads to maturity: microRNA biogenesis pathways and their regulation. *Nat Cell Biol* 11: 228-234.

[50]   Kim J, Bartel DP (2009) Allelic imbalance sequencing reveals that single-nucleotide polymorphisms frequently alter microRNA-directed repression. *Nat Biotechnol* 27: 472-477.

[51]   Arasu P, Wightman B, Ruvkun G (1991) Temporal regulation of lin-14 by the antagonistic action of two other heterochronic genes, lin-4 and lin-28. *Genes & development* 5: 1825-1833.

[52]   Wightman B, Burglin TR, Gatto J, Arasu P, Ruvkun G (1991) Negative regulatory sequences in the lin-14 3'-untranslated region are necessary to generate a temporal switch during Caenorhabditis elegans development. *Genes & development* 5: 1813-1824.

[53]   Pasquinelli AE, Reinhart BJ, Slack F, Martindale MQ, Kuroda MI, et al. (2000) Conservation of the sequence and temporal expression of let-7 heterochronic regulatory RNA. *Nature* 408: 86-89.

[54]   Reinhart BJ, Slack FJ, Basson M, Pasquinelli AE, Bettinger JC, et al. (2000) The 21-nucleotide let-7 RNA regulates developmental timing in Caenorhabditis elegans. *Nature* 403: 901-906.

[55]   Vasudevan S, Tong Y, Steitz JA (2007) Switching from repression to activation: microRNAs can up-regulate translation. *Science* 318: 1931-1934.

[56]   Buchan JR, Parker R (2007) Molecular biology. The two faces of miRNA. *Science* 318: 1877-1878.

[57]   Delcuve GP, Khan DH, Davie JR (2012) Roles of histone deacetylases (HDACs) in epigenetic regulation: emerging paradigms from studies with inhibitors. *Clinical epigenetics* 4: 5.

[58]   Esteller M (2011) Non-coding RNAs in human disease. *Nature reviews Genetics* 12: 861-874.

[59]   Scott MS, Ono M (2011) From snoRNA to miRNA: Dual function regulatory non-coding RNAs. *Biochimie* 93: 1987-1992.

[60]   Hu S, Dong TS, Dalal SR, Wu F, Bissonnette M, et al. (2011) The microbe-derived short chain fatty acid butyrate targets miRNA-dependent p21 gene expression in human colon cancer. *PLoS One* 6: e16221.

[61]   Iorio MV, Piovan C, Croce CM (2010) Interplay between microRNAs and the epigenetic machinery: An intricate network. *Biochim Biophys Acta*.

[62]   Leder A, Leder P (1975) Butyric acid, a potent inducer of erythroid differentiation in cultured erythroleukemic cells. *Cell* 5: 319-322.

[63]   Gallinari P, Di Marco S, Jones P, Pallaoro M, Steinkuhler C (2007) HDACs, histone deacetylation and gene transcription: from molecular biology to cancer therapeutics. *Cell research* 17: 195-211.

[64]   Khan O, La Thangue NB (2012) HDAC inhibitors in cancer biology: emerging mechanisms and clinical applications. *Immunology and cell biology* 90: 85-94.

[65]   Suliman BA, Xu D, Williams BR (2012) HDACi: molecular mechanisms and therapeutic implications in the innate immune system. *Immunology and cell biology* 90: 23-32.

[66]   Leggatt GR, Gabrielli B (2012) Histone deacetylase inhibitors in the generation of the anti-tumour immune response. *Immunology and cell biology* 90: 33-38.

[67] Woan KV, Sahakian E, Sotomayor EM, Seto E, Villagra A (2012) Modulation of antigen-presenting cells by HDAC inhibitors: implications in autoimmunity and cancer. *Immunology and cell biology* 90: 55-65.

[68] Andrews KT, Haque A, Jones MK (2012) HDAC inhibitors in parasitic diseases. *Immunology and cell biology* 90: 66-77.

[69] Fairlie DP, Sweet MJ (2012) HDACs and their inhibitors in immunology: teaching anticancer drugs new tricks. *Immunology and cell biology* 90: 3-5.

[70] Uffenbeck SR, Krebs JE (2006) The role of chromatin structure in regulating stress-induced transcription in Saccharomyces cerevisiae. *Biochem Cell Biol* 84: 477-489.

[71] Jaattela M (1999) Heat shock proteins as cellular lifeguards. *Ann Med* 31: 261-271.

[72] Lindquist S (1986) The heat-shock response. *Annu Rev Biochem* 55: 1151-1191.

[73] Collier RJ, Dahl GE, VanBaale MJ (2006) Major advances associated with environmental effects on dairy cattle. *J Dairy Sci* 89: 1244-1253.

[74] Fujita J (1999) Cold shock response in mammalian cells. *J Mol Microbiol Biotechnol* 1: 243-255.

[75] Sonna LA, Fujita J, Gaffin SL, Lilly CM (2002) Invited review: Effects of heat and cold stress on mammalian gene expression. *J Appl Physiol* 92: 1725-1742.

[76] Pirkkala L, Nykanen P, Sistonen L (2001) Roles of the heat shock transcription factors in regulation of the heat shock response and beyond. *FASEB J* 15: 1118-1131.

[77] Sonna LA, Gaffin SL, Pratt RE, Cullivan ML, Angel KC, et al. (2002) Effect of acute heat shock on gene expression by human peripheral blood mononuclear cells. *J Appl Physiol* 92: 2208-2220.

[78] C. David Allis TJaDR, editor (2006) *Epgenetics*. New York: Cold Spring Harbor Laboratory Press.

[79] Zheng C, Hayes JJ (2003) Intra- and inter-nucleosomal protein-DNA interactions of the core histone tail domains in a model system. *J Biol Chem* 278: 24217-24224.

[80] Zheng C, Hayes JJ (2003) Structures and interactions of the core histone tail domains. *Biopolymers* 68: 539-546.

[81] Mikkelsen TS, Ku M, Jaffe DB, Issac B, Lieberman E, et al. (2007) Genome-wide maps of chromatin state in pluripotent and lineage-committed cells. *Nature* 448: 553-560.

[82] Bernstein BE, Meissner A, Lander ES (2007) The mammalian epigenome. *Cell* 128: 669-681.

[83] Goldberg AD, Allis CD, Bernstein E (2007) Epigenetics: a landscape takes shape. *Cell* 128: 635-638.

[84] Boulant JA, Hardy JD (1974) The effect of spinal and skin temperatures on the firing rate and thermosensitivity of preoptic neurones. *J Physiol* 240: 639-660.

[85] Nakayama T (1985) Thermosensitive neurons in the brain. *Jpn J Physiol* 35: 375-389.

[86] Kouzarides T (2007) Chromatin modifications and their function. *Cell* 128: 693-705.

[87] Kisliouk T, Ziv M, Meiri N (2010) Epigenetic control of translation regulation: alterations in histone H3 lysine 9 post-translation modifications are correlated with the expression of the translation initiation factor 2B (Eif2b5) during thermal control establishment. *Dev Neurobiol* 70: 100-113.

[88] Kisliouk T, Meiri N (2009) A critical role for dynamic changes in histone H3 methylation at the Bdnf promoter during postnatal thermotolerance acquisition. *Eur J Neurosci* 30: 1909-1922.

[89] Fritah S, Col E, Boyault C, Govin J, Sadoul K, et al. (2009) Heat-shock factor 1 controls genome-wide acetylation in heat-shocked cells. *Mol Biol Cell* 20: 4976-4984.

[90] Ruden DM, Xiao L, Garfinkel MD, Lu X (2005) Hsp90 and environmental impacts on epigenetic states: a model for the trans-generational effects of diethylstibesterol on uterine development and cancer. *Hum Mol Genet* 14 Spec No 1: R149-155.

[91] Ruden DM, Lu X (2008) Hsp90 affecting chromatin remodeling might explain transgenerational epigenetic inheritance in Drosophila. *Curr Genomics* 9: 500-508.

[92] Sims RJ, 3rd, Reinberg D (2004) From chromatin to cancer: a new histone lysine methyltransferase enters the mix. *Nat Cell Biol* 6: 685-687.

[93] Rakyan VK, Blewitt ME, Druker R, Preis JI, Whitelaw E (2002) Metastable epialleles in mammals. *Trends Genet* 18: 348-351.

[94] Rutherford SL, Lindquist S (1998) Hsp90 as a capacitor for morphological evolution. *Nature* 396: 336-342.

[95] Sollars V, Lu X, Xiao L, Wang X, Garfinkel MD, et al. (2003) Evidence for an epigenetic mechanism by which Hsp90 acts as a capacitor for morphological evolution. *Nat Genet* 33: 70-74.

[96] Martinez-Arguelles DB, Papadopoulos V (2010) Epigenetic regulation of the expression of genes involved in steroid hormone biosynthesis and action. *Steroids* 75: 467-476.

[97] Carone BR, Fauquier L, Habib N, Shea JM, Hart CE, et al. (2010) Paternally induced transgenerational environmental reprogramming of metabolic gene expression in mammals. *Cell* 143: 1084-1096.

[98] Seong KH, Maekawa T, Ishii S (2012) Inheritance and memory of stress-induced epigenome change: roles played by the ATF-2 family of transcription factors. *Genes to cells : devoted to molecular & cellular mechanisms* 17: 249-263.

[99] Shin JH, Li RW, Gao Y, Baldwin Rt, Li CJ (2012) Genome-wide ChIP-seq mapping and analysis reveal butyrate-induced acetylation of H3K9 and H3K27 correlated with transcription activity in bovine cells. *Functional & integrative genomics* 12: 119-130.

[100] D'Haeseleer P (2006) What are DNA sequence motifs? *Nature biotechnology* 24: 423-425.

[101] Ohta T (2011) Near-neutrality, robustness, and epigenetics. *Genome biology and evolution* 3: 1034-1038.

[102] Li RW, Connor EE, Li CJ, Baldwin Vi RL, Sparks ME (2012) Characterization of the rumen microbiota of pre-ruminant calves using metagenomic tools. *Environmental microbiology* 14: 129-139.

[103] Gregg K (1995) Engineering gut flora of ruminant livestock to reduce forage toxicity: progress and problems. *Trends in biotechnology* 13: 418-421.

[104] Sirohi SK, Pandey N, Goel N, Singh B, Mohini M, et al. (2009) Microbial activity and ruminal methanognesis as affected by plant secondary metabolites in different plant extracts. *International Journal of Civil and Environmental Engineering* 1: 52-58.

[105] Li RW, Wu S, Baldwin RL, Li W, Li CJ (2012) Perturbation dynamics of the rumen microbiota in response to exogenous butyrate. *PLoS One* 7: e29392.

In: Cattle: Domestication, Diseases and the Environment
Editor: George Liu

ISBN: 978-1-62417-820-7
© 2013 Nova Science Publishers, Inc.

Chapter 5

ENDOCRINE CONTROL OF BULL FERTILITY

Katherine L. Gilbert[1,], Eric A. Gilbert[1,*],
Aruna Govindaraju[2,*], Lyndi L. Jury[2,*],
Melissa C. Mason[2,*], Kathryn E. Pfeiffer[2,*],
Tricia M. Rowlison[3,*], Lori Ward[2,*], Abdullah Kaya[4],
Jamie Larson[2] and Erdogan Memili[2,†]*

[1]Departments of Agriculture and Biomedical Engineering, [2]Animal and Dairy
Sciences, [3]Biochemistry Molecular Biology Entomology and Plant Pathology,
Mississippi State University, Mississippi State, MS, US
[4]Alta Genetics, Inc., Watertown, WI, US

ABSTRACT

Male fertility—the ability to produce viable sperm that are able to support
fertilization and oocyte activation and to sustain development during embryogenesis and
beyond—is essential for success of mammalian reproduction and development.
Production of quality semen depends on the existence of an effective male reproduction
system that is consistently able to produce viable gametes. This requires a male with a
fertility phenotype that has evolved under the influence of its genetics, environment, and
epistasis to a high degree of efficacy. As the sperm from one bull can be used to
inseminate tens of thousands of cows, bull fertility has an enormous influence on the
efficiency and success of the cattle breeding and reproduction. Even among bulls that
produce ample amounts of sperm having apparent normal morphology, some of these
animals will still not exhibit high fertility. Despite large investments to study the causes
of low fertility as well as research on methods to prevent, diagnose, and treat subpar male
fertility, only limited success has been achieved, and the problem remains poorly defined.
The objectives of this paper are to review the male reproductive system and the endocrine
regulation of male fertility. It will explore the functions of specific hormones regulating
male fertility, hormonal control of sperm viability, as well as environmental factors

---

[*] Equal contributions by students who developed this review while taking the graduate course "PHY 8133
Endocrine Secretions" at Mississippi State University.
[†] Corresponding author: Erdogan Memili; em149@ads.msstate.edu.

influencing male fertility. The bovine will be the species of focus, but key aspects of male fertility of other mammals (pigs, goats, horses, monkeys and humans) will be included. This review is intended to be a useful source of information for both basic and applied research, as well as for animal production and human andrologists.

Keywords: Hormones, Male Fertility, Sperm, Environment

MALE REPRODUCTIVE SYSTEM

Genesis of Maleness

Development of the mammalian male is specified genetically at conception when a sperm bearing a Y chromosome fertilizes the oocyte. This leads to development of testes, designating the phenotypic sex. Expression of the sex-determining region Y gene (SRY) on the Y chromosome initiates the testis determining factor (TDF), which transforms genital ridges into testes at seven weeks of gestation in humans. Morphologically, the testis consists of the Leydig cells and seminiferous tubules. Located in the seminiferous tubules of the testis, are the somatic sertoli cells, which nurse germ cells including spermatogonial stem cells from which sperm cells are produced throughout life. Testes descend from the peritoneal cavity into the scrotum via the inguinal canal by mid-gestation, late gestation and just prior to parturition in bulls and rams, boars, and stallions, respectively. Testes come into maturity based on the endocrine and gametogenic potential for reproductive function. This action is referred to as puberty and may be controlled partly by melatonin, which is synthesized and secreted by the pineal gland. Bucks reach puberty at 4-5 months, bulls and stallions at approximately 1 year, boars at approximately 6 months, and men at approximately 14 years of age. Along with the sperm, testes via Leydig cells also produce sex hormones, primarily testosterone, which causes the wolffian ducts to progress in the male. Testosterone via its metabolite dihydrotestosterone, also causes development of external genitalia in males and causes male-like behavior. Estrogens metabolized from testosterone, defeminize the brain, and play important roles in sperm physiology.

In addition to testes, the male reproductive system also includes other components that are vital for production of viable sperm. The scrotum surrounds the testes and provides temperature control, support, and protection. The spermatic cord supports the testes and aids in temperature control. The epididymis functions to concentrate, store, mature, and transport spermatozoa; the vas deferens transports sperm to the penis. Accessory glands empty their secretions, seminal plasma, into the urethra which transports semen in addition to urine. In most species, the vesicular gland contributes fluid, energy substrates, and buffers to semen. In bulls, these glands contribute well over half of the total fluid volume of semen. While the prostate gland also contributes fluid and inorganic ions to semen, the bulbourethral gland flushes urine residue from the urethra before ejaculation. Bulls, boars, and rams have a sigmoid flexure and a retractor muscle is attached to their penis, the organ of copulation in males. Supplied with sensory nerves, the prepuce encloses the free end of the penis. The bull penis has a twisted groove, ram and buck have a filiform appendage, the boar has a spiral corkscrew, and the stallion has a flattened end. The prepuce or sheath is an invagination of skin that completely encloses the free end of the penis. The boar has a pouch dorsal to the orifice that may contribute to boar odor due to secretion build up (Bearden et al., 2004).

Spermatogenesis

Production of male gametes (Figure 1) is highly conserved across all mammalian species. The process begins in the testes where luteinizing hormone (LH) released from the anterior pituitary gland (AP), binds to receptors located on the Leydig cells. The Leydig cells produce testosterone which enters the seminiferous tubules where the spermatogonial stem cells both replenish themselves and produce spermatogonia by mitosis for continuation of the germ line, which allows sustained spermatogenesis for the entirety of the life of a male. The spermatogonia then divide into spermatocytes, which undergo meiosis I and meiosis II in the seminiferous tubules to form spermatids. Sertoli cells in the seminiferous tubules are joined by tight junctions that function to create a blood/testis barrier. The blood/testis barrier protects the spermatocytes and spermatozoa from the male's own immune system since they are viewed as a foreign body because these cells did not exist in fetal life when the immune system determines self from non-self. The Sertoli cells also usher the developing spermatozoa along the tubules toward the rete testis, a network that forms a conduit to the efferent ducts, which exit the testis to the head of the epididymis.

As developing spermatid cells travel through the seminiferous tubules, they undergo a conformational change from their early spherical conformation to their more functional conformation of a head with a flagellum. During the conformational change of the sperm, the DNA of the sperm cell condenses and moves to one end of the cell. Centrioles start to elongate at the other end resulting in the flagellum of the sperm. Mitochondria of the sperm cell align along the base of the flagella. The Golgi transforms into a single globule adjacent to the tip of the condensed genetic material and forms the acrosome. The acrosome, a specialized lysosome, contains enzymes that will assist the sperm to penetrate the zona pellucida of the oocyte during fertilization. With the rearranging of the contents of the sperm cell into a more functional conformation, a small portion of the cytoplasm (cytoplasmic droplet) gets pushed to the side of the cell into a small pouch that initially rests where the flagellum attaches to the head of the cell.

Once the sperm cells reach the epididymis they continue to develop and mature, gaining motility and losing cytoplasmic droplets. The epididymis functions to help concentrate the seminal fluid. When the sperm enter the epididymis from the seminiferous tubules, the sperm cells are relatively dilute having a concentration of approximately 100 million cells/mL (Bearden et al., 2004). The first part of the epididymis absorbs seminal fluid to a final sperm concentration of up to 4 billion cells/mL. Another function of the epididymis is storage; sperm are made continuously, therefore have to be stored until needed. The epididymal tail, the final portion of this duct, creates an environment conducive to the storage of sperm cells. The environment of the epididymis has many characteristics such as low pH, high carbon dioxide concentration, high viscosity and other components that slow the metabolic rate of the spermatozoa and prolong longevity for up to 60 days. It is in the epididymis that the sperm continue to mature and is also a site for abnormalities to develop. While the spermatozoa gain motility in the epididymis, the sperm cells can also be rendered useless due to bent flagellum. Changes in the osmolarity of the epididymal environment could cause the flagella of the sperm to become permanently angled in such a way that linear motility is not possible (Cooper, 2007). Males could produce sperm, but without proper epididymal maturation the sperm would be unable to achieve fertilization.

Hormones Regulating Reproduction in Males

Balanced production of male reproductive hormones is essential in development of spermatozoa. Misregulation of hormones in the male body can impair proper production of spermatozoa and other aspects of male fertility. Measurements of semen quality, such as sperm concentration and seminal volume have decreased in human males, possibly leading to decreased fertility since the 1940's (Giwercman et al., 1993). Many factors including environmental contaminants and physical abnormalities such as testicular germ cell cancer and cryptorchidism can lead to the improper production of reproductive hormones, which are essential for maintaining male fertility. Men with testicular germ cell tumors have shown decreased fertility (Giwercman et al., 1993; Fraietta et al., 2010). It is unknown whether the tumor itself imparts a detrimental effect or if infertility is a result of treatment (DeSantis et al., 1999). Regardless of the cause, an altered testis leads to reduced fertility (Petersen et al., 1998). This physical abnormality leads to improper production of many key reproductive hormones such as testosterone, LH, and estradiol. In this section we will review these hormones that are essential to spermatogenesis and abnormal hormonal regulations that may cause male infertility.

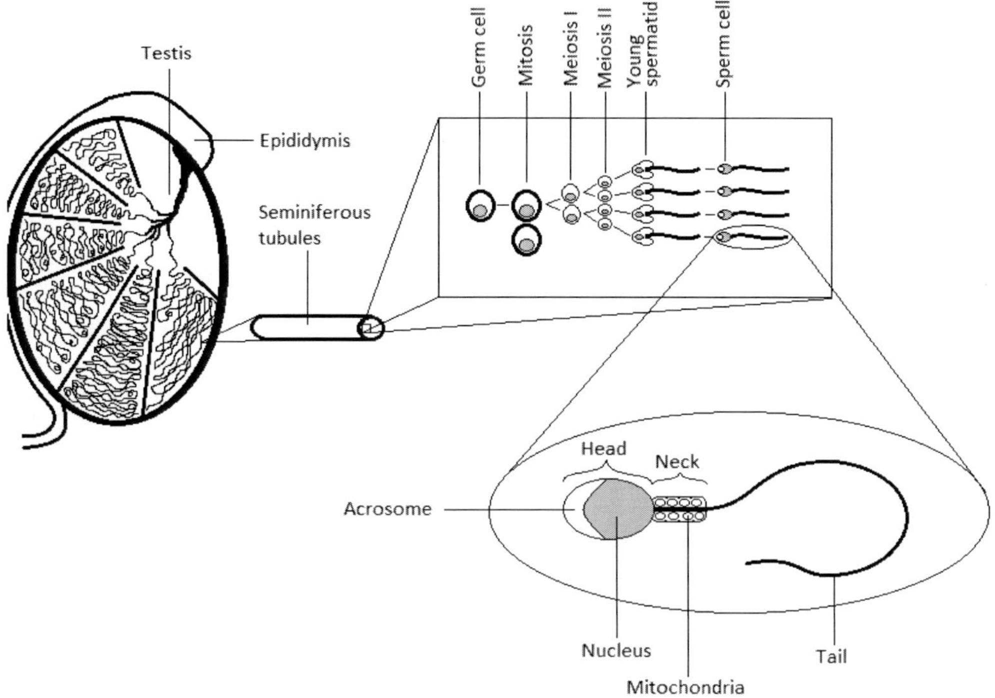

Figure 1. Flow chart of spermatogenesis.

Gonadotropin-releasing Hormone (GnRH)

Gonadotropin releasing hormone (GnRH) is synthesized by neurons within the hypothalamus and is essential for reproduction. GnRH induces the release of follicle stimulating hormone (FSH) and luteinizing hormone (LH); GnRH is also sometimes termed luteinizing-hormone-releasing hormone (LHRH). Since the discovery of the amino acid make up of GnRH by Nobel laureates Roger Guillemin and Andrew V. Schally (Raju, 1999), the specific role and control mechanisms of GnRH have been investigated. Gonadotropin releasing hormone is released from the hypothalamus and acts on the anterior pituitary (AP). In males, there is a steady pulsatile release of GnRH, which is controlled through a negative feedback mechanism regulated by steroids. Testosterone is the primary steroid that regulates GnRH production in males; concentrations of these two hormones are inversely related. Testosterone feeds back on both the hypothalamus and the AP to regulate the release of FSH and LH. Gonadotropin releasing hormone neurons do not have steroid receptors; therefore, the steroids work through other pathways to deactivate production of GnRH, such as through afferent neurons that secrete kisspeptin.

Production of GnRH is essential for sperm production and alterations in the secretion of GnRH will have a direct effect on fertility. Hypogonadotropic hypogonadism is a disorder that can lead to decreased hormone production from reproductive glands (Trabado et al., 2011). It is typically a result of decreased hormone production from the hypothalamus and/or AP. Hormonal treatments, such as GnRH, can be administered to remedy the disorder in humans (Sykiotis et al., 2010). Another method that has been employed by fertility clinics, but is less practical, is the administration of FSH and LH to bypass the AP.

GnRH agonists can inhibit or stimulate the production or secretion of GnRH, depending on the dose. Administration of a GnRH agonist pre-pubertally demonstrated that bulls receiving the GnRH agonist had an increased production of LH which stimulates testosterone production. Young bulls receiving the GnRH agonist had increased circulating testosterone concentrations in the blood and inside the testes (Jimenez-Severiano, 2003). Misregulation of GnRH can have vast repercussions on male fertility. Since GnRH stimulates the AP to secrete FSH and LH, its misregulation can affect many different reproductive pathways (Mortimer and Yeo, 1976). Typically, the production of sex hormones (such as FSH, LH, and testosterone) has a negative feedback effect on the production of GnRH. Impairing any of these feedback systems can cause a cascade effect on the reproductive system and could potentially lead to infertility.

Kisspeptins are neuropeptides synthesized in neural cells of the hypothalamus and play important roles in regulating expression of GnRH. Once secreted from the kisspetin neurons, kisspeptins bind to their receptors on the surface of GnRH neurons in the pituitary and thereby stimulate secretion of LH and FSH which in turn signal the gonads to produce testosterone (Hameed et al., 2011). Kisspeptin signaling is also important in prepubertal development and seasonal reproductive activity because people with mutations in kisspeptin receptor do not enter puberty (Topaloglu et al., 2012). Additionally, kisspeptins are affected by nutritional status because leptin, produced by adipose tissue, is involved in regulating fertility. Humans with mutations in leptin or its receptor display hypogonadotrophic hypogonaidism and hypoleptinemia. The reproductive abnormalities in these people are reversed through leptin therapy (Welt et al., 2004). Administration of kisspeptin-10 to prepubertal male and female cattle stimulated secretion of LH and FSH but not growth hormone (Ahmed et al., 2011). Research thus far shows that kisspeptins play vital roles in hormonal regulation of the hypothalamic-pituitary-gonadal axis.

Follicle Stimulating Hormone

Follicle stimulating hormone (FSH) is a glycoprotein and is released from the AP in response to GnRH. It travels through the blood, from the brain into the gonads, where it stimulates spermatogenesis. Follicle stimulating hormone is essential during early gamete development and can improve the ultrastructure and morphology of the developing sperm. Follicle stimulating hormone binds to Sertoli cells of the seminiferous tubules and acts to nurse sperm cell development during the early stages (Paola et al., 2009). Males require FSH to begin sperm production, which makes it a critical hormone in reproduction and fertility. FSH works through a feedback mechanism similar to GnRH. The feedback mechanism for FSH involves inhibin, which is secreted from the Sertoli cells in the testes. When FSH is sufficiently increased and many receptors are activated, inhibin is produced and acts on the AP to decrease production of FSH.

Improper production of FSH can impair spermatogenesis. Decreased FSH production has been correlated with decreased numbers of Sertoli cells present in the male testes. Subsequently, defects in sperm production in multiple species were noted (Dorrington et al., 1975; Johnson and Thompson, 1983). The effects of FSH on Sertoli cell development is most critical during early fetal development (Orth, 1984). Improper secretion of FSH during this time can alter the formation of Sertoli cells, causing life-long repercussions. Impairing the number and function of Sertoli cells can lead to improper spermatogenesis and ultimately be a cause of infertility.

Luteinizing Hormone

Released from the AP in response to GnRH, luteinizing hormone (LH) is transported through the blood to act on the interstitial cells called Leydig cells in the testes to initiate the production of testosterone. Similar to FSH, LH is a glycoprotein composed of an alpha and beta sub-unit. Luteinizing hormone is released from the AP due to pulses of GnRH acting on the AP. Luteinizing hormone causes the interstitial cells of the testes to produce testosterone, and therefore is essential in males to form masculine characteristics and is also very important for fertility because it aids in sperm production. Luteinizing hormone is a member of the hypothalamus-pituitary-gonadal feedback mechanism, which regulates the production of GnRH. When LH is high, testosterone is high, and GnRH production is slowed, so an inverse relationship exists. Low GnRH signals the AP to stop producing LH. When testosterone is low, this indicates to the AP and hypothalamus that there is not enough LH in the blood; therefore the AP increases production of LH mostly due to GnRH stimulation. As a result of these delicate feedback mechanisms, the body maintains homeostasis, which is pivotal for fertility.

Luteinizing hormone receptors are an important part in the pathway to fertile sperm. LH binds to specific LH receptors located on the Leydig or interstitial cells, residing in the testicles. Luteinizing hormone is acquired by the Leydig cells for the production of testosterone. If LH is lacking, there will be insufficient production of testosterone. The male reproductive system needs to maintain a proper balance of these hormones. Misregulation of hormones or mutations in receptors can lead to infertility. In males, mutations in LH receptors are thought to cause an underestimated number of cases of male hypogonadism and reduced spermatogenesis (Brustyers et al., 2008).

Males with Kallmann syndrome have insufficient LH, FSH, testosterone, and GnRH levels. This disease causes males to lack sexual maturation as well as other characteristics which set it apart from hypogonadism. Men with an abnormal testis, such as in cryptorchidism patients, have abnormal production of estradiol, LH and testosterone (Giwercman et al., 1993; Petersen et al., 1998). Estradiol is related to the incidence of germ cell tumors and can negatively impact the production of other reproductive hormones. Production of LH from the AP is specifically down regulated by estradiol.

Misregulation of production of LH affects the subsequent secretion of testosterone from the Leydig cells. Removing the negative feedback on the AP's release of LH can result in an excess production of testosterone (Katongole et al., 1971; Eacker et al., 2008). Insufficient production of LH has been correlated with decreased production of testosterone in many species.

As discussed later on, many sexual repercussions can arise from defective testosterone production in male reproduction. It is vital that LH production be successfully regulated for proper male reproduction.

Testosterone

Testosterone is a steroid hormone produced in the Leydig cells and has secondary sex characteristics effects on the male body. It enhances muscle and bone density growth, and it initiates development of the penis and testis, as well as hair growth. Testosterone is formed through chemical changes to cholesterol. It activates genes in Sertoli cells in the testes, and is essential for sperm production (Walker, 2010).

Testosterone has a role in the negative feedback system involving FSH, LH, and GnRH. When testosterone is low, GnRH is released from the hypothalamus, which acts on the AP to produce FSH and LH. FSH and LH, in turn, cause an increase in secretion of testosterone in the body. When testosterone is increased, it signals the hypothalamus and AP to reduce the production of GnRH and FSH/LH, respectively. This feedback system allows the body to maintain proper amounts of each hormone for normal physiology.

With a lack of testosterone, germ cells that are beyond the meiosis stage will not progress, and they ultimately die. Sperm cells matured without testosterone will not be released from the Sertoli cells, which ultimately cause infertility. Testosterone acts through classical and non-classical pathways to maintain spermatogenesis and male fertility (Walker, 2010).

Reduced amounts of testosterone can be caused by a problem in the hypothalamus-pituitary-gonadal axis or by testicular dysfunction. The first occurs when there is an error that causes the feedback mechanism to fail. Castration or other types of trauma to the testis could cause testicular dysfunction in males.

Progesterone

In males, progesterone is essential for the formation of proper sperm molecular makeup (Gadkar et al., 2002). It is produced in the testes and adrenal glands. One of the key functions of progesterone is to help balance production of estradiol. This is essential for properly functioning sperm because a large increase in estradiol can impair proper sperm development. Progesterone is also a precursor to testosterone and estradiol (Winters et al., 1999). If progesterone is too low, testosterone production will decrease, which in turn will cause male infertility. If progesterone levels were high, this would cause testosterone production to increase. An increase in testosterone would alert the feedback system causing the brain to decrease production of GnRH, FSH, and LH. All the hormones in the male reproductive system work together to create an organism that can reproduce effectively, and any hormone imbalance will threaten to disrupt this process, causing infertility.

Inhibins

A glycoprotein member of the transforming growth factor-β superfamily and produced in Sertoli cells of the testis (Ling et al., 1985), inhibin consists of an α and a β subunit. Two isoforms of inhibin exist, differing by the β subunit, and have been established as inhibin A (β_A) and inhibin B (β_B). Inhibin B is the prevalent form expressed in male mammals and is considered to be the significant physiological form in regards to testicular function (Meachem et al., 2001). The production of inhibin B is dependent on concentrations of FSH and spermatogenesis (Meachem et al., 2001). An inverse relationship between concentrations of FSH and inhibin has been established, regulating the production of FSH (Anderson et al., 1997) through a negative feedback mechanism. The production of FSH is stimulatory to the production of inhibin B, and increased concentrations of inhibin B down regulate the subsequent secretion of FSH (Meachem et al., 2001). This mechanism has also been postulated in regulation of spermatogenesis, specifically in primates (Ramaswamy et al., 2000). Prior to spermatogenesis, concentrations of inhibin B in serum increase neonatally. This increase is concurrent with an increase in serum concentrations of FSH and the development of Sertoli cells. Concentrations of inhibin B then decrease until puberty, when increased concentrations of FSH are prevalent and spermatogenesis is occurring. Following the attainment of pubescence, concentrations of inhibin B are expressed in a diurnal pattern with a reduction in the concentration occurring in the night. This expression is similar to the secretion of testosterone and related to the stage of spermatogenesis (Meachem et al., 2001).

Inhibin B can be used diagnostically to identify primary testicular disorders or testicular damage and can be considered a measure of testicular function. Concentrations of inhibin B in serum have been positively correlated to testicular volume and sperm counts in males (Byrd et al., 1998; Andersson et al., 1998; Pierik et al., 1998). In regards to infertility, a decrease in concentrations of inhibin B and testosterone are evident in males. Decreased inhibin B is also associated with increased FSH caused by spermatogenic dysfunction (Meachem et al., 2001). In contrast, inhibin B cannot be used to identify the presence of sperm in individual testicular tube samples (von Eckardstein et al., 1999) or spermatogenic damage. Regulation of inhibin is dependent on FSH production in response to GnRH (Welt et al., 2002). This has been established as the concentrations of GnRH and subsequent concentrations of inhibin are increased during pubescence (Byrd et al., 1998). In addition, administration of GnRH increases the concentration of inhibin (Seminara et al., 1996). Specifically, FSH is involved in the proliferation of Sertoli cells and the process of spermatogenesis. In prepubertal males, in which Sertoli cell development is occurring, FSH administration increases inhibin levels (Raivio et al., 1997). In adult males the proliferation of Sertoli cells has concluded and changes in concentrations of inhibin are produced during spermatogenesis. In males with hypospermatogenesis, administration of FSH increases inhibin. In males that exhibit normal spermatogenesis, administration of FSH does not cause subsequent increases in inhibin.

Prolactin (PRL)

Secretion of PRL occurs in the lactotropic cells of the AP, and regulation originates in both the gonads and hypothalamus. Production of PRL is regulated by the gonadal steroids, testosterone and estradiol. Testosterone inhibits while estradiol stimulates production of PRL, by means of a feedback mechanism of the hypothalamic-pituitary-gonadal axis (Gill-Sharma, 2009). Prolactin has also been hypothesized to have an autoregulatory mechanism whereby autoreceptor neurons in the hypothalamus release dopamine in response to PRL (Moore and Demarest, 1982). Dopamine inhibits the release of PRL (Kelly et al., 1997) by acting on the dopaminergic receptors on the lactotrophs of the AP (Anderson et al., 2006). The defined physiological mechanism of PRL in male reproduction has not been elucidated, but is hypothesized to be stimulatory or latent, depending on the concentrations of PRL (Bartke, 1999). Prolactin has been postulated to have an effect on testicular function and is involved with the synthesis of testosterone through the possible up regulation of LH receptors on Leydig cells (Purvis et al., 1979). In contrast, increases in concentrations of PRL have also been reported to suppress LH and FSH (Bartke, 1999).

Hyperprolactinemia may lead to decreased libido and infertility in males by reducing the production of GnRH. A reduced release of GnRH subsequently affects the production of the gonadotropins and testosterone. This negatively impacts spermatogenesis affecting sperm quality and motility. Hyperprolactinemia produces hypogonadism by acting on PRL receptors and ultimately decreases fertility (Masud et al., 2007). Hyperprolactinemia has been reported to suppress synthesis of testosterone by inhibiting the secretion of GnRH (Bartke, 1986; Albertson et al., 1987). In contrast, the reduction in fertility observed in male mice was not dependent on concentrations of testosterone. However, decreased concentrations of LH and decreased weights of accessory reproductive glands have been observed (Steger et al., 1998). The most physiologically significant contribution of PRL is control of gonadotropin release and regulation of growth and function of male accessory reproductive glands. PRL is not specifically required for gametogenesis, androgen production, or fertility in the male mouse (Bartke, 1999).

Growth Hormone (GH)

Growth hormone is produced in somatotrophic cells of the AP and is found in free form or bound to GH binding protein in blood plasma. The pulsatile release of GH is mediated by releasing factors in the hypothalamus, known as GH-releasing hormone and somatostatin. These factors work inversely to regulate the production of GH. Significant target tissues of GH in male reproduction include the Leydig and Sertoli cells of the testis (Lobie et al., 1990). Both cell types possess receptors for GH (Tres et al., 1986). The possible correlation of quantitative aspects of spermatogenesis and GH involves the proliferation of Sertoli cells.

Although deficiency of GH does not directly alter fertility, it does have an effect on development of the reproductive system, the attainment of puberty, and produces a subsequent reduction in sexual behavior of mice (Bartke, 1999). Changes in concentrations of GH are postulated to be associated with hypothalamic neurons that are involved in copulatory behavior and gonadotropin secretion from the AP. Growth hormone transgenic mice expressed an increased rate of neurotransmitter turnover in the hypothalamic region (Bartke et al., 1994). Regulation of hypothalamic-pituitary axis by the negative feedback of gonadal steroids has been hypothesized to be altered by both increased and decreased concentrations of GH (Childs et al., 1994). In GH defiant mice, LH and FSH concentrations are decreased, and administration of GH increased LH binding in the testis of the rat (Zipf et al., 1978) and golden hamster (Bex et al., 1978). However, treatment with GH did not affect LH, FSH, or concentrations of testosterone in either normal or GH-deficient men (Ovesen et al., 1993; Juul et al., 1998) and appears to be dependent on the species. In summary, further research is necessary to establish the mechanism of action of GH on fertility.

Estradiol 17β

Hundreds of substances have estrogenic activity, but by far the most important for reproductive function is estradiol 17β, often just termed estradiol or estrogen. Estradiol is synthesized by Sertoli cells of immature and post-pubertal males (van der Molen et al., 1981). Leydig cells also are involved in the production of estrogens in the adult male (Rommerts et al., 1982), and increased concentrations of estrogen are prevalent in the rete testis. Estrogen receptors are also present in the testes, efferent ductules and epididymis (Hess, 2003). The receptors in the efferent ductules are involved in fluid reabsorption by regulating the expression of proteins. This is one important function of estrogen in male fertility. Estrogen is also important in the regulation of other parts of the male reproductive tract and has significant activity in establishing Sertoli cell function (O'Donnell et al., 2001). It has been hypothesized that estrogen regulates gonadotropin secretion through the hypothalamic-pituitary-gonadal axis, and in male mice that do not possess estrogen increased concentrations of LH are prevalent (Smith et al., 1994; Morishima et al., 1995). Specifically, regulation of AP gonadotropin secretion requires aromatization of testosterone to produce estrogen (Lindzey et al., 1998). This is further supported by reports of aromatase-deficient males expressing increased concentrations of FSH and LH (Smith et al., 1994; Morishima et al., 1995).

Exposure to a high dose of estrogen causes malformation of the male reproductive tract. In contrast, low levels of estrogen cause decreased concentrations of sperm in the epididymis, disruption of sperm morphology, and inhibition of sodium transport. Homeostasis of fluid balance by estrogen is altered, causing subsequent physiological dysfunction. The mechanisms by which estrogen acts on male reproduction and fertility are being developed, but further research in this area is still necessary to fully understand this concept.

ENVIRONMENT, HORMONES AND INFERTILITY

Endocrine Disruptors

The endocrine system maintains the critical balance between cellular requirements and concentrations of hormones. Endocrine disruptors are chemicals that act as agonists or antagonists to hormones and interfere with hormonal balance. These chemicals may alter homeostasis of the body fluids, sexual development, cognition and behavior as well as other aspects of animal development. The disruptions may also cause tumors, birth defects, and other developmental disorders. A variety of chemical classes including drugs, pesticides, pollutants (including toxins produced by fungi and other microbes), compounds used in the plastics industry, and industrial by-products can be categorized as endocrine disruptors.

Many commonly used pesticides such as dichlorodiphenyltrichloroethane (DDT), glycol ethers, dibromocholoropropane (DBCP) (Sharpe, 2010), and methoxychlor (Uzumcu et al., 2006) are known to disrupt the reproductive function as well as embryo development (Hall et al. 1997) by mimicking the steroidal hormones. Apart from these known chemicals many other synthetic and naturally occurring compounds are suspected to alter normal concentrations of hormones by either halting or stimulating the production of hormones, or changing the way hormones travel through the body, thus affecting the normal hormonal functions.

In most cases, the estrogenic activity of these chemicals is responsible for reproductive malfunction. However, disruption can be anti-estrogenic, androgenic, or anti-androgenic, depending on the compound. Prenatal exposure of mice with estrogenic chemicals such as diethylstilbestrol (DES), bisphenol A (BPA) and aroclor has affected male sexual differentiation by increasing anogenital distance, increasing prostate development with increasing androgen receptor binding activity and reducing epididymis weight (Gupta, 2000). Song et al tested the effects of BPA on several nuclear receptor gene expressions and found that the gene for nuclear receptor Nur77 (NR4A1) is induced and as a result, increased steroidogenesis is observed in mouse testicular Leydig cells. Previously only LH was shown to induce the Nur77 gene (Song et al., 2002).

Endocrine disruptors of environmental sources may affect descent of the testis, leading to cryptorchidism. Histological analyses confirmed the lack of gubernaculum development in prenatal DES-exposed animals (Emmen et al., 2000). Alkaloids from fungus may also be endocrine disruptors. Tall fescue (*Festuca arudinacea* Shreb) infected with *Neotyphodium coenophialum* fungus produces alkaloids such as ergovaline and other toxins that are harmful to animals, which feed on them. A decrease in concentration of PRL in serum was observed in livestock that consumed endophyte-infected fescue (Ross et al., 2004). A significant decrease in total testes weight, epididymis weight and sperm motility was measured in mice fed with 50% (w/w) infected tall fescue seed (Zavos et al., 1990).

Integrity of the genome is questioned when mammals are exposed to toxins, drugs and other environmental pollutants. Similarly, endocrine disruptors have been implicated in the alteration of the germ line at the genomic level. Transient exposure of gestating female rats to the endocrine disruptors such as vinclozolin or methoxychlor during the period of gonadal sex determination resulted in an F1 generation with decreased sperm cell numbers and viability and increased incidence of male infertility. In addition, these effects were transferred to subsequent generations (F1 to F4) through the male germ line. These reproduction abnormalities were associated with altered DNA methylation, indicating endocrine disruptors can alter the epigenetic regulation in a transgenerational fashion (Anway et al., 2005).

Decoding the pathways and mechanisms by which these disruptors cause hormonal imbalance may help in the development of therapies. Identification of nuclear receptor Nr0b2 as a mediator of the adverse effects of DES on fertility has the potential as a possible therapeutic target. The decreased capacity for fertilization associated with neonatal DES exposure in male mice is not observed in the case of $Nr0b2^{-/-}$ mice. Post-natal DES exposure will cause an inhibition in germ cell differentiation, whereas $Nr0b2^{-/-}$ mice do not show such inhibition upon exposure to this chemical (Decourteix and Volle, 2010).

Nutrition

Increasing rates of obesity and body mass index (BMI) among humans have become a growing concern because of reduced sperm count and male infertility. Jensen et al. (2004) studied the association between BMI and semen quality. Overweight as well as slim men had decreased concentrations of sperm and decreased sperm counts compared to men with ideal weights. With increasing BMI, serum T, sex hormone-binding globulin and inhibin B were decreased, and free androgen index and concentration of estradiol were increased. Serum FSH was increased among slim men (Jensen et al., 2004). Obesity was associated with increased sperm DNA damage, and assessed by the comet assay (Chavarro et al., 2010). Increased estradiol and reduced sperm quality were observed in rats fed with a high-fat diet (Fernandez et al., 2011).

To evaluate whether the phytoestrogens in soy affected male reproductive development, offspring of rats fed with a soy diet and a soy-free diet were compared. The presence of soy in the diet or the direct administration of genistein (an active ingredient of soy) to neonatal rats resulted in retarded spermatogenesis. Rats that received a soy-free diet had significantly larger testes and decreased FSH in adulthood. Elevated FSH as a result of soy could form the etiology of early male puberty (Atanassova et al., 2000). It has been shown that isoflavone phytoestrogens in soybeans could cause adverse effects on the testicular and reproductive functions in males. This dietary phytoestrogen down-regulates androgen-response genes and the spermatozoa glycolysis genes as evident from their decreased transcription in the testes of soy-fed animals (Cederroth et al., 2010).

Stress Caused by Management, Heat and other Environmental Factors

Many factors affect semen quality of bulls including management, environmental stress, thermoregulation, body condition, and season. Semen quality, volume and sperm concentration of the ejaculate, and motility of sperm increased over time when transitioning from colder months (January and February) to warmer months (May and June) in areas with very cold winters. This suggests that a combination of short photoperiod, cold stress, and reduced feed quality can have detrimental effects on semen quality and spermatogenesis in bulls (Barth and Waldner, 2002). It is well established that threshold concentrations of testosterone in blood and testes are necessary for normal spermatogenesis (Courot et al.,

1979; Zirkin et al., 1989). Photoperiod may have an effect on semen quality as it has been reported that seasonal variations in LH and testosterone exist (Welsh et al., 1981). Many of the environmental factors observed in bulls also occur in other species. Pigs have little ability to sweat which makes them making them more susceptible to decreased reproductive performance when thermally stressed. This could be as a combined result of heat and humidity (Kunavongkrit et al., 2005).

Cold stress may be more severe in bulls without adequate body fat, while excess body fat can also have undesirable effects. Excess fat accumulation around the scrotal neck increases scrotal/testicular temperature affecting the body's ability to cool the testes. This results in decreased seminal quality and sperm production (Coulter et al., 1997). Physical abnormalities such as scrotal frostbite can result from cold and windy weather, and create unwanted side effects. The most likely mechanism for the interruption of spermatogenesis in cases of frostbite is an increase in temperature of the testis as a result of inflammation of the scrotum. Severe frostbite affects semen quality; however, bulls typically recover over a period of time. Paying close attention to body condition and providing adequate bedding, such as hay, and shelter from wind and weather during the winter months will help prevent losses of bull breeding capability (Barth and Waldner, 2002).

The semen quality of a bull generally increases with age (Almquist et al., 1976; Fuente et al., 1984) with season having an increased significance in all semen traits of young bulls. Ejaculate sperm concentration and total number of cells were generally improved during the winter and spring compared to summer and fall months (Mathevon et al., 1998). This coincides with findings by Fuerst-Waltl et al. (2006) that temperature on the day of semen collection or during epididymal maturation or spermatogenesis had important effects on semen production and sperm quality. Ambient temperatures ranging from 5°C to 15°C were optimal for semen production (Fuerst-Waltl et al., 2006). The effect of season on semen production seems to be somewhat inconsistent as no clear pattern has been established to explain this effect on young bulls and older bulls that have produced the most motile spermatozoa during the summer and fall (Mathevon et al., 1998).

Trends have been seen in morphological abnormalities of sperm with differences between seasons and physiological states. Abnormal sperm heads have the greatest prevalence in the spring while abnormal sperm tails are most abundant in the winter (Phillips et al., 1943). Distal midpiece reflexes increase dramatically in response to stress, such as winter (Barth and Waldner, 2002). However, the significant influence of season, ambient temperature, photoperiod, and feed quality on sperm quality should be interpreted carefully. Sperm in the ejaculate sperm have been produced and matured over the previous 6 to 8 weeks in the male reproductive tract and traits observed may reflect conditions present two months prior to collection (Mathevon et al., 1998). It is important that cattle producers evaluate cold stress, body condition, and feed quality to ensure that bulls are receiving the proper management throughout the year to avoid decreasing semen quality prior to or during the breeding season (Barth and Waldner, 2002). Thermoregulation of the testes is essential for production of viable sperm in mammalian species (Waites, 1970; Setchell, 1978). In bulls, the testes must be 2 to 5°C cooler than the body temperature (38°C). Elevated scrotal temperature can have adverse effects on semen quality (Ross and Entwistle, 1979; Vogler et al., 1993) and male fertility. Bulls with inferior seminal quality produce semen with reduced motility and sperm with morphological defects, as indicated with abnormal scrotal thermograms (Lunstra and Coulter, 1997). In the bovine, the scrotum and testes have opposing temperature gradients that work in concert with one another to obtain a uniform intra-testicular temperature. The testicular artery runs from the top of the testes to the bottom, divides into several offshoots and separates dorsally and laterally before entering the testicular parenchyma; this contributes to the temperature gradient (Kastelic et al., 1997). Maloney and Mitchell (1996) confirmed that scrotal temperature is regulated in rams. Although body temperature increased during exercise and exposure to heat, scrotal temperature remained constant. Scrotal temperature regulated the tunica dartos muscle, which contracts or relaxes to move the testes closer to or further from the body, but was modulated by core body temperature (Maloney and Mitchell, 1996).

Semen quality decreases more readily in *Bos taurus* than in *Bos indicus* bulls that are exposed to warmer ambient temperatures (Johnston et al., 1963; Skinner and Louw, 1966). This may be attributed to the decreased ratio of testicular artery length and volume to the volume of testicular tissue observed in *B. taurus* bulls making them more susceptible to warmer ambient temperatures (Brito et al., 2003). The distance between the testicular artery and vein from the pampini form plexus increases the efficiency of heat exchange. The thickness of the testicular artery wall and the distance of the artery from the lumen of the nearest vein in the testicular vascular cone decreased with proximity to the testes (Cook et al., 1994; Hees et al., 1984). In *B. indicus* bulls, a greater proximity between the arterial and venous blood can be observed and as a result there is a more drastic cooling of the arterial blood after it passes through the testicular vascular cone. This may contribute to their tolerance of increased environmental temperatures when compared to crossbred or *B. taurus* bulls (Brito et al., 2003). A pendulous scrotum favors a greater surface for exposure of the testicular vascular cone area, and as a result may increase testicular cooling, or heat dissipation (Coulter and Kastelic, 1994). This may contribute to decreased arterial temperature as well as testes and epididymal temperature since arterial blood is the main source of heat entering the testes (Barros et al., 1999). Bulls with an increased or positive top-to-bottom temperature gradient (determined with infrared thermography) had fewer proportions of sperm defects and increased sperm motility and epididymal sperm reserves than bulls that did not have a clear positive temperature gradient nor had "hot spots" in the scrotum (Cook et al., 1994; Lunstra and Coulter, 1997). Over the past several decades, a decrease in sperm count and fertility has been noted in human European males. When compared to rodents, spermatogenesis in human males is inefficient and asynchronous. As a result, humans are forced to cope with lifestyle and environmental factors that could affect spermatogenesis. Like the bull, obesity in humans negatively affects sperm production and quality. Obese men have fat accumulation around the scrotal neck which causes inefficient cooling of the testes.

HORMONAL DYSFUNCTIONS CAUSING MOLECULAR DAMAGE TO SPERM

DNA Integrity

DNA integrity of sperm is associated with male infertility (O'Brien and Zini, 2005) preventing fertilization or early embryonic development. Sperm DNA integrity can be compromised by reactive oxygen species (ROS) and condensation defects (Agarwal and Allamneni, 2004). Reactive oxygen species are naturally produced in sperm mitochondria as a result of the electron transport chain, and the potentially damaging result is oxidative stress that can cause damage to the DNA of sperm (Dizdaroglu, 1992). Antioxidants, such as uric acid and catalase that are found in the body convert ROS to non-damaging molecules. However, oxidative stress occurs when either an excessive amount of ROS is being produced and the antioxidants are outnumbered, or, on the contrary, if there is an underproduction of antioxidants, and the normal amount of ROS has become damaging (Dobrzynska et al., 2004). Infertile males may have more condensation defects that can cause damage to DNA integrity when the packaging of the DNA that is normally very organized and compact becomes degraded and loosens (Manicardi et al., 1998) due a to an imbalance of protamines (Aoki and Carrell, 2003). Reactive oxygen species attack the polyunsaturated fatty acids of the sperm head causing alterations in the fatty acid pattern of the membrane (Lenzi et al., 1996), and cause damage to the sperm plasma membrane halting fertilization. Deficiencies in sperm chromatin packaging due to malfunctions in the replacement of histones with protamines or altered P1 and P2 protamines can also cause infertility (Blanchard et al., 1990; Olivia, 2006).

Endogenous hormones are considered important factors in affecting the integrity of the DNA of sperm; however, no studies have been able to elucidate how or what specific hormones have the most impact on male infertility. The mechanisms of FSH, LH, and testosterone and the hypothalamus-pituitary-gonadal axis in male reproduction are understood, however, it is apparent that other hormones may also play a role in stabilizing the DNA of sperm. If these hormonal changes could be understood and documented they could possibly be used as markers for male infertility. Meeker et al. (2008) discovered that there is an inverse relationship between estradiol and thyroid hormone compared to sperm DNA damage in which they suggest that both hormones may play protective roles against DNA damage by controlling calcium. In contrast, Appasamy et al. (2007) suggested that overall there was no significant relationship between the male reproductive hormones, FSH, inhibin B, anti-Muellerian hormone, and testosterone with oxidative stress damage in the DNA of sperm. In a more recent study, Palomba et al. (2011) determined that the treatment of FSH in men with known idiopathic infertility reduced the ROS and DNA damage in the sperm. There are still unknown aspects between the potential roles of hormones and DNA integrity, and additional studies are required to determine the relationship between the two.

Apoptosis

Apoptosis is the natural process of programmed cell death that occurs in germ cells and regulates their size and quality. Apoptosis ensures that undamaged DNA sperm cells are selected, although sperm with DNA damage that are not eliminated by apoptosis can still fertilize ova (Martincic et al., 2001). Sperm apoptosis occurs extrinsically by means of the Fas model (Lee et al., 1997) where a Fas receptor (Fas-R) binds to the Fas ligand (Fas-L) when a cell gives out a signal for the activation of Fas. The interaction between the Fas-R and the Fas-L creates a death inducing signaling complex (DISC) that activates caspase 8 (Sinha and Swerdloff, 1999). Caspase 8 activates other proteins of the caspase family, directly or indirectly that eventually cause the degradation of a cell (Guixiang et al., 2009). Increased percentages of Fas positive sperm are found in infertile men, indicating that the correct amount of spermatozoa undergoing apoptosis is not occurring (McVicar et al., 2004) and that Fas positivity in sperm indicates DNA damage and infertility (Chen et al., 2006).

Spermatogenesis is controlled by the reproductive hormones GnRH, FSH, LH, and testosterone. Apoptosis is a process that is constantly occurring to ensure that spermatogenesis stays in homeostasis; therefore, it would be natural to assume that some relationship must take place between endogenous hormones and apoptosis. It has been suggested that apoptosis keeps spermatogenesis in homeostasis by balancing germ cells and Sertoli cells, which contain FSH and testosterone receptors as well as the Fas receptor and Fas Ligand (Kierszenbaum, 2001). As discussed previously, estrogen plays a vital role in the reproductive process of males. Animals exposed to treatments with estrogen had decreased fertility rates by estrogen inducing apoptosis in the germ cell (Nikula et al., 1999). The reduction in FSH or LH increased the apoptotic signal, and FSH and testosterone must obstruct the DISC signal for the germ cell (Pareek et al., 2007). This deduction is also supported by Ruwanpura et al. (2008) who concluded that FSH helped control both apoptotic pathways during spermatogenesis and by Yang et al. (2006) who discovered that decreased LH increased apoptosis in sperm cells and thereby increased male infertility.

Advancing age and gonadotoxins have been associated with reduced germ cell apoptosis in the testicle and an increased percentage of ejaculated spermatozoa with DNA damage, which suggests that both spermatogenesis and apoptosis have been disrupted (Zini and Libman, 2006). Male infertility appears to be positively correlated with increased numbers of sperm with apoptotic markers (Wang et al., 2003). There is also a decrease in apoptosis with increasing age, suggesting an increase in damaged DNA of sperm from older men because apoptosis is not operating as efficiently (Singh et al., 2003). Apoptosis and oxidative stress are closely related. Therefore, the precautions and preventions that should be taken to decrease oxidative stress through antioxidants could possibly be used to decrease the damage from the improper functioning of apoptosis (Zini and Agarwal, 2011). However, decreased apoptosis is also related to age, which is an unstoppable effect. Further studies are required to understand the complexity of how hormones play a role in apoptosis and how age increases natural cell death.

CONCLUSION

Semen quality has the vital role in animal fertility, which is an economically important and complex. In addition to genetics, other conditions such as environmental factors can influence endocrine homeostasis by the misregulation of specific hormones that control male fertility. Despite considerable progress in the search for underlying mechanisms and new factors regulating male fertility, research at the critical intersection between hormones and sperm viability has been limited. This gap in the knowledge base is important, in fact urgent, because it is preventing progress in the basic science of reproductive biology and in improvements in the understanding of male fertility. Many aspects of male fertility among species are similar; however, significant differences exist in the actions of specific hormones and how they regulate male fertility in different mammals. This study reviewed male reproductive systems, endocrine regulation of male fertility, influence of external environmental factors on fertility, and pointed out specific challenges and much needed research in each area. Such research has the potential for social and financial benefits for families and man, and economic importance for the primary focus of this report, that is, on agriculture animals, through improving fertility and reproduction of farm animals. Any measure of progress or success among these needs will be profound.

ACKNOWLEDGMENTS

The authors thank Drs. Graham and Martha Wells for their critical review of this manuscript. We also would like to thank Dr. George Seidel of Colorado State University for his valuable guidance in development of this paper.

REFERENCES

Agarwal, A; Allamaneni, SSR. The effect of sperm DNA damage on assisted reproduction outcomes. *Minerva Ginecol,* 2004, 56, 235-24.

Ahmed, AE; Saito, H; Sawada, T; Yaegashi, T; Yamashita, T; Hirata, TI; Sawai, K; Hashizume, T. Characteristics of the stimulatory effect of kisspeptin-10 on the secretion of luteinizing hormone, follicle-stimulating hormone and growth hormone in prepubertal male and female cattle. *J Reprod Dev,* 2009, 55(6), 650-654.

Albertson, BD; Sienkiewicz, M; Kimball, D; Munabi, AK; Cassorla, F; Loriaux, DL. New evidence for a direct effect of prolactin on rat adrenal steroidogenesis. *Endoc Res,* 1987, 13, 317-333.

Almquist, JO; Branas, RJ; Barber, KA. Post-pubertal changes in semen production of Charolais bulls ejaculated at high frequency and the relation between testicular measurements and sperm output. *J Anim Sci,* 1976, 42, 670-676.

Anderson, RA; Wallace, EM; Groome, NP; Bellis, AJ; Wu, FC. Physiological relationships between inhibin B, follicle stimulating hormone secretion and spermatogenesis in normal men and response to gonadotrophin suppression by exogenous testosterone. *Hum Reprod,* 1997, 12, 746-751.

Anderson, ST; Barclay, JL; Fanning, KJ; Kusters, DHL; Waters, MJ; Curlewis, JD. Mechanisms underlying the diminished sensitivity to prolactin negative feedback during lactation: reduced STAT5 signaling and upregulation of cytokine inducible SH2 domain containing protein (CIS) expression in tuberoinfundibular dopaminergic neurons. *Endocrinology,* 2006, 147, 1195-1202.

Andersson, AM; Toppari, J; Haavisto, AM; Petersen, JH; Simell, T; Simell, O. Longitudinal reproductive hormone profiles in infants: peak of inhibin B levels in infant boys exceeds levels in adult men. *J Cli Endoc Metab,* 1998, 83, 675-681.

Anway, MD; Cupp, AS; Uzumcu, M; Skinner, MK. Epigenetic transgenerational actions of endocrine disruptors and male fertility. *Science,* 2005, 308, 1466-1469.

Aoki, VW; Carrell, DT. Human protamines and the developing spermatid: their structure, function, expression and relationship with male infertility. *A J Androl,* 2003, 5, 315-324.

Appasamy, M; Muttukrishna, S; Pizzey, AR; Ozturk, O; Groome, NP; Serhal, P; Jauniaux, E. Relationship between male reproductive hormones, sperm DNA damage, and markers of oxidative stress in infertility. *Reprod BioMed Online,* 2007, 14, 15-165.

Atanassova, N; McKinnell, C; Turner, KJ; Walker, M; Fisher, JS; Morley, M; Millar, MR; Groome, NP; Sharpe, RM. Comparative effects of neonatal exposure of male rats to potent and weak (environmental) estrogens on spermatogenesis at puberty and the relationship to adult testis size and fertility: evidence for stimulatory effects of low estrogen levels. *Endocrinology,* 2000, 141, 3898-3907.

Barros, CMQ; Oba, E; Brito, LFC; Cook, RB; Coulter, GH; Groves, G; et al. Testicular blood flow and oxygen evaluation in Aberdeen Angus bulls. *Rev Bras Reprod Anim,* 1999, 23, 218-20.

Barth, AD; Waldner, CL. Factors affecting breeding soundness classification of beef bulls examined at the Western College of Veterinary Medicine. *Can Vet J,* 2002, 43, 274-284.

Bartke, A; Cecim, M; Tang, K; Steger, RW; Chandrashekar, V; Turyn, D. Neuroendocrine and reproductive consequences of overexpression of growth hormone in transgenic mice. *Proc Soc Exp Biol Med,* 1994, 206, 345-359.

Bartke, A. Hyperprolactinemia and male reproduction. *And, Male Fert and Ster,* 1986, 101-123.

Bartke, A. Role of growth hormone and prolactin in the control of reproduction: What are we learning from transgenic and knock-out animals? *Steroids,* 1999, 64, 598-604.

Bearden, HJ; Fuquay, J; Willard, S. *App Anim Reprod,* 2004, 22-32.

Bex, F; Bartke, A; Goldman, BD; Dalterio, S. Prolactin, growth hormone, luteinizing hormone receptors, and seasonal changes in testicular activity in the golden hamster. *Endocrinology,* 1978, 103, 2069-2080.

Blanchard, Y; Lescoat, D; Le Lannou, D. Anomalous distribution of nuclear basic proteins in round-headed human spermatozoa. *Andrologia,* 1990, 22(6), 549-55.

Brito, LF; Silva, AE; Barbosa, RT; Kastelic, JP. (2003) Testicular thermoregulation in *Bos indicus,* crossbred and *Bos taurus* bulls: relationship with scrotal, testicular vascular cone and testicular morphology, and effects on semen quality and sperm production. *Theriogenology,* 2003, 61, 511-528.

Bruysters, M; Christin-Maitre, S; Verhoef-Post, M; Sultan, C; Auger, J; Faugeron, I; Larue, L; Lumbroso, S; Themmen, AP; Bouchard, P. A new LH receptor splice mutation responsible for male hypogonadism with subnormal sperm production in the propositus, and infertility with regular cycles in an affected sister. *Hum Reprod,* 2008, 23, 1917-1923.

Byrd, W; Bennett, MJ; Carr, BR; Dong, Y; Wians, F; Rainey, W. Regulation of biologically active dimeric inhibin A and B from infancy to adulthood in the male. *J Clin Endoc Metab,* 1998, 83, 2849-2854.

Cederroth, CR; Zimmermann, C; Beny, JL; Schaad, O; Combepine, C; Descombes, P; Doerge, DR; Pralong, FP; Vassalli, JD; Nef, S. Potential detrimental effects of a phytoestrogen-rich diet on male fertility in mice. *Mol Cell Endoc,* 2010, 321,152-160.

Chavarro, JE; Toth, TL; Wright, DL; Meeker, JD; Hauser, R. Body mass index in relation to semen quality, sperm DNA integrity, and serum reproductive hormone levels among men attending an infertility clinic. *Fert Steril,* 2010, 93, 2222-2231.

Chen, Z; Hauser, R; Trobvich, A; Shifren, JL; Dorer, DJ; Godfrey-Bailey, L; Singh, N. The Relationship Between Human Semen Characteristics and Sperm Apoptosis: A Pilot Study. *J Androl,* 2006, 27, 112-120.

Childs, GV; Unabia, G; Rougeau, D. Cells that express luteinizing hormone (LH) and follicle-stimulating hormone (FSH) subunit messenger ribonucleic acids during the estrous cycle: the major contributors contain LH, FSH, and/or growth hormone. *Endocrinology,* 1994, 134, 990–997.

Cook, RB; Coulter, GH; Kastelic, JP. The testicular vascular cone, scrotal thermoregulation and their relationship to sperm production and seminal quality in beef bulls. *Theriogenology,* 1994, 41, 453-71.

Cooper, T. Sperm maturation in the epididymis: a new look at an old problem. *A J Androl,* 2007, 9, 533-539.

Coulter, GH; Cook, RB; Kastelic, JP. Effects of dietary energy on scrotal surface temperature, seminal quality, and sperm production in young beef bulls. *J Anim Sci,* 1997, 75, 1048-1052.

Coulter, GH; Kastelic, JP. Testicular thermoregulation in bulls. In: Proceedings to the 15th Technical Conference of Artificial Insemination and Reproduction. *Nat Assoc Anim Breed,* 1994, 28-34.

Courot, M, Hochereau de Reviers, MT; Monet-Kuntz, C; et al. Endocrinology of spermatogenesis in the hypophysectomized ram. *Reprod Ret Suppl,* 1979, 26, 165-173.

Decourteix, M; Volle, DH. Endocrine disruptors and fertility: NR0B2, a new therapeutic target? *Med Sci (Paris),* 2010, 26, 359-361.

DeSantis, M; Albrecht, W; Höltl, W; Pont, J. Impact of cytotoxic treatment on long-term fertility in patients with germ-cell cancer. *Int J Can J Intl Du Cancer,* 1999, 83, 864-865.

Dizdaroglu, M. Oxidative damage to DNA in mammalian chromatin. *Mut Res,* 1992, 275, 331-342.

Dobrzynska, MM; Baumgartner, A; Anderson, D. Antioxidants modulate thyroid hormone- and noradrenaline-induced DNA damage in human sperm. *Mutagenesis,* 2004, 19, 325-330.

Dorrington, JH; Roller, NF; Fritz, IB. Effects of follicle-stimulating hormone on cultures of sertoli cell preparations. *Mol Cell Endoc,* 1975, 3, 57-70.

Eacker, S; Agrawal, MN; Qian, K; Dichek, HL; Gong, EY; Lee, K; Braun, R.E. Hormonal regulation of testicular steroid and cholesterol homeostasis. *Mol Endoc,* 2008, 22, 623-635.

Emmen, JM; McLuskey, A; Adham, IM; Engel, W; Verhoef-Post, M; Themmen, AP; Grootegoed, JA; Brinkmann, AO. Involvement of insulin-like factor 3 (Insl3) in diethylstilbestrol-induced cryptorchidism. *Endocrinology,* 2000, 141, 846-849.

Fernandez, CD; Bellentani, FF; Fernandes, GS; Perobelli, JE; Favareto, AP; Nascimento, AF; Cicogna, AC; Kempinas, WD. Diet-induced obesity in rats leads to a decrease in sperm motility. *Reprod Biol Endocrinol,* 2011, 9, 32.

Fraietta, R; Spaine, DM; Bertolla, RP; Ortiz, V; Cedenho, AP. Individual and seminal characteristics of patients with testicular germ cell tumors. *Fert and Steril,* 2010, 94, 2107-2112.

Fuente, LF; anchez-Garcia, L; Vallejo, M. Reproductive characters in Galician Blonds. I. Characters of semen used for artificial insemination. *Anal Fac Vet Leon,* 1984, 30,119-125.

Fuerst-Waltl, B; Schwarzenbacher, M; Perner, C; Sölkner, J. Effects of age and environmental factors on semen production and semen quality of Austrian Simmental bulls. *Anim Reprod Sci*, 2006, 95, 27-37.

Gadkar, S; Shah, CA; Sachdeva, G; Samant, U; Puri, CP. Progesterone Receptor as an Indicator of Sperm Function. *Biol Reprod*, 2002, 67, 1327-1336.

Gill-Sharma, MK. Prolactin and Male Fertility: The Long and Short Feedback Regulation. *Int J Endocrinol*, 2009, 1-13.

Giwercman, A; Carlsen, E; Keiding, N; Skakkebaek NE. Evidence for increasing incidence of abnormalities of the human testis: a review. *Env Health Pers 101 Suppl,* 1993, 2, 65-71.

Guixiang Ji, G; Gu, A; Hu, F; Wang, S; Liang, J; Xia, Y; Lu, C; Song, L; Fu, G; Wang, X. Polymorhpisms in cell death pathway genes are associated with altered sperm apoptosis and poor semen quality. *Hum Reprod*, 2009, 2, 2439–2446.

Gupta, C. (2000) Reproductive malformation of the male offspring following maternal exposure to estrogenic chemicals. *Proc Soc Exp Biol Med*, 2000, 224, 61-68.

Hall, DL; Payne, LA; Putnam, JM; Huet-Hudson, YM. (1997) Effect of methoxychlor on implantation and embryo development in the mouse. *Reprod Toxicol*, 1997, 11, 703-708.

Hameed, S; Jayasena, CN; Dhillo, W. (2011) Kisspeptin and fertility. *J Endocrinol*, 2011, 2008, 97-105.

Hees, H; Leiser, R; Kohler, T; Wrobel. KH. Vascular morphology of the spermatic cord and testis I. Light- and scanning electron-microscopic studies on the testicular artery and pampiniform plexus. *Cell Tissue Res.*, 1984, 237, 31-38.

Hess, RA. Estrogen in the adult male reproductive tract: A review. *Reprod Biol Endocrinol*, 2003, 1-14.

Jensen, TK; Andersson, AM; Jorgensen, N; Andersen, AG; Carlsen, E; Petersen, JH; Skakkebaek, NE. Body mass index in relation to semen quality and reproductive hormones among 1,558 Danish men. *Fertil Steril*, 2004, 82, 863-870.

Jiménez-Severiano, H; D'Occhio, MJ; Lunstra, DD; Mussard, ML; Koch, JW; Ehnis, LR; Enright, WJ; Kinder, JE. Effect of chronic treatment with the gonadotrophin-releasing hormone agonist azagly-nafarelin on basal concentrations of LH in prepubertal bulls. *Reproduction*, 2003, 125(2), 225-32.

Johnson, L; Thompson DL Jr. Age-related and seasonal variation in the sertoli cell population, daily sperm production and serum concentrations of follicle-stimulating hormone, luteinizing hormone and testosterone in stallions. *Biol Reprod*, 1983 29, 777-789.

Johnston, JE; Naelapaa, H; Frye, JB. Physiological responses of Holstein, Brown Swiss and Red Sindhi crossbreed bull exposed to high temperatures and humidities. *J Anim Sci*, 1963, 22, 432-6.

Juul, A; Andersson, AM; Pedersen, SA; Jorgensen, JOL; Christiansen, JS; Groome, NP, Skakkebaek, NE. Effects of growth hormone replacement therapy on IG related parameters and on the pituitary-gonadal axis in GH-deficient males a double blind, placebo controlled crossover study. *Hormone Res*, 1998, 49, 269–278.

Kastelic, JP; Cook, RB; Coulter, GH. (1997) Contribution of the scrotum, testes, and testicular artery to scrotal/testicular thermoregulation in bulls at two ambient temperatures. *Anim Reprod Sci,* 1997, 45, 255-261.

Katongole, CB; Naftolin, F; Short, RV. Relationship between blood levels of luteinizing hormone and testosterone in bulls, and the effects of sexual stimulation. *J Endocrinol*, 1971, 50, 457-466.

Kelly, MA; Rubinstein, M; Asa, SL. Pituitary lactotroph hyperplasia and chronic hyperprolactinemia in dopamine D2 receptor-deficient mice. *Neuron*, 1997, 19, 103–113.

Kierszenbaum, AL. Apoptosis during spermatogenesis: the thrill of being alive. *Mol Reprod Dev*, 2001, 58, 1–3.

Kunavongkrit, A; Suriyasomboon, A; Lundeheim, N; Heard, TW; Einarsson, S. Management of sperm production of boars under differing environmental conditions. *Theriogenology*, 2005, 63, 657-667.

Lee, J; Richburg, JH; Younkin, SC; Boekelheide, K. The Fas system is a key regulator of germ cell apoptosis in the testis. *Endocrinology*, 1997, 138, 2081-2088.

Lenzi, A; Picardo, M; Gandini, L; Dondero, F. Lipids of the sperm plasma membrane from polyunsaturated fatty acids considered as markers of sperm function to possible scavenger therapy. *Hum Reprod*, 1996, 2, 246-256.

Lindzey, J; Wetsel, WC; Couse, JF; Stoker, T; Cooper, R; Korach, KS. Effects of castration and chronic steroid treatments on hypothalamic gonadotropin releasing hormone content and pituitary gonadotropins in male wild type and estrogen receptor knockout mice. *Endocrinology*, 1998, 139, 4092–4101.

Ling, N; Ying, SY; Ueno, N; Esch, F; Denoroy, L; Guillemin, R. Isolation and partial characterization of a Mr 32000 protein with inhibin activity from porcine follicular fluid. *PNAS*, 1985, 82, 7217-7221.

Lobie, PE; Breipohl, W; Aragon, JG; Waters, MJ. Cellular localization of the growth hormone receptor binding protein in the male and female reproductive systems. *Endocrinology*, 1990, 126, 2214–2221.

Lunstra, DD; Coulter, GH. Relationship between scrotal infrared temperature patterns and natural-mating fertility in beef bulls. *J Anim Sci*, 1997, 75, 767-774.

Maloney, SK; Mitchell, D. Regulation of ram scrotal temperature during heat exposure, cold exposure, fever and exercise. *J Physiol*, 1996, 496.2, 421-430.

Manicardi, GC; Tombacco, A; Bizzaro, D; Bianchi, U; Bianchi, P; Sakkas, D. DNA

Martincic, DS; Klun, IV; Zorn, B; Vrtovec, HM. Germ cell apoptosis in the human testis. *Pflugers Arch*, 2001, 442, 159–60.

Masud, S; Mehboob, F; Bappi, MU. Severe hyperprolactinemia directly depresses the gonadal activity causing infertility. *Esc J Serv Inst Med Sci*, 2007, 2, 25-27.

Mathevon, M; Buhr, MM; Dekkers, JCM. Environmental, Management, and Genetic Factors Affecting Semen Production in Holstein Bulls. *J Dairy Sci*, 1998, 81, 3321-3330.

McVicar, CM; McClure, N; Williamson, K; Dalzell, LH; Lewis, SE. Incidence of Fas positivity and deoxyribonucleic acid double-stranded breaks in human ejaculated sperm. *Fert Steril*, 2004, 81, 767–774.

Meachem, SJ; Nieschleg, E; Simoni, M. Inhibin B in male reproduction: pathophysiology and clinical relevance. *Eu J Endocrinol*, 2001, 145, 561-577.

Meeker, JD; Singh, NP; Hauser, R. Serum concentrations of estradiol and free T4 are inversely correlated with sperm DNA damage in men from an infertility clinic. *J Androl*, 2008, 29, 379-388.

Moore, KE; Demarest, KT. Tuberoinfundibular and tuberohypophysial dopaminergic neurons. *Front Neuroendocrinol*, 1982, 7, 161-190.

Morishima, A; Grumbach, MM; Simpson, ER; Fisher, C; Qin, K. Aromatase deficiency in male and female siblings caused by a novel mutation and the physiological role of estrogens. *J Cli Endoc Met*, 1995, 80, 3689–3698.

Mortimer, CH; Yeo, T. (1976) Gonadotrophin-releasing hormone. *J Cli Path. Supp (Association Of Clinical Pathologists)*, 1976, 7, 46-54.

Nikula, H; Talonpoika, T; Kaleva, M; Toppari, J. Inhibition of hCG-stimulated steroidogenesis in cultured mouse Leydig tumor cells by bisphenol A and octylphenols. *Toxicol App Pharm*, 1999, 157, 166-173.

O'Donnell, L; Robertson, KM; Jones, ME; Simpson, ER. *Estrogen and spermatogenesis. Endoc Rev*, 2001, 22, 289-318.

O'Brien, J; Zini, A. Sperm DNA integrity and male infertility. *Urology*, 2005, 65, 16-22.

Olivia, R. Protamines and male infertility. *Hum Reprod Update*, 2006, 12, 417-435.

Orth, JM. The role of follicle-stimulating hormone in controlling Sertoli cell proliferation in testes of fetal rats. *Endocrinology*, 1984, 115, 1248-1255.

Ovesen, P; Moller, J; Jorgensen, JO; Moller, N; Christiansen, JS. Effect of growth hormone administration on circulating levels of luteinizing hormone, follicle stimulating hormone and testosterone in normal healthy men. *Hum Reprod*, 1993, 8, 1869–1872.

Palomba, S; Falbo, A; Espinola, S; Rocca, M; Capasso, S; Cappiello, F; Zullo, F. Effects of highly purified FSH on sperm DNA damage in men with male idiopathic subfertility: a pilot study. *J Endoc Inv*, 2011, [Epub ahead of print].

Paola, P; Francesca, S; Laura, G; Concetta, M; Giulia, C; Giuseppe, C;Vincenzo De, L. Sperm aneuploidies after human recombinant follicle stimulating hormone therapy in infertile males. *Reprod BioMed Onl*, 2009, 18:622-629.

Pareek, TK; Joshi, AR; Sanyal, A; Dighe, RR. Insights into male germ cell apoptosis due to depletion of gonadotropins caused by GnRH antagonists. *Apoptosis*, 2007, 12, 1085-1100.

Petersen, PM; Skakkebaek, NE; Giwercman, A. Gonadal function in men with testicular cancer: Biological and clinical aspects. *APMIS*, 1998, 106, 24-36.

Phillips, RW; Bradforn Jr., K; Heemstra, LC; Eaton, ON. Seasonal variation in the semen of bulls. *Am J Vet Res*, 1943, 4, 115-119.

Pierik, FH; Vreeburg, JTM; Stijnen, T; De Jong, FH; Weber, RFA. Serum inhibin B as a marker of spermatogenesis. *J Cli Endoc Met*, 1998, 83, 3110 –3114.

Purvis, K; Clausen, OPF; Olsen, A; Haug, E; Hansson, V. Prolactin and Leydig cell responsiveness to LH/hCG in the rat. *Arch Andr*, 1998, 3, 219-230.

Raivio, T; Toppari, J; Perheentupa, A; McNeilly, AS; Dunkel, L. Treatment of prepubertal gonadotrophin deficient boys with recombinant human follicle stimulating hormone. *Lancet*, 1997, 350, 263-264.

Raju, TN. The Nobel Chronicles. 1977: Roger Charles Louis Guillemin (b 1924); Andrew Victor Schally (b1926); Rosalyn S Yalow (b 1921). *Lancet* 1999, 20, 354(9192), 1828.

Ramaswamy, S; Plant, TM; Marshall, GR. Pulsatile stimulation with recombinant single chain human luteinizing hormone elicits precocious Sertoli cell proliferation in the juvenile male rhesus monkey (Macaca mulatta). *Biol Reprod*, 2000, 63, 82–88.

Rommerts, FF; de Jong, FH; Brinkmann, AO; van der Molen, HJ. Development and cellular localization of rat testicular aromatase activity. *J Reprod Fert*, 1982, 65, 281-288.

Ross, AD; Entwistle, KW. The effect of scrotal insulation on spermatozoal morphology and the rates of spermatogenesis and epididymal passage of spermatozoa in the bull. *Theriogenology*, 1979, 11, 111-129.

Ross, MK; Hohenboken, WD; Saacke, RG; Kuehn, LA. Effects of feeding endophyte-infected fescue seed on reproductive traits of male mice divergently selected for resistance or susceptibility to fescue toxicosis. *Theriogenology*, 2004, 61, 651-662.

Ruwanpura, SM; McLachlan, RI; Stanton, PG; Loveland, KL; Meachem, SJ. Pathways involved in testicular germ cell apoptosis in immature rats after FSH suppression. *J Endoc,* 2008, 197, 35-43.

Seminara, SB; Boepple, PA; Nachtigall, LB; Pralong, FP; Khoury, RH; Sluss. Inhibin B in males with gonadotropin-releasing hormone (GnRH) deficiency: changes in serum concentration after short term physiologic GnRH replacement. *J Cli Endoc Met*, 1996, 81, 3692-3696.

Setchell, BP. (1978) The scrotum and thermoregulation. In: *The Mammalian Testis* (1st Ed.) p 90. Cornell Univ. Press, Ithaca, NY.

Sharpe, RM. Environmental/lifestyle effects on spermatogenesis. *Phil Trans R Soc B*, 2010, 365, 1697-1712.

Singh, N; Nuller, C; Berger, R. Effects of age on DNA double strand breaks and apoptosis in human sperm. *Fert Steril*, 2003, 80, 420-1430.

Sinha Hikim, AP; Swerdloff, RS. Hormonal and genetic control of germ cell apoptosis in the testis. *Rev Reprod*, 1999, 4, 38 -47.

Skinner, JD; Louw, GN. Heat stress and spermatogenesis in *Bos indicus* and *Bos taurus* cattle. *J. Appl Phys*, 1966, 21, 1784-90.

Smith, EP; Boyd, J; Frank, GR; Takahashi, H; Cohen, RM; Specker, B; Williams, TC; Lubhan, DB; Korach, KS. Estrogen resistance caused by a mutation in the estrogen receptor gene in a man. *New Eng J Med*, 1994, 331, 1056–1061.

Song, KH; Lee, K; Choi, HS. Endocrine disrupter bisphenol a induces orphan nuclear receptor Nur77 gene expression and steroidogenesis in mouse testicular Leydig cells. *Endocrinology*, 2002, 143, 2208-2215.

Steger, RW; Chandrashekar, V; Zhao, W; Bartke, A; Horseman, ND. Neuroendocrine and reproductive functions in male mice with targeted disruption of the prolactin gene. *Endocrinology*, 1998,139, 3691–3695.

Sykiotis, GP; Hoang, XH; Avbelj, M; Hayes, FJ; Thambundit, A; Dwyer, A; Au, M; Plummer, L; Crowley, WF Jr; Pitteloud N. Congenital idiopathic hypogonadotropic hypogonadism: evidence of defects in the hypothalamus, pituitary, and testes. *J Clin Endocrinol Metab*, 2010, 95(6), 3019-27. Epub 2010 Apr 9.

Topaloglu, AK; Tello, JA; Kotan, LD; Ozbek, MN; Yilmaz, MB; Erdogan, S; Gurbuz, F; Temiz, F; Millar, RP; Yuksel, B. Inactivating KISS1 mutation and hypogonadotropic hypogonadism. *N England J Med*, 2012, 16, 629-635.

Trabado, S; Maione, L; Salenave, S; Baron, S; Galland, F; Bry-Gauillard, H; Guiochon-Mantel, A; Chanson, P; Pitteloud, N; Sinisi, AA; Brailly-Tabard, S; Young, J. Estradiol levels in men with congenital hypogonadotropic hypogonadism and the effects of different modalities of hormonal treatment. *Fertil Steril*, 2011, 95(7), 2324-9, 2329.e1-3. Epub 2011 May 4.

Tres, LL; Smith, EP; Van Wyk, JJ; Kierszenbaum, AL. Immunoreactive sites and accumulation of somatomedin C in rat Sertoli spermatogenic cell cocultures. *Exp Cell Res*, 1986, 162, 33–50.

Uzumcu, M; Kuhn, PE; Marano, JE; Armenti, AE; Passantino, L. Early postnatal methoxychlor exposure inhibits folliculogenesis and stimulates anti-Mullerian hormone production in the rat ovary. *J Endoc*, 2006, 191, 549-558.

van der Molen, HJ; Brinkmann, AO; de Jong, FH; Rommerts, FF. Testicular oestrogens. *J Endoc*, 1981, 89, 33P-46P.

Vogler, CJ; Bame, JH; DeJarnette, JM; McGilliard, ML; Saacke, RG. Effects of elevated testicular temperature on morphology characteristics of ejaculated spermatozoa in the bovine. *Theriogenology*, 1993, 40, 1207-1219.

von Eckardstein, S; Simoni, M; Bergmann, M; Weinbauer, GF; Gassner, P; Schepers, AG. Serum inhibin B in combination with serum follicle stimulating hormone (FSH) is a more sensitive marker than serum FSH alone for impaired spermatogenesis in men, but cannot predict the presence of sperm in testicular tissue samples. *J Cli Endoc Metab*, 1999, 84, 2496-2501.

Waites, GMH. Temperature regulation and the testis. In: A. D. Johnson, W.R. Gomes and N.L. VanDemark (Ed.), 1970, *The Testis*, 1, 241-265. Academic Press, New York, NY.

Walker, WH. Non-classical actions of testosterone and spermatogenesis. *Philos Trans R Soc Lond B Biol Sci*, 2010, 365(1546), 1557-69.

Wang, X; Sharma, RK; Sikka, SC; Thomas, AJ Jr; Falcone, T; Agarwal, A. Oxidative stress is associated with increased apoptosis leading to spermatozoa DNA damage in patients with male factor infertility. *Fert Steril*, 2003, 80, 531 -535.

Welsh, TH Jr.; Randel, RD; Johnson, BH. Interrelationships of serum corticosteroids, LH and testosterone in the male bovine. *Arch Androl*, 1981, 6, 141-150.

Welt, C; Sidis, Y; Keutmann, H; Schneyer, A. Activins, Inhibins, and Follistatins: From Endocrinology to Signaling. A Paradigm for the New Millennium. *Exp Biol Med*, 2002, 227, 724-752.

Welt, CK; Chan, JL; Bullen, J; Murphy, R; Smith, P; DePaoli, AM; Karalis, A; Mantrozos, CS. Recombinant human leptin in women with hypothalamic amenorrhea. *New Eng J Med*, 2004, 351, 987-997.

Winters,SJ; Takahashi, J; Troen, P. Secretion of Testosterone and Its Δ4Precursor Steroids into Spermatic Vein Blood in Men with Varicocele-Associated Infertility. *JCEM,* 1999, 84, 997.

Yang, MG; Yang, Y; Huang, P; Hao, XK; Zhang, ZY; Zheng, SL; Fan, AL; Rao, GZ; Wei, XM. Sexual hormone levels in semen and germ cell apoptosis. *Zhonghua Nan Ke Xue*, 2006, 12, 432-434.

Zavos, PM; Siegel, MR; Grove, RJ; Hemken, RM; Varney, DR. Effects of feeding endophyte-infected tall fescue seed on reproductive performance in male CD-1 mice by competitive breeding. *Theriogenology*, 1990, 33, 653-660.

Zini, A; Agarwal, A. Sperm Chromatin: Biological and Clinical Applications in male infertility and assisted reproduction. *ISBN:978-1-4419-1781-2*, 2011.

Zini, A; Libman, J. Sperm DNA damage: clinical significance in the era of assisted reproduction. *Can Med As J,* 2011, 175, 495-500.

Zipf, WB; Payne, AH; Kelch, RP. Prolactin, growth hormone, and luteinizing hormone in the maintenance of testicular luteinizing hormone receptors. *Endocrinology*, 1978, 103, 595–600.

Zirkin, BR; Santulli, R; Awoniyi, CA; Ewing, LL. Maintenance of advanced spermatogenic cells in the adult rat testis: quantitative relationship to testosterone concentration within the testis. *Endocrinology*, 1989, 124, 2043-2049.

In: Cattle: Domestication, Diseases and the Environment   ISBN: 978-1-62417-820-7
Editor: George Liu   © 2013 Nova Science Publishers, Inc.

Chapter 6

OZONE AS A NOVEL TREATMENT MODALITY FOR UROVAGINA, ENDOMETRITIS AND RETAINED PLACENTA IN CATTLE

R. Zobel and Z. Tuček

Centre for Animal Reproduction of Croatia, Zagreb, Croatia

ABSTRACT

Urovagina, endometritis and retained placenta are detrimental to the health and fertility of cows worldwide. Different treatment options for urovagina, so far, included only surgical modifications of vaginal tissue. Treatments of endometritis and retained placenta included antibiotics applied parenteraly and/or into the uterus as well as prostaglandin and oxytocin analogues administered parenteraly. Recently, infusion of collagenase into the umbilical arteries in animals with retained placenta was introduced. Efficacy of many of these treatments is questionable and others are too expensive and inappropriate for daily field practice. Urovagina, endometritis and retained placenta can be successfully treated by the ozone flush applied into the uterus and vagina. The ozone flush was found to be the most effective treatment modality for investigated fertility issues in cattle with an advantage of no milk and meat withdrawal period.

Keywords: Cattle, urovagina, endometritis, treatment, ozone

INTRODUCTION

Urovagina is a pathological condition characterized by urine accumulation in the cranial portion of the vagina resulting in vaginitis and endometritis [1,2]. The etiology of urovagina is poorly understood, however, the disease has been correlated with stretching of the suspensory apparatus as a result of dystocia, twinning and successive pregnancies [3,4]. Available treatment options include complex and invasive surgical interventions through the remodelling of the vaginal tissue to reduce or eliminate the backflow of urine [1,5,6].

Mentioned procedures are expensive, require a prolonged recovery period, and have limited success in returning the animal back to full reproductive capabilities [7]. Consequently, urovagina often goes untreated in cows and frequently results in reduced health and reproductive success or culling. Practical alternatives to surgical treatment of urovagina in cows have been investigated by [8] and included ozone flush of vagina and uterus prior the artificial insemination in Simmental cattle. According to [9], one of the most important causes of subfertility in dairy cows is endometritis. Clinical endometritis (CE) can be defined as the presence of purulent or mucopurulent uterine discharge detectable externally or in the anterior vagina and/or with a cervical diameter greater than 7.5 cm, uterine-horn diameter > 8 cm after 30 days in milk [10]. As reported by [11,12], various treatment approaches have been used, including parenteral administration or intrauterine infusion of antibiotics and intramuscular administration of prostaglandin analogues. A variety of antibiotics have been infused into the uterus of cows in attempts to treat postpartum infections. In adition, [12] suggested ceftiofur as an alternative if the animal does not appear to respond to penicillin administration. Alternatives to reported treatments have been investigated by [13] including prostaglandins applied parenteraly simultaneously with antibiotics and ozone administered into the uterus.

The definition of Retention of Fetal Membranes (RFM) is varied, ranging from retention of the fetal membranes for 8 hours [14], 8 - 12 hours [15], 12 - 24 hours [16] to up to 48 hours [17] post calving, while the majority of cattle will pass the fetal membranes within 6 hours after parturition [14]. Many common therapies for RFM have not been shown to be effective, and some could actually have a negative impact on future reproduction [18]. A variety of methods have been used in the treatment of bovine RFM, although efficacy of many of these treatments is questionable. Local antimicrobials, given as uterine infusions or boluses, have not been shown to reduce the incidence of endometritis or improve fertility [19]. Although occasional reports exist, immediate post partum administration of prostaglandins, oxytocin or calcium have generally showed low efficacy in preventing the retained placenta or hastening the expulsion of retrained fetal membranes [20]. The aim of the study conducted by [21] was to assess and compare different treatment options, including ozone flush, prostaglandins and antibiotics in cows with retained placenta.

Ozone (O_3) is unstable natural gas and a potent bactericide with efficacy equal to or greater than iodine and chlorine [22,23]. Ozone therapy was reported as a successful treatment option in medicine and dentistry due to its potent antimicrobial activity for a wide range of microorganisms, and based on its high oxidation potential and its fast transformation into free oxygen (within a few minutes) that has no negative impact on the spermatozoa [24,25]. Ozone also stimulates host immunity by activating erythrocyte metabolism and local tissue immunity through an increase in lysozyme activity, IgA and cervical mucus myeloperoxidases levels, with a simultaneous decrease in IgM and IgG resulting in a balanced coefficient of local immunity factors [26,27].

RESULTS AND DISCUSSION

In search of a practical means to reduce economic losses associated with urovagina, the ability of antibiotic and O_3 therapy, as a novel treatment option, was tested to improve conception and term-pregnancy rates in dairy cows diagnosed with urovagina [8]. As shown in Table 1, the most successful therapy was achieved for the group of animals where O_3 was infused into the uterine corpus and vagina prior to artificial insemination. In this group, the overall success of O_3 therapy, regardless of the level of disease (mild, moderate, and severe), was considered effective as the average number of artificial inseminations and days open were significantly reduced in comparison to other treatment groups. Of major significance, it was found that O_3 therapy out-performed antibiotic treatment at all reproductive stages in cows exhibiting mild, moderate and severe cases of urovagina. These findings are the first to suggest that the single vaginal infusion of O_3 in dairy cows reduces the reproductive losses associated with urovagina when followed by a deep intracornual insemination. As cows treated with O_3 showed increased conception rates, this is likely due to its disinfecting effect coupled with an immunomodulative capacity of the ozone at the level of contact with vaginal and cervical mucosa [28]. Therefore, O_3 is likely to provide a more favourable environment for insemination and fertilization by reducing the spermicidal effect and urovagina-related inflammation. In summary, the results of the study conducted by [8] suggest that non-surgical treatment options are effective in managing clinical signs of urovagina in cows and allowing females to conceive and carry offspring to term. In addition, ozone therapy offers a practical and relatively inexpensive treatment option for urovagina by its one-time application, non-spermicidal action, and lack of negative effect on the host regarding residues.

When it comes to clinical endometritis (CE) in cows 30 - 40 days in milk, the best therapy results were achieved in animals treated with prostaglandin analogues parenteraly and ozone product (as a novel treatment option) applied into the uterus, as reported by [13]. Results are presented in Table 1. This treatment option resulted with the highest number of cow's concieved following the first post treatment artificial insemination and the lowest number of days open. Slightly less effective, although not significantly, was the treatment combining prostaglandin analogues and antimicrobials applied into the uterus. The lowest therapy success was achieved in the group of animals where only prostaglandins were given in 11 day periods. This study results are similar to those of [29] who reported that treatment with prostaglandin analogues has no effect on the incidence of CE. The poor therapy result in the group of animals treated with prostaglandins only could be the consequence of the ovarian status with the small number of cows having corpus luteum on the ovaries, thus ineffective prostaglandin treatment. Obviously, some kind of treatment of the endometrium should be used in the treatment of the CE, coupled with hormone administration. As cows treated with O_3 showed increase in the number of cow's concieved following the first AI and decreased number of days open, this is likely due to its disinfecting effect coupled with an immunomodulative capacity of the ozone at the level of contact with uterine mucosa as already described. Therefore, O_3 is likely to provide a more favourable uterine environment for insemination and fertilization by reducing the spermicidal effect and CE related inflammation. Ozone products, combined with prostaglandins, are slightly more effective than the cephapirin in the postpartal CE treatment with an advantage of no milk (and meat) withdrawing period [13]. In cows with RFM, O_3 was found again as a most effective treatment modality resulting in the lowest number of animals having clinical endometritis 30 - 40 days post calving, the lowest number of animals having fever inside 10 days after calving and the lowest number of days open, if compared to the other treatment options (prostaglandins applied parenteraly, antimicrobials applied parenteraly and into the uterus), again with an advantage of no milk and meat withdrawing period [21]. It can be speculated that the O_3, thanks to it's various mechanisms of action, increases local uterine immunity, acts anti-inflammatory and antimicrobial resulting with less number of animals developing fever (within 10 days after calving) and clinical endometritis (30 to 40 days after calving), thus improve puerperal health and fertility in RFM cows.\

Table 1. The summary results of ozone treatment compared to the other treatment modalities of urovagina, endometritis and Retention of foetal membranes in cattle

RFM						
Group	A (n=40)	B (n=40)	C (n=40)	D(n=40)	E (n=40)	F (n=200)
DO	82.8^a	83^a	116.8^b	129^c	157.6^d	78.7^a
nAI	2.1±1.22^a	2.3±1.34^a	3.3±1.42^b	3.9±0.78^c	4.55±0.98^d	1.8±1.18^a
F	2 (5%)^a	3 (7.5%)^a	9 (22.5%)^b	14 (35%)^c	20 (50%)^d	3 (7.5%)^a
UROVAGINA						
Group	X (n=400)	XY (n=400)	Y (n=419)			
DO	95^a	85^b	79^c			
nAI	2.38±1.26^a	1.84±1.01^b	1.63±0.67^c			
CLINICAL ENDOMETRITIS						
Group	W (n=101)	Z (n=96)	WZ (n=103)			
CP	108^a	85^b	80^b			
DO	51^a	85^b	91^b			

Legend: RFM = Retention of fetal membranes; DO = days open expressed as average and range (±); nAI = average number of artificial inseminations until pregnancy; F = number of animals having fever (>40°C) within 10 days post calving expressed with the total number and percentage from the number of animals within the group; Group A = ozone intrauterine and antibiotics parenterally; Group B = ozone only; Group C = antibiotics into the uterus and parenterally; Group D = antibiotics into the uterus; Group E = prostaglandins parenterally in 11 days periods; Group Z = controls (cows gave birth without assistance and with no RFM diagnose); Urovagina = cows with urovagina condition; Group X = saline infused into the uterus and vagina; Group XY = antibiotic solution (streptomycin) infused into the uterus and vagina; Group Y = ozone produvt infused into the uterus and vagina; Clinical Endometritis = cows diagnosed with clinical endometritis; Group W = prostaglandins injected parenterally in 11 days intervals; Group Z = cephapirin administered into the uterine corpus simultaneously with the first two doses of prostaglandins; first two doses of prostaglandins were followed by the ozone product applied into the uterus
[a,b,c,d] Values in each row marked with different leter in superscript differ significantly (p < 0.05).

Finally, the ozone therapy offers a practical and relatively inexpensive treatment option for urovagina, clinical endometritis and retained placenta in cows due to its simple administration and lack of negative effect on the host regarding residues.

REFERENCES

[1]   Gilbert, R.O.; Wilson, D.G.; Levine, S.A. & Bosu, W.T. (1989). Surgical Management of Urovagina and Associated Infertility in a Cow. *J. Am. Vet. Med. Assoc., 194*, 931–9322.

[2]   Gautam, G. & Nakao, T. (2009). Prevalence of urovagina and its effects on reproductive performance in Holstein cows. *Theriogenology, 71*, 1451-1461.

[3]   St. Jean, G.; Hull, B.L.; Robertson, J.T.; Hoffsis, G.F. & Haibel, G.K. (1988) Urethral Extension for Correction of Urovagina in Cattle: A Review of 14 Cases. Vet. Surg. 17 258–62.

[4]   Fubini, S.L. & Ducharme, N.G. (2004). *Farm Animal Surgery*. 1st Edition. New York: Saunders, Elsevier.

[5]   Hudson, R.S. (1986). Current Therapy in Theriogenology: Genital Surgery of the Cow. (Morrow, DA. vol. 2.). New York, WB Saunders.

[6]   González -Martin, J.V.; Astiz, S.; Elvira, L. & López-Gatius, F. (2008). New Surgical Technique to Correct Urovagina Improves the Fertility of Dairy Cows. *Theriogenology, 69*, 360-365.

[7]   Prado, T.M.; Schumacher, J.; Hayden, S.S.; Donnell, R.R. & Rohrbach, B.W. (2007) Evaluation of a Modified Surgical Technique to Correct Urine Pooling in Cows. *Theriogenology 67*, 1512–1517.

[8]   Zobel, R.; Tkalčić, S.; Štoković, I.; Pipal, I. & Buić, V. Efficacy of Ozone as a Novel Treatment Option for Urovagina in Dairy Cows. Available from: URL: http://onlinelibrary.wiley.com/doi/10.1111/ j.1439-0531.2011.01857.x/abstract

[9]   Parkinson, T.J.: Infertility. In: Noakes, D.E., Parkinson, T.J., England, G.C.W., Eds. Arthur's Veterinary Reproduction and Obstetrics. 8th edn., Saunders Company, USA. 2001; 463-464.

[10] LeBlanc, S.J.; Duffield, T.F.; Leslie, K.E.; Bateman, K.G.; Keefe, G.P.; Walton, J.S. & Johnson,W.H. (2000). Defining and diagnosing postpartum clinical endometritis and its impact on reproductive performance in dairy cows. *J. Dairy Sci., 285*, 2223-2236.

[11] LeBlanc, S.J.; Duffield, T.F.; Leslie, K.E.; Bateman, K.G.; Keefe, G.P.; Walton, J.S. & Johnson, W.H. (2002). The effect of treatment of clinical endometritis on reproductive performance in dairy cows. *J. Diary Sci., 85*, 2237-2249.

[12] Kasimanickam, R.; Duffield, T.F.; Foster, R.A.; Gartley, C.J.; Leslie, K.E.; Walton, J.S. & Johnson, W.H. (2005). The effect of a single administration of cephapirin or cloprostenol on the reproductive performance of dairy cows with subclinical endometritis. *Theriogenology, 63*, 818-830.

[13] Zobel, R. (2012). Endometritis in Simmental Dairy Cows: Incidence, Causes and Therapy Options. T. *J. Vet. Anim. Sci.* 2012 (accepted)

[14] Van Werven, T.; Schukken, Y.H.; Lloyd, J., Brand, A.; Heeringa, H.T. & Shea, M. (1992). The effects of duration of retained placenta on reproduction, milk production, postpartum disease and culling rate. *Theriogenology 37*, 1191–1203.

[15] Drillich, M.; Pfutzer, A.; Sabin, H.J.; Sabin, M. & Heuwieser, W. (2003). Comparison of two protocols for treatment of retained fetal membranes in dairy cattle. *Theriogenology, 59*, 951–960.

[16] Roberts, S.J. 1986: Veterinary Obstetrics and Genital Diseases. *Woodstock, VT: SJ Roberts*, pp. 373–393.

[17] Lee, L.A.; Ferguson, J.D. & Galligan, D.T. (1989). Effect of disease on days open assessed by survival analysis. *J. Dairy Sci. 22*, 1020–1026.

[18] Drillich, M.; Klever, N. & Heuwieser, W. (2007). Comparison of two management strategies for retained fetal membranes on small dairy farms in Germany. *J. Dairy Sci., 90*, 4275–4281.

[19] Peters, A.R. & Laven, R.A. (1996). Treatment of bovine retained placenta and its effects. *Vet. Rec. 139*, 539–541.

[20] LeBlanc, S.J. (2008). Postpartum uterine disease and dairy herd reproductive performance: A review. *Vet. J. 176*, 102–114.

[21] Zobel, R. & Tkalčić, S. (2012). Efficacy of Ozone and Other Treatment Modalities for Retained Placenta in Dairy Cows. Rep. Dom. Anim. (accepted)

[22] Mehlman, M.A. & Borek, C. (1987). Toxicity and biochemical mechanisms of ozone. *Environ. Res. 42*, 36-53.

[23] Silva, R.A.; Garotti, J.E.G.; Silva, R.S.; Navarini, A. & Pacheco, Jr. A. (2009). Analysis of the bactericidal effect of ozone pneumoperitoneum. *Acta Cir. Bras. 24*, 124-127.

[24] Ogata, A. & Nagahata, H. (2000). Intramammary aplication of ozone therapy to acute clinical mastitis in dairy cows. *J. Vet. Med. Sci. 62*, 681-686.

[25] Bialoszewski, D.; Bocian, E.; Bukowska, B.; Czajkowska, M.; Sokół-Leszczyńska, B. & Tyski, S. (2010). Antimicrobial activity of ozonated water. *Med. Sci. Monit., 16*, 71-75.

[26] Terasaki, N.; Ogata, A.; Ohtsuka, H.; Tamura, K.; Hoshi, F.; Koiwa, M. & Kawamura, S. (2001) Changes of immunological response after experimentally ozonated autohemoadministration in calves. *J. Vet. Med. Sci. 63*, 1327-1330.

[27] Guennadi, O.G.; Katchalina, O.V.; El-Hassoun, H. (2008). *The New Method of Treatment of Inflammatory Diseases of Lower Female Genital Organs.* Congreso Mundial Ozono Londres.

[28] Jakab, G.J.; Spannhake, E.W.; Canning, B.J.; Kleeberger, S.R. & Gilmour, M.I. (1995). The effects of ozone on immune function. *Environ. Health Perspect., 103*, 77–89.

[29] Hendricks, K.E.M.; Bartolome, J.A.; Melendez, P.; Risco, C. & Archbald, L.F. (2006). Effect of repeated administration of PGF2a in the early post partum period on the prevalence of clinical endometritis and probability of pregnancy at first insemination in lactating dairy cows. *Theriogenology, 65,* 1454-1464.

Reviewed by Mario Matković, Biol., PhD, Centre for Animal Reproduction of Croatia, Zagreb, Croatia; marmatko@vef.hr.

In: Cattle: Domestication, Diseases and the Environment
Editor: George Liu

ISBN: 978-1-62417-820-7
© 2013 Nova Science Publishers, Inc.

Chapter 7

THE USE OF CLINOPTILOLITE AS FEED ADDITIVE FOR THE PREVENTION AND TREATMENT OF CERTAIN DISEASES IN CATTLE

P. D. Katsoulos, M. A. Karatzia and H. Karatzias

Clinic of Farm Animals, Faculty of Veterinary Medicine, Aristotle University of
Thessaloniki, Thessaloniki, Greece

ABSTRACT

Clinoptilolite is a natural clay mineral that is part of the zeolite group. Zeolites are crystalline, hydrated aluminosilicates of alkali and alkaline earth cations that have infinite structures which are three-dimensional. These materials have unique properties and are characterized by their ability to lose and gain water reversibly, to absorb molecules of appropriate diameter (adsorption property or acting as molecule sieves) and to exchange their constituent cations without major change of their structure (ion-exchange property). Because of these properties, zeolites are used as feed additives, mainly in order to improve performance traits. In the last decade a there has been much interest in the investigation of whether the unique properties of clinoptilolite can be used for the prevention of certain diseases in dairy cattle. A series of experiments has been conducted in this direction. The results indicated that the dietary administration of clinoptilolite at a rate of 2.5% in the concentrate mixture during the last month of the dry period is effective in preventing milk fever and ketosis after calving. It was further proved that the daily addition of 200gr clinoptilolite in the ration enhances the immune response of cattle vaccinated against E. coli and prevents the reduction of ruminal pH in cattle that are fed high concentrate diets. As far as calves are concerned, the results of many experiments concluded that the addition of clinoptilolite in the colostrum of newborn animals increases the intestinal absorption of immunoglobulins and reduces the incidence and the duration of diarrhea syndrome. The objective of this chapter is to review the experimental results that concern the efficacy of clinoptilolite on the prevention of the aforementioned diseases in dairy cattle and calves and to suggest possible focus topics for further research.

Keywords: Clinoptilolite, cattle health, prevention, treatment

INTRODUCTION

Clinoptilolite is a crystalline, hydrated alluminosilicate which is encountered worldwide. It belongs to natural zeolites, a group of minerals that have unique physico-chemical properties. The most important of their properties are their ability to selectively exchange cations of their structure with cations from their environment (cation exchange capacity-CEC) and to adsorb substances with appropriate cross-sectional diameter (adsorption property) (Mumpton and Fishman 1977). Based on these properties and taking into account the first experimental results, zeolites and especially clinoptilolite, have been used as feed additives in order to ameliorate mycotoxicosis and to improve animals' performance (Mumpton 1999, Papaioannou et al. 2005). Recently, clinoptilolite has been approved as feed additive by the European Committee at the highest inclusion rate of 2% of dry matter. The effectiveness of clinoptilolite on mycotoxins' binding, as well as the increased interest for the production of organic animal products that favors the use of feed additives that do not have residuals on the animal products that may reach the final consumers, are expected to increase the use of clinoptilolite as feed additive.

Many researchers have proved that the dietary inclusion of clinoptilolite improves average daily gain and/or feed conversion in calves (Mumpton and Fishman 1977, Nestorov 1984), and increase the milk yield of dairy cows (Garcia-Lopez et al. 1992, Katsoulos et al. 2006). However, the extent of performance enhancement effects is related to the purity of the clinoptilolitic material that is used, its particle size and to the supplementation level selected in the diets.

Apart from the positive effects on animals' performance, dietary supplementation of clinoptilolite appears to represent an efficacious, complementary, as well as supportive strategy in the prevention of certain diseases and the improvement of animals' health status. During the last decade, the research was focused on the safety of using clinoptilolite as feed additive in cattle and on the potential beneficial effects of clinoptilolite feeding on the health status of these animals. The results of these researches have proved that the administration of clinoptilolite is not only safe in cattle but is also beneficial for the prevention of certain diseases in dairy cattle, such as milk fever, ketosis, ruminal acidosis and diarrhea syndrome in calves. Moreover, it was shown that clinoptilolite enhances antibody production in cattle that have been vaccinated against E. coli. The aim of the present chapter is to address the data concerning the influence of the in-feed inclusion of natural zeolite clinoptilolite on certain diseases of cattle, to summarize the proposed mechanisms of clinoptilolite's effects and to suggest possible focus topics for further research in selected areas.

STABILITY OF CLINOPTILOLITE IN THE GASTROINTESTINAL LUMEN

The main issue that arises from the use of clinoptilolite as feed additive in ruminants is whether it remains stable or is hydrolyzed through its passage from the rumino-intestinal tract. If a considerable amount of clinoptilolite is hydrolyzed, the released aluminium (Al) may interfere with the utilization of several minerals, with phosphorus absorption and metabolism being the most affected. The stability of zeolites on the acidic pH is directly related with their silicon to aluminium ratio (Si:Al), as they are more stable when this ratio is higher. Synthetic zeolites such as zeolite A that have an Si:Al equal to 1:1 (Holmes 1994) are hydrolyzed in cows' gastrointestinal tract (Grabherr et al. 2009) and significantly decrease the blood serum levels of inorganic phosphorus (Thilsing-Hansen et al. 2002, Thilsing-Hansen et al. 2003, Grabherr et al. 2009). Clinoptilolite has an Si:Al ratio equal to 5 and its stability in the gastrointestinal lumen of cattle was evaluated by Karatzia et al. (2011) using dairy cows with permanent external fistulas of the rumen. Then, it was observed that the administration of 200g clinoptilolite per day for a 12 week period had no significant effect, neither on the average ruminal and blood serum concentration of Al nor on the blood serum levels of phosphorus, thus proving that clinoptilolite remains practically stable in the gastrointestinal lumen of dairy cows.

PREVENTION OF AMMONIA TOXICITY

White and Ohlrogge (1975) were the first to state that ammonium ions formed by the enzyme decomposition of non-protein nitrogen were immediately ion exchanged into the zeolite structure and held there for several hours until they are released by the regenerative action of Na+, entering the rumen in saliva during the after-feeding fermentation period. From both in vitro and in vivo experiments they found that up to 15% of the NH_4^+ in the rumen could be taken up by the zeolite. These observations were the causation for the conduction of a great number of experiments with the aim of determining the influence of zeolites on rumen NH_4^+ concentration and their potential use for the counteraction of the toxic effects of urea inclusion in ruminants' rations.

At the early experiments high inclusion rates of clinoptilolite were used. Hemken et al. (1984) first showed that a supplementation of 6% clinoptilolite, in the ration of dairy cows containing 2% urea, significantly reduced rumen NH_3 concentration. The same trend was observed in steers by the dietary addition of 5% clinoptilolite (Sweeney et al. 1984). In a more recent study, Sadeghi and Shawrang (2006), while using lower levels of clinoptilolite, proved that the addition of 3% clinoptilolite in the diet of steers which is containing 2% urea significantly decreased the ruminal ammonia nitrogen concentration and the plasma urea nitrogen levels in comparison to the controls. They further noticed that the highest plasma urea nitrogen levels in the clinoptilolite group were recorded 6h post feeding and not at 3h post feeding as in the control group, confirming the statement of White and Ohlrogge (1975) that clinoptilolite releases NH_4^+ in the rumen gradually.

The effectiveness of clinoptilolite in reducing rumen ammonia concentration has also been proven even in cases when no urea was present in the ration. McCollum and Gallyean (1983) observed that the addition of 2.5% clinoptilolite in the ration of steers receiving a high concentrate diet not only reduced rumen ammonia but also that this reduction was associated in a linear way to the percentage of clinoptilolite inclusion. In contrast to the former observations, Bergero et al. (1997) and Bosi et al. (2002) found that daily administration of 250 g or 200 g of clinoptilolite in dairy cows, respectively, did not affect rumen NH_4^+ concentration. However, it has to be emphasized that the clinoptilolite content of the zeolitic materials used in both experiments was low.

PREVENTION OF MILK FEVER

In practice, most dairy cows experience some degree of subclinical hypocalcaemia during the periparturient period. There are some cases where serum calcium concentrations become too low to support nerve and muscle function, resulting in a clinical disease commonly known as milk fever (Goff and Horst 1997). Results of numerous studies support the idea that a reduction of dietary calcium during the dry period, will improve cows' resistance to milk fever (Wiggers et al. 1975, Yarrington et al. 1977, Green et al. 1981, Kichura et al. 1982). However, the formulation of rations with very low calcium is very difficult when using ordinary feedstuffs (Goff et al. 1987). Hence, research efforts were focused on the reduction of dietary calcium availability in the gastrointestinal tract using materials that have the ability to act as calcium binders. Initially, a series of experiments has been conducted so that the potential use of synthetic zeolite A for the prevention of milk fever in dairy cows could be studied. The objective of these experiments was to reduce the bioavailability of dietary Ca in the gastrointestinal tract by the administration of synthetic zeolite A. The results obtained were satisfactory as the administration of synthetic zeolite A, either as an oral drench or supplemented to the total mixed ration, during the dry period reduced the bioavailability of dietary Ca and efficiently protected the cattle against milk fever, by stimulating Ca-homeostatic mechanisms prior to parturition (Jorgensen et al. 2001, Thilsing-Hansen et al. 2001, Thilsing-Hansen et al. 2002, Jorgensen et al. 2003, Thilsing-Hansen et al. 2003, Enemark et al. 2003).

Taking under consideration that clinoptilolite has similar ion-exchange properties with zeolite A, Katsoulos et al. (2005a) evaluated the effectiveness of using clinoptilolite for the same purpose. They used 52 clinically healthy dairy cows that were assigned into 3 groups. The first group was consisting of 17 cows that were offered a concentrate diet supplemented with clinoptilolite at the rate of 1.25%, the second group was consisted of 17 cows that were fed concentrates supplemented with 2.5% clinoptilolite and the control group was consisted of 18 cows that were fed a concentrate diet without any clinoptilolite supplementation. The experiment started one month before the expected parturition and lasted until the onset of the new dry period. The results proved that clinoptilolite feeding during the transition period can be used as a preventive measure against periparturient paresis. They also observed that the incidence of milk fever was significantly lower in cows that were receiving a concentrate feed supplemented with clinoptilolite at the level of 2.5% (5.9%) during the last month of the dry period and on the onset of lactation, compared to the animals in the control group (38.9%), whereas the incidence was not significantly different than in those animals that were receiving 1.25% clinoptilolite (17.6%) at the same period. The authors suggested that clinoptilolite might have had a similar effect with the one zeolite A has, in activating Ca homeostatic mechanisms prior to parturition. As a consequence, the animals receiving 2.5% clinoptilolite responded faster and more efficiently in the drop of serum Ca levels observed at the day of calving and did not show any clinical signs of milk fever in the following days. However, the exact mechanism for this positive effect of clinoptilolite supplementation is currently unknown and should be further investigated.

PREVENTION OF KETOSIS

The critical period for the development of ketosis is the first month of lactation due to the elevated amount of energy that is required for the increased milk production and maintenance of body tissues, which exceeds significantly the amount of energy the cow, can obtain via dietary sources. According to Goff and Horst (1997), the concentration of AcAc and β-HBA increase during early lactation and may reach levels that are indicative of clinical ketosis, mainly in the period from 10 days to 3 weeks after calving. The best strategy to prevent ketosis in dairy cows is to improve the energy uptake both in the dry period, as well as on the onset of lactation (Goff and Horst 1997). Katsoulos et al. (2006) proved that the use of clinoptilolite during the transition period was effective in improving the energy balance at this critical period. They observed that feeding dairy cows on a diet supplemented with clinoptilolite at the level of 2.5% of the concentrate feed, resulted in significantly lower incidence of ketosis (5.9%) during the first month after parturition, compared to the control group (38.9%) and the group of the animals receiving a concentrate supplemented with 1.25% clinoptilolite (35.3%). These researchers suggested two mechanisms by which clinoptilolite had improved the energy status of the cows at this critical period that may act alone or in combination.

The first was that clinoptilolite may have increased the production of propionate in the rumen. It was based on the proved antiketogenic action of propionate (Grummer 1993) and on the observations that clinoptilolite increases the molar proportion of propionate in the rumen when added in the ration of steers (Mc Collum and Galyean 1983). The second explanation was that clinoptilolite may have improved the post ruminal digestion of starch. At an earlier point, Garcia-Lopez et al. (1992), had supported that zeolite alters post ruminal pH levels, which becomes more receptive to the action of alpha amylase pancreatic enzyme in the digestion of compounds containing starch. In accordance to this point of view, increased fecal pH levels -which indicate more complete digestion of dietary starch (Hemken and others 1984)- and decreased fecal grain loses had been observed when clinoptilolite was incorporated in the ration of dairy cattle (Hemken et al. 1984, Pond and Lee 1984, Garcia-Lopez et al. 1992) and steers (Galyean and Chabot 1981).

PREVENTION OF RUMINAL ACIDOSIS

Clinoptilolite acts as a regulatory factor when it is added to acidic or basic aqueous solutions (Filippidis et al. 1996). On the basis of this property, the effect of clinoptilolite feeding on rumen pH of dairy cattle was tested in order for it to be used as a buffer for the prevention of ruminal acidosis. At the first experiments that zeolitic materials with a low content of clinoptilolite were used, it was observed that the administration of 250g (Bergero et al. 1997) and 200g (Bosi et al. 2002) clinoptilolite per cow per day had no significant effect on ruminal pH values.

However, the most recent studies suggest clinoptilolite exhibits buffering effects. In the study conducted by Karatzia et al. (2011) it was proved that the administration of 200g clinoptilolite in dairy cows on a daily basis, resulted in significantly higher pH values in all test days in comparison to the controls throughout the experimental period of 12 weeks.

Similar results were obtained by Dschaak et al. (2010). They observed that dairy cows receiving clinoptilolite at the rate of 1.4% dry matter had higher ruminal pH values than the control animals. They further observed that the pH values of the cows fed clinoptilolite were comparable to those obtained from cows consuming equal amounts of sodium bicarbonate. Taking into account the above, they concluded that clinoptilolite can cost-effectively replace sodium bicarbonate as a ruminal buffer.

PREVENTION OF NEONATAL DIARRHEA

Neonatal diarrhea in calves is a syndrome that occurs frequently in many countries worldwide and is considered as an important cause of financial losses (Barragry, 1997). Enterotoxigenic strains of Escherichia coli (ETEC) consistute one of the main causative agents of diarrhea in calves during the first days of their life. The prevention of this syndrome in commercial dairy farms relies on adequate levels of passive immunity, acquired by the absorbion of immunoglobulins from the colostrum. Research results have shown that the use of clinoptilolite as a feed additive can effectively prevent ETEC diarrhea acting in two ways; by enhancing the antibody production of dairy cattle vaccinated against E. coli while, at the same time, increasing the intestinal immunoglobulins' absorption in newborn calves.

Karatzia (2010) first evaluated the effect of clinoptilolite feeding on the immune response demonstrated by dairy cows vaccinated against certain pathogens, using first-calf heifers. The results of this study showed that the dietary administration of clinoptilolite at the rate of 200g per day in heifers vaccinated against *E. coli*, is associated with a significant increase in antibody titres against *E. coli* in blood serum and in colostrum likewise, compared to their vaccinated controls. This increase was proved to be even higher when clinoptilolite was combined with the intramuscular administration of selenium at the day of vaccination. The enhancement of the antibody production against *E. coli* by dairy cows after vaccination was attributed to the improved energy status of the animals that received clinoptilolite as a supplement.

There is an abundance of published data which indicate that the dietary use of clinoptilolite enhances the intestinal absorption of the colostral immunogloboulins. Fratric et al. (2005 and 2007) observed that the administration of clinoptilolite at the rate of 5g/kg of body weight along with the colostrum significantly increases the degree of absorption of colostral IgG, as well as the blood serum concentrations of IgG in dairy calves. Similar results were obtained from Gvozdic et al. (2008) using a liquid suspension of clinoptilolite. They also observed that the addition of 25ml of a clinoptilolite suspension (20% in distilled water) in the colostrum significantly increased the apparent intestinal absorption of colostral IgG and the blood serum concentration of IgG in newborn calves. In a more recent study, Pourliotis et al. (2012) reached the same results using lower levels of clinoptilolite. They proved that the administration of clinoptilolite with the colostrum initially, and milk afterwards, at the rate of 1 g/kg of body weight and 2 g/kg of body weight per day during the first 10 days of their life is associated with significantly higher antibody titres against *E. coli* in blood serum of calves compared to the control animals after the first colostrum feeding. These researchers suggested that clinoptilolite could have increased the intestinal absorption of immunogloboulins through the following mechanisms. Either by increasing the pinocytotic activity of intestinal epithelial cells or by retarding the intestinal passage rate and increasing in that way the time that the immunoglobulins are available to the specific receptors of the epithelial cells, or by binding some degradation products of the colostral proteins in the intestine that have negative effect on the intestinal epithelial cells, such as ammonia.

At the same study it was further proved by Pourliotis et al. (2012) that the incidence of ETEC diarrhea was significantly lower in calves that were receiving clinoptilolite compared to the controls. This indicates that these calves, due to the higher blood serum antibody titres against ETEC, could respond faster and more efficiently to the infection with ETEC. The shorter duration of the illness in these animals was further attributed to the alteration of metabolic acidosis caused by clinoptilolite, through its effects on osmotic pressure in the intestinal lumen and to the absorption by clinoptilolite of bile acids, one of the endogenic causes of diarrhea and of glucose whose high content in intestinal fluid acts as an irritant factor while its transport through the intestinal cells is reversed during diarrhea.

BLOOD SERUM VITAMINS, MACRO- AND TRACE ELEMENTS

One of the major concerns that arise from the use of absorbents such as clinoptilolite as feed additives is whether they interact or not with nutrients like vitamins or macro- and trace elements and reduce their bioavailability. If large quantities of these nutrients are rendered unavailable to the animals via feed in the long-term, the consequent nutritional imbalances might have an undesirable effect on both animal performance and preservation of its health status.

In long-term experiments it has been proved that the administration of clinoptilolite at the rates of 1.25% or 2.5% for a whole productive period (starting one month before the expected calving date until the onset of the new dry period) in dairy cattle had not adverse effects on the blood serum concentrations of fat-soluble vitamins (β-carotene and vitamins A and E; Katsoulos et al. 2005b), of macroelements (calcium, phosphorus, magnesium, sodium and potassium; Katsoulos et al. 2005a) and of trace elements (iron, copper, zinc; Katsoulos et al. 2005c). It was further proved that clinoptilolite feeding does not negatively affect the liver function of dairy cows and has no influence on the blood serum concentrations of glucose, blood urea nitrogen and total proteins (Katsoulos et al. 2006). In a long-term study in calves, Pourliotis (2009) observed that the addition of clinoptilolite in the colostrum initially and milk afterwards, at the rate of 1g/kg or 2g/kg of body weight during the first two months of their life had no significant effect on the blood serum concentrations of the macro- (calcium, phosphorus, magnesium, sodium and potassium) and trace elements (iron, copper, zinc) tested. This researcher further proved that the administration of clinoptilolite not only has no adverse effects, on the contrary it significantly increases the blood serum concentrations of vitamin A.

PERFORMANCE

Concerning the effect of clinoptilolite feeding on the performance of dairy cattle, recent research results have shown that it has beneficial effects on the milk production and the reproductive traits. Two experiments have been conducted in order to assess the effects of clinoptilolite on milk production. At the first one (Katsoulos et al. 2006), adult cows were receiving clinoptilolite at the level of 2.5% of the concentrate feed from the last month of the dry period until the end of the lactation period. According to the results of this experiment the cows that were receiving clinoptilolite had significantly higher mean daily milk yield during the first six months of the lactation period and significantly higher 305-days total milk yield compared to the controls. Similar results were obtained at the second experiment (Karatzia unpublished data) where first calf heifers were receiving 200g clinoptilolite per day starting feeding two months before the expected parturition and until the end of lactation. The increased milk production in both experiments was attributed to the improved energy status of the animals that were receiving clinoptilolite. This is further confirmed by the fact that the cows fed clinoptilolite at the second experiment had significantly higher body condition scores throughout the lactation period in comparison to the controls.

These heifers that were receiving clinoptilolite in the latter experiment had significantly improved reproductive traits compared to the controls. They had lower calving to first heat, calving to first service, calving to new conception, and calving intervals and required a significantly lower number of services per conception. The improvement of the reproductive parameters was also attributed to the enhanced energy status of the animals receiving clinoptilolite with their diets.

CONCLUSION

All these studies proved that the use of clinoptilolite as a feed additive in cattle can have a significant contribution on the prevention and the treatment of certain diseases. Taking into account its low market price in combination to the beneficial effects on the animals' performance without having residuals on the animal products, clinoptilolite is considered without a doubt as one of the safest materials that can be used for the improvement of cattles' health.

REFERENCES

Barragry, T. (1997). Calf diarrhoea. *Irish Vet. J. 50,* 49–58.

Bergero, D., Rumello, G., Sara, C. & D' Angelo, A. (1997). Effect of natural clinoptilolite or phillipsite in the feeding of lactating dairy cows. In: Kirov, G., Filizova, L. & Petrov O. (Eds.), *Natural zeolites – Sofia '95* (pp 67-72). Sofia-Moscow, Pensoft Publishers.

Bosi, P., Creston, D. & Casini, L. (2002). Production performance of dairy cows after the dietary addition of clinoptilolite. *Italian J. Anim. Sci., 1,* 187-195.

Dschaak, C.M., Eun, J.-S., Young, A.J., Stott, R.D. & Peterson S. (2010). Effects of supplementation of natural zeolite on intake, digestion, ruminal fermentation, and lactational performance of dairy cows. *Prof. Anim. Sci., 26,* 647-654.

Enemark, J.M., Frandsen ,A.M., Thilsing-Hansen, T. & Jorgensen R.J. (2003). Aspects of physiological effects of sodium zeolite A supplementation in dry non-pregnant dairy cows fed grass silage. *Acta Vet. Scand. Suppl., 97,* 97-117.

Filippidis, A., Godelitsas, A., Charistos, D., Misaelides, P. & Kassoli-Fournaraki, A. (1996). The chemical behaviour of natural zeolites in aquaeous environments: interactions between low-silica zeolites and 1M NaCl solutions of different initial pH-values. *Appl. Clay Sci., 11*, 199-209.

Fratric, N., Stojic, V., Jankovic, D., Samanc, H. & Gvozdic, D. (2005). The effect of a clinoptilolite based mineral adsorber on concentrations of immunoglobulin G in the serum of newborn calves fed different amounts of colostrum. *Acta Vet- Beograd, 55,* 11-21.

Fratric, N., Stojic, V., Rajcic, V. & Radojicic, B. (2007). The effect of mineral adsorbent in calf diet colostrum on the levels of serum immunoglobulin g, protein and glucose. *Acta Vet-Beograd, 57,* 169-180.

Galyean, M.L. & Chabot, R.C. (1981). Effect of sodium bentonite, buffer salts, cement kiln dust and clinoptilolite on rumen characteristics of beef steers fed a high roughage diet. *J. Anim. Sci., 52,* 1197-1204.

Garcia-Lopez, R., Elias, A. & Menchaca, M.A. (1992). The utilization of zeolite by dairy cows. 2. Effect on milk yield. *Cuban J. Agric. Sci., 26,* 131-133.

Goff, J.P. & Horst, R.L. (1997). Physiological changes at parturition and their relationship to metabolic disorders. *J. Dairy Sci., 80,* 1260-1268.

Goff, J.P., Horst, R.L. & Reinhardt, T.A. (1987). The pathophysiology and prevention of milk fever. *Vet. Med., 9,* 945-950.

Grabherr, H., Spolders, M., Lebzien, P., Huther, L., Flachowsky, G., Furll, M. & Grun, M. (2009). Effect of zeolite A on rumen fermentation and phosphorus metabolism in dairy cows. *Arch. Anim. Nutr., 63,* 321-336

Green, H.B., Horst, R.L., Beitz, D.C. & Littledike, E.T. (1981). Vitamin D metabolites in plasma of cows fed low-calcium diet for prevention of parturient hypocalcemia. *J. Dairy Sci., 64,* 217-226.

Grummer, R.R. (1993). Etiology of lipid-related metabolic disorders in periparturient dairy cows. *J. Dairy Sci., 76,* 3882-3896

Gvozdic, D., Stojic, V., Samanc, H., Fratric, N. & Dacovic, A. (2008). Apparent efficiency of immunoglobulin absorption in newborn calves orally treated with zeolite. *Acta Vet-Beograd, 58,* 345-355.

Hemken, R.W., Harmon, R.J. & Mann, L.M. (1984). Effect of clinoptilolite on lactating dairy cows fed a diet containing urea as a source of protein. In Pond, W.G. & Mumpton, F.A. (Eds.), *Zeo-Agriculture: Use of natural zeolites in agriculture and aquaculture* (pp. 175-181). Boulder, CO: Westview Press Inc.

Holmes, D.A. (1994). Zeolites. In Carr D.D. (Ed.), *Industrial Minerals and Rocks* (pp. 1129-1158). Littleton, CO: Society for Mining, Metallurgy and Exploration, Inc..

Jorgensen, R.J., Bjerrum, M.J., Classen, H. & Thilsing-Hansen, T. (2003). A short introduction to the new principle of binding ration calcium with sodium zeolite. *Acta Vet. Scand. Suppl., 97,* 83-86.

Jorgensen, R.J., Hansen, T., Jersen, M.L. & Thilsing-Hansen, T. (2001). Effect of oral drenching with zinc oxide or synthetic zeolite A on total blood calcium in dairy cows. *J. Dairy Sci., 84,* 609-613.

Karatzia, M.A., 2010. Effect of dietary inclusion of clinoptilolite on antibody production by dairy cows vaccinated against Escherichia coli. *Livestock Sci., 128,* 149-153.

Karatzia, M.A., Pourliotis, K., Katsoulos, P.D. & Karatzias H. (2011). Effects of in-feed inclusion of clinoptilolite on blood serum concentrations of aluminium and inorganic phosphorus and on ruminal pH and volatile fatty acid concentrations in dairy cows. *Biol. Trace Elem. Res., 142,* 159-66.

Katsoulos, P.D., Panousis, N., Roubies, N., Christaki, E. & Karatzias, H. (2005b). Effects on blood concentrations of certain serum fat-soluble vitamins of long-term feeding of dairy cows on a diet supplemented with clinoptilolite. *J. Vet. Med. A, 52,* 157–161.

Katsoulos, P.D., Panousis, N., Roubies, N., Christaki, E., Arsenos, G. & Karatzias, H. (2006). Effects of long-term feeding of a diet supplemented with clinoptilolite to dairy cows on the incidence of ketosis, milk yield, and liver function. *Vet. Rec., 159,* 415–418.

Katsoulos, P.D., Roubies, N., Panousis, N. & Karatzias, H. (2005c). Effects of long-term feeding dairy cows on a diet supplemented with clinoptilolite on certain serum trace elements. *Biol. Trace Elem. Res., 108,* 137–145.

Katsoulos, P.D., Roubies, N., Panousis, N., Arsenos, G., Christaki, E. & Karatzias, H. (2005a). Effects of long-term dietary supplementation with clinoptilolite on incidence of parturient paresis and serum concentrations of total calcium, phosphate, magnesium, potassium, and sodium in dairy cows. *Am. J. Vet. Res., 66,* 2081–2085.

Kichura, T.S., Horst, R.L., Beitz, D.C. & Littledike E.T. (1982). Relationships between prepartal dietary calcium and phosphorus, vitamin D metabolism and parturient paresis in dairy cows. *J. Dairy Sci., 65,* 480-487.

McCollum, M.I. & Galyean, M.I. (1983). Effects of clinoptilolite on rumen fermentation, digestion and feedlot performance in beef steers fed high concentrate diets. *J. Anim. Sci., 56,* 517-524.

Mumpton, F.A. & Fishman, P.H. (1977). The application of natural zeolites in animal science and aquaculture. *J. Anim. Sci., 45,* 1188–1203.

Mumpton, F.A. (1999). La roca magica: Uses of natural zeolites in agriculture and industry. *Proc. Natl. Acad. Sci. USA, 96,* 3463-3470.

Nestorov, N. (1984). Possible applications of natural zeolites in animal husbandry. In Pond, W.G. & Mumpton, F.A. (Eds.), *Zeo-Agriculture: Use of natural zeolites in agriculture and aquaculture* (pp. 167-174). Boulder, CO: Westview Press Inc.

Papaioannou, D., Katsoulos, P.D., Panousis, N. & Karatzias, H. (2005). The role of natural and synthetic zeolites as feed additives on the prevention and/or the treatment of certain farm animal diseases: A review. *Microporous Mesoporous Mater., 84,* 161–170.

Pond, W.G. & Lee, J. (1984). Physiological effects of clinoptilolite and synthetic zeolite in animals. In Pond, W.G. & Mumpton, F.A. (Eds.), *Zeo-Agriculture: Use of natural zeolites in agriculture and aquaculture* (pp. 129-145). Boulder, CO: Westview Press Inc.

Pourliotis, K, Karatzia, M.A., Florou-Paneri, P., Katsoulos, P.D. & Karatzias, H. (2012). Effects of dietary inclusion of clinoptilolite in colostrum and milk of dairy calves on absorption of antibodies against Escherichia coli and the incidence of diarrhea. *Anim. Feed Sci. Technol., 172,* 136-140.

Pourliotis, K. (2009). The effect of zeolite inclusion in colostrum and milk on the absorption of antibodies against Escherichia coli, health status and performance of dairy calves fed exclusively colostrum and milk. *PhD Thesis,* Clinic of Farm Animals, Faculty of Veterinary Medicine, Aristotle University of Thessaloniki, Thessaloniki, Greece. Available in: http://phdtheses.ekt.gr/eadd/handle/10442/19234.

Sadeghi, AA. & Shawrang, P. (2006). The effect of natural zeolite on nutrient digestibility, carcass traits and performance of Holstein steers given a diet containing urea. *Anim. Sci., 82,* 163-167.

Sweeney, T.F., Cervantes, A., Bull ,L.S. & Hemken R.W. (1984). Effect of dietary clinoptilolite on digestion and rumen fermentation in steers. In Pond, W.G. & Mumpton, F.A. (Eds.), *Zeo-Agriculture: Use of natural zeolites in agriculture and aquaculture* (pp. 183-193). Boulder, CO: Westview Press Inc.

Thilsing-Hansen, T. & Jorgensen, R.J. (2001). Hot topic: Prevention of parturient paresis and subclinical hypocalcemia in dairy cows by zeolite A administration in dry period. *J. Dairy Sci. 84,* 691-693.

Thilsing-Hansen, T., Jorgensen, R.J., Enemark, J.M.D. & Larsen T. (2002). The effect of zeolite A supplementation in the dry period on periparturient calcium, phosphorus and magnesium homeostasis. *J. Dairy Sci., 85,* 1855-1862.

Thilsing-Hansen, T., Jorgensen, R.J., Enemark, J.M.D., Zelvyte, R. & Sederevicius A. (2003). The effect of zeolite A supplementation in the dry period on blood mineral status around calving. *Acta Vet. Scand., 97,* 87-93

White, J.L. & Ohlrogge, A.J. (1974). Ion exchange materials to increase consumption of non protein nitrogen in ruminants. *Canadian Patent 939186, Jan.2.*

Wiggers, K.D., Nelson, D.K. & Jakobsen, N.L. (1975). Prevention of parturient paresis by a low-calcium diet prepartum. *J. Dairy Sci., 58,* 430-431.

Yarrington, J.F., Cappen, C.C., Black, H.E., & Re R. (1977). Effects of a low calcium prepartum diet on calcium homeostatic mechanisms in the cow: morphological and biochemical studies. *J. Nutr. 107,* 2244-2256.

In: Cattle: Domestication, Diseases and the Environment   ISBN: 978-1-62417-820-7
Editor: George Liu   © 2013 Nova Science Publishers, Inc.

Chapter 8

OCCURRENCE, ETIOLOGY AND PREVENTION OF ABOMASAL DISPLACEMENT IN DAIRY CATTLE

H. Karatzias, M. A. Karatzia and P. D. Katsoulos
Clinic of Farm Animals, Faculty of Veterinary Medicine,
Aristotle University of Thessaloniki, Thessaloniki, Greece

ABSTRACT

Displaced abomasum (DA), either to the left (LDA) or to the right (RDA) side of the abdomen, is one of the most important diseases that are commonly observed in dairy cattle. It is encountered worldwide and represents the most common reason for abdominal surgery in dairy cattle, especially in cows of high-producing dairy breeds, such as Holstein. The incidence rate of DA in dairy herds varies between 1 and 15%, with LDA being more frequent than RDA. The peak of DA occurrence is during the first 4-6 weeks post partum and is commonly observed in first-calf heifers. DA is a multifactorial disease and its exact causes are still unclear. Nutritional factors, such as rations with high quantities of concentrates and reduced forage to concentrate ratio, seem to be of great importance. Metabolic diseases such as hypocalcaemia and ketosis, as well as other concomitant diseases or situations like retained placenta, metritis, mastitis or high body condition score, fatty liver and endotoxaemia can cause abomasal hypomobility, increased gas production within the abomasum and displacement. Another important factor for the development of DA is the increased stress due to calving and the beginning of lactation. Certain anatomical and physiological factors, such as location and loose wall structure promote gas collection, distention and finally, displacement of the abomasum. In the last thirty years (1981-2011) the etiological factors of DA were investigated in about 10, 000 cows. DA prevention is based on administering sufficient quantities of roughage in the ratio, avoiding abrupt ratio changes-particularly puerperium and on prevention or early treatment of postpartum diseases.

Keywords: Cattle, abomasal displacement, etiology, prevention, treatment

INTRODUCTION

Abomasal displacement occurs worldwide affecting mainly high producing dairy cattle. Nowadays the disease is detected with increased frequency, with left abomasal displacement in particular being so ordinary that is considered as the most common gastrointestinal disease of cattle. The prevalence of abomasal displacement in countries with developed dairy industry ranges between 1.7% and 2.3% of the total dairy population (Wolf et al. 2001), whereas the incidence rate in individual farms ranges between 0% and 20%. In Greece, according to the authors' data based on records of considerable amount of dairy farms of northern Greece for over 30 years, the annual incidence rate of abomasal displacement ranges between 3% and 20% (Karatzias and Panousis 2003). It is easy to comprehend that the disease causes significant financial losses due to the lower milk production and the treatment costs. This chapter reviews the current knowledge and the authors' experience on the etiopathogenesis, treatment and prevention options of the disease in dairy cattle based on the data of about 10, 000 cases of abomasal displacement.

ETIOLOGY – PATHOGENESIS

The results of recent investigations that are still in progress in many veterinary clinics mainly in Europe and North America, suggest that before right or left displacement of the abomasum, atony or hypotony, gas accumulation and distension of the organ occur (Dirksen 1961). Gas accumulation is considered as the dynamic factor that causes the displacement of the abomasum. The major question that arises is where the gases originate from. The possibility of origin from the fore stomachs is considered low. Most of the researchers suggest that the gases are produced within the abomasal lumen because of increased fermentation of the content that remains for a longer period in the lumen due to the atony of the abomasum and the low flow rate of the abomasal content to the duodenum. The increased gas production causes abomasal distension and worsens the atony. As a result, any factor that causes abomasal atony is considered a predisposing factor for left and right abomasal displacement with or without torsion.

I. Anatomical Factors

a. The loose construction of the abomasal wall, which is characterized by increased connective and low muscle tissue, allows the atony of the organ to occur easily (Dirksen 1962).
b. The presence of the abomasomasal orifice on the side of the abomasal body results in the development of an "empty space" between this position and the abomasal bottom where the first gases that cause the distension of the abomasum are accumulated (Dirksen 1962).
c. The junction of the abomasun with the omentum allows the abomasum to move in the abdominal cavity and is considered a significant factor for the displacement of the abomasums (Pinsent et al. 1961, Hull and Wass 1973, Ide and Henry 1984).

d. The accumulation of fat on the abomasal wall in overconditioned cattle that are on dry period for long time and consume high quantities of concentrates, facilitates the abomasal atony (Ide and Henry 1984).

e. According to our observations and those of other researchers, abomasal displacement occurs more frequently in large cows in comparison to smaller ones of the same farms. The deeper thorax, as defined by the vertical axis between the withers and the xiphoid process, allows more room in the abdomen for the abomasum to move, thus permiting its displacement to the left (Stober and Saratsis 1974).

II. Nutritional Factors

The higher incidence of abomasal displacement in the countries of North Europe and North America during winter time when the cows are housed and fed mainly with concentrates, suggests that feeding mistakes as the following, play important role on the pathogenesis of the disease.

a. The administration of rations rich in concentrates and poor in forages, especially in the post-partum period in order to meet the increased requirements for milk production, results in a rapid flow of poorly ingested feed from the fore stomachs to the abomasum, causing some degree of abomasitis and abomasal atony. Along with the poorly ingested feed, large amounts of volatile fatty acids are transferred in the abomasum. Volatile fatty acids affect the abomasal wall and cause atony. The atony retards the flow rate of the abomasal content to the duodenum resulting in abnormal fermentation of the abomasal content causing gas production, mainly methane (Grymer et al. 1981, Furll and Kruger 1999, Van Winden 2002).

b. Feeding cows only twice a day, a usual management practice in many farms, increases the flow rate of the fore stomachs to the abomasum causing abomasal atony and gas accumulation (Dirksen 1962).

c. The administration of over chopped corn silage with particle size less than 3cm, without the concurrent administration of forages increases the incidence rate of abomasal displacement (Karatzias and Panousis 2003).

III. Stress Factors

a. Parturition and the onset of lactation, especially in first-calf heifers, are recognized as stress factors that can possibly cause abomasal atony. It has been observed that abomasal displacement occurs at a rate of 90-95% during the first 3-4 weeks after calving. The hypotony of the gastrointestinal tract that occurs a few hours before calving and lasts for about 1-4 days after parturition is considered as the most important predisposing factor for the abomasal atony (Hultgren and Pehrson 1996, Furll and Kruger 1999).

b. Diseases such as primary ketosis, milk fever, periparturient hemoglobinuria, retained fetal membranes, septic metritis, acute mastitis, traumatic reticuloperitonitis, abomasal ulcers and lower limb diseases that affect cows during the transition period are considered as predisposing factors for the abomasal atony (Poike and Furll 2000, Wolf et al. 2001, Stengarde and Pehrson 2002, LeBlanc et al. 2005).

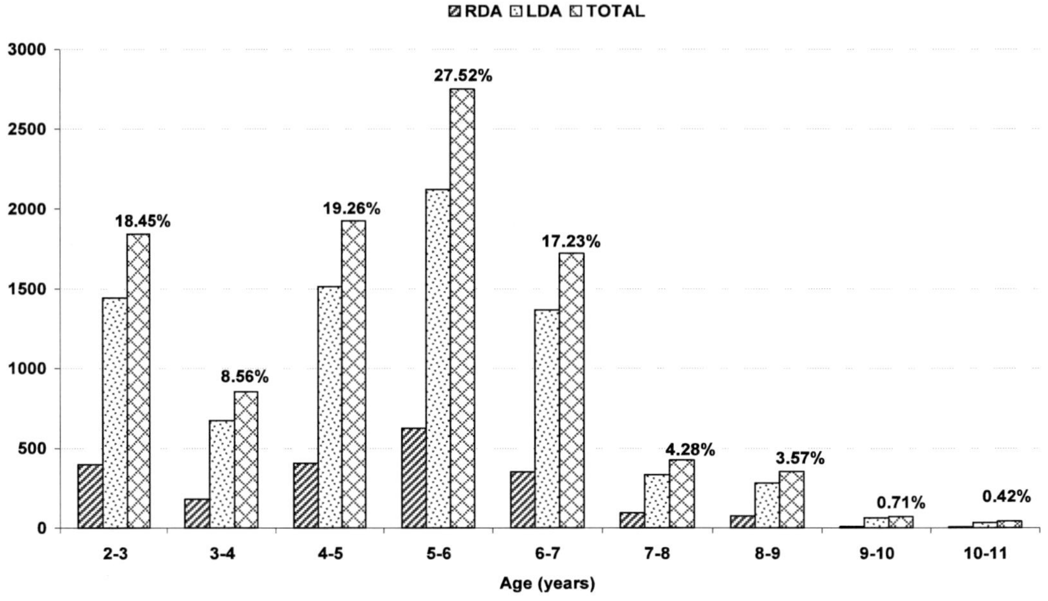

Figure 2. Age distribution of abomasal displacement cases in 9986 cattle evaluated. Right displaced abomasum (RDA) was recorded in 7834 cases and left displaced abomasum (LDA) in 2152 cases.

IV. Mechanical Factors

a. The distended uterus at late stages of gestation lifts the rumen from the bottom of the abdominal cavity and moves the abomasum anteriorly facilitating its passage below the rumen and the displacement of the abomasum on the left. The same conditions occur during calving and the empty space that is created in the abdominal cavity immediately after calving, especially in large sized dairy cattle, allows the displacement of the abomasum to the left or to the right (Moore et al. 1954, Nilsson 1962).

b. The transportation of cows for long distances, rolling of the cattle to correct uterine torsion and holding in lateral recubency for relatively long period of time are factors that if practiced just before or after calving can cause abomasal displacement.

Apart from the aforementioned factors, it is believed that pyloric stenosis (Hoflund syndrome) and the accumulation of foreign bodies (sand, soil, nylon bags) in the abomasum can also cause right abomasal displacement.

Based on the abundance of factors contributing to the disease, it can be concluded that the etiopathogenesis of abomasal displacement is not fully understood. The simultaneous action of more than one factor characterizes the abomasal displacement as a "multifactorial syndrome".

Table 1. Causative factors of abomasal displacement in 9986 cattle evaluated

Causative factor	Parity													
	1		2		3		4		5		6		7	
	n	%	n	%	n	%	n	%	n	%	n	%	n	%
Dystocia (n=1109)	1059	56.83	41	4.94	9	0.45	-	-	-	-	-	-	-	-
Retained placenta (n=1760)	326	17.49	153	18.52	543	28.12	483	1541	142	10.29	61	11.32	52	16.66
Milk fever (n=2919)	-	-	-	-	69	3.57	1308	41.78	967	69.85	367	67.92	208	66.66
Primary ketosis (n=1341)	10	0.55	41	4.94	353	18.3	794	25.34	92	6.62	51	9.43	-	-
Ration changes (n=288)	132	7.10	10	1.23	104	5.38	32	1.02	10	0.73	-	-	-	-
Vagal problems (n=114)	-	-	-	-	26	1.34	32	1.02	20	1.46	10	1.88	26	8.34
Transportation (n=90)	31	1.65	-	-	17	0.89	32	1.02	-	-	10	1.88	-	-
Other factors (n=2365)	305	16.38	580	70.37	809	41.95	451	14.41	153	11.05	41	7.57	26	8.34
Total (n=9986)	1863	100	825	100	1930	100	3132	100	1384	100	540	100	312	100

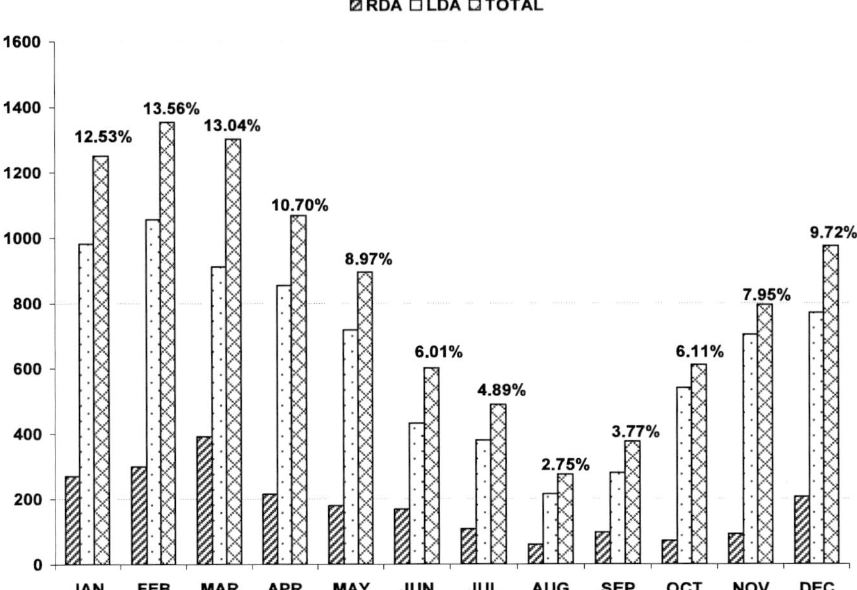

Figure 1. Monthly distribution of abomasal displacement cases throughout the year in 9986 cattle evaluated. Right displaced abomasum (RDA) was recorded in 7834 cases and left displaced abomasum (LDA) in 2152 cases.

In order to study the epidemiology of abomasal displacement in Greece, the data of 9986 dairy cattle with abomasal displacement from central and northern Greece during the last 30 years were evaluated. These data contained information about the age of the animals, parity, nutrition, housing conditions, month of the year and possible etiological factors for abomasal displacement. According to our results, 78.45% of these animals had left abomasal displacement and 21.55% had right abomasal displacement. The incidence of the disease was higher during February and March, a period during which the animals are kept indoors, consuming large amounts of concentrates (Figure 1). The highest incidence of abomasal displacement was recorded in cows at the 3rd and the 4th parity, i.e. at the age of 5-6 years old (Figure 2). Almost 60% of the animals were fed with corn silage and concentratres and the remaining 40% with wheat straw, alfalfa hay, industrial by-products and concentrates. As far as potential etiological factors are concerned, dystocia was recorded at the 56.8% of the first-calf cows, whereas in animals over the 3rd parity milk fever and primary ketosis were the most common causative factors (Table 1).

CLINICAL SIGNS

Dairy cattle with left or right abomasal displacement lose their appetite for concentrate high-energy feed and prefer forages. They also have significant drop of the milk production. The body temperature and the respiratory rate are normal. The pulse rate is also normal, except at the early stages of left abomasal displacement where bradycardia is usually observed, due to the stimulation of the vagal nerve. Rumen contractions are present and moderate in strength. The simultaneous auscultation and percussion reveals the presence of a high-pitched tympanic resonance sound ("ping") under the rib cage on the left or the right side, corresponding to the location of displaced abomasum. It is recommended that clinical evaluation should be focused along a line drawn from the left elbow to the left tuber coxae between ribs 9 and 13 (Cockcroft and Jackson 2004). Abomasal volvulus exhibits more severe clinical signs. Affected cattle have dramatically decreased milk production, are off-feed, depressed, dehydrated and may have colic at the first stages lasting for few hours. Physical examination reveals normal temperature or hypothermia, tachycardia, tachypnoea, cool peripheral parts and anxious expression. The most common laboratory data on these animals include hemoconcentration and severe hypochloremic, hypokalemic alkalosis.

DIAGNOSIS

Recent parturition, partial anorexia and decreased milk production provide the first signs of abomasal displacement. The diagnosis is based on the presence "pings" produced during simultaneous auscultation and percussion. In cases of right abomasal displacement the diagnosis is confirmed by rectal palpation that reveals a tense, gas-filled viscus at arm's length laterally on the right. Left abomasal displacement can be confirmed by abomasocentesis and measurement of pH at the obtained fluid. If the pH is in the range of 2 to 4, this is consistent with the presence of a left displaced abomasum (Cockcroft and Jackson 2004). Furthermore, the characteristic hypochloremic and hypokalemic alkalosis typically observed in cows with left or right abomasal displacement are indicative of the disease.

PROGNOSIS

The prognosis of left displaced abomasum is good if the disease is early diagnosed and surgically treated by an experienced veterinarian and there are not other concurrent diseases (Karatzias 1992, Goerigk et al. 2012). Although the course of the disease is slow, delayed intervention results in extended recovery time due to damage caused in the internal organs and mainly of the liver. The prognosis is poor in cases with hepatic jaundice. Abomasal volvulus is an emerging condition that should be surgically treated within a 48h period from the onset of the clinical signs. Animals with severe cardiovascular signs such as tachycardia with more than 120 heart beats per min, arrhythmias and coincidence of the first and second heart sounds, should be euthanized.

TREATMENT

Left Abomasal Displacement

The treatment of left abomasal displacement aims to the repositioning of the abomasum and its stabilization at its normal position to avoid reoccurrence. The suggested treatment options vary from conservative treatment (casting and rolling) to surgical intervention.

Casting and rolling was first described by Begg and Whiteford in 1956 (Begg & Whiteford, 1956). Permanent cure rate, however, was judged to be less than 25%. Furthermore, right torsion of the abomasum was described as a complication of casting and rolling (St-Jean *et al.* 1989). More recently, casting and rolling was combined with blind percutaneous toggle-pin abomasopexy (Grymer & Sterner, 1982). However the disadvantages of this procedure are numerous and include missing the abomasum, suturing the abomasum in malposition, allowing leakage from the abomasal lumen in the peritoneal cavity, puncturing the wrong organ, phlevitis from injury to the mammary vein and risking peritonitis via endogenous (abomasal contents) or exogenous (skin, hair, environment) means of contamination of the abdominal cavity (Divers and Peek 2008).

According to our opinion the best treatment option for cows with left abomasal displacement is surgical intervention and the best method is the right flank omentopexy as described by Dirksen (1967). According to this method, a standing laparotomy is performed in the right paralumbar fossa after local anesthesia with either proximal paralumbar block or topical infiltration along the incision site. The abdomen is entered through a 20 cm vertical incision standing 4 to 5 cm ventral to the transverse processes of the lumbar vertebrae. When the peritoneal cavity is entered, the left hand of the surgeon is directed behind the omentum and over the dorsal sac of the rumen and then to the left of the animal, cranially and ventrally in order to palpate the distended abomasum between rumen and the left abdominal wall. The surgeon checks for the presence of adhensions and evaluates the degree of the abomasal tension. If the abomasal tension is significant, the gases are removed with the aid of a hypodermic needle with a length of sterile tubing attached until no palpable gas is left in it. Afterwards, the surgeon's left hand, following the abdominal wall, passes below rumen and between the left of the rumen and the abomasum. At this position, the hand is used to sweep the abomasum back to its normal position at the right side of the abdomen. Subsequently, the omentum is grasped and pulled out through the incision. It is gently retracted dorsally and caudally until the pylorus can be visualized. The omentum is then fixed on the abdominal wall by a suture which is placed on the omentum 5-10 cm caudal to the pylorus and after passing through the abdominal wall at the lower site of the incision. Post-operative management includes the administration of broad-spectrum antibiotics for 3-4 days and the treatment of secondary diseases such as fatty liver. The cow should be fed with roughage diet for 5-6 days and the concentrates should be gradually offered after the 7th day.

Abomasal Volvulus

The abomasal volvulus is surgically treated with right-flank omentopexy. The restrain, the anesthesia and the laparotomy are the same as in left abomasal displacement. Entering the peritoneal cavity care should be taken not to incise the dilated abomasum. Replacement of the abomasum is attempted after the removal of excess gas with a hypodermic needle. Sometimes, the accumulation of large amount of fluids in the abomasum makes the repositioning difficult, so some researchers suggest relieving fluid distension via abomasotomy (Dirksen 1970). However, the recovery is better in animals that the abomasal fluid is not removed compared to those that it is removed (Karatzias 1991). This is due to the fact that the abomasal fluid has high concentrations of K, Na and Cl that are necessary for the correction of the electrolytic and acid-base imbalances such as the hypokalemic and the hypochloremic alkalosis that is a constant finding in these animals. Once the abomasum is returned to its normal position, the duodenum resumes its normal position and is commonly observed to fill with gas. To avoid relapse, omentopexy is performed as described above. The post-operative management is similar with that of left abomasal displacement.

PREVENTION

Prevention of abomasal displacement is difficult due to the great number of factors that act simultaneously. Based on the fact that a higher incidence of the disease occurs around calving, the preventive measures should be focused on that period. The measures suggested are related with correcting nutritional mistakes and reducing the stress factors around calving.

a. During dry period cows should receive a balanced diet with increased quantities of forages and should not be overconditioned.

b. The quantity of concentrates offered should be gradually increased during the last two weeks before calving.

c. At least 40% of the ration's dry matter should come from high quality forages.

d. During the first days after calving and until the normalization of gastrointestinal function, a ration with high forage and low concentrates content should be offered.

e. Any change in the ration's ingredients should be avoided during the first month after calving.

f. The total amount of concentrates offered should be divided into three or four feedings.

g. The ration should contain adequate amounts of vitamins, macro- and trace elements whereas rations with high contents of crude proteins and fat should be avoided.

h. The metabolic diseases that occur during the transition period should be treated immediately.

i. The cattle should not be fallen down or transported immediately during the first two weeks after calving.

j. According to our observations, the administration of clinoptilolite at the rate of 200g/animal/day seems to reduce the incidence of abomasal displacement. Of course, further investigation is required.

REFERENCES

Begg, H. & Whiteford, W. (1956). Displacement of abomasum in the cow. *Vet. Rec., 63,* 122.

Cockcroft, P. & Jackson, P. (2004). Clinical examination of the abdomen in adult cattle. *In Practice, June,* 304-317.

Dirksen, G. (1961). Die Erweiterung, Verlagerung und Drehung des Labmagens beim Rind. *Zentralbl. Veterinarmed, 8,* 934–1015.

Dirksen, G. (1962). Die Erweiterung, Verlagerung und Drehung des Labmagens beim Rind. Habil.-Schr., Hannover.

Dirksen, G. (1967). Present state of diagnosis, treatment and prophylaxis of left displacement of bovine abomasum. *Dtsch. Tierärz. Wschr., 74,* 625-633.

Divers, T.J. & Peek, S.F. (2008). *Rebuhn's Diseases of Dairy Cattle* (2nd Edition). St. Louis, MO: Elsevier.

Furll, M. & Kruger, M. (1999). Alternative Moglichkeiten zur Prophylaxe der Dislocatio abomasi (DA) beim Rind. *Praktischer Tierarzt.* 80, 81–90.

Goerigk, D., Muller, M. & Furll, M. (2011). Dislicatio abomasi – und was kommt danach? In Furll, M. (Ed.), *Internationale Konferenz Prophylaxe von Herden- bzw. Produktionskrankheiten, Leipzig, 7 und 8 Oktober 2011* (pp. 49-50). Leipzig, Germany: Merkur.

Grymer, J. & Sterner, K.E. (1982). Percutaneous fixation of left displaced abomasum, using a bar suture. *J. Am. Vet. Med. Assoc., 180,* 1458-1461.

Grymer, J., Hesselholt, M. & Willeberg, P. (1981). Feed composition and left abomasal displacement in dairy cattle A case-control study. *Nord. Veterinarmed. 33,* 306–309.

Hull, B.L. & Wass, W.M. (1973). Causative factors in abomasal displacement: 1st literature review. Vet. Med. Small Anim. Clin., 68, 283-287.

Hultgren, J. & Pehrson, B. (1996). Risk factors of displaced abomasum in Wisconsin dairy herds. *Bovine Pract. 32,* 56–57.

Ide, P.R. & Henry, J.H. (1984). Abomasal abnormalities in dairy cattle. A review of 90 clinical cases. *Can. Vet. J., 5,* 46-55.

Karatzias, H. & Panousis, N. (2003). A study on the occurrence and aetiology of abomasal displacement in dairy cattle in Greece. *Cattle Pract., 11,* 135-139.

Karatzias, H. (1992). Untersuchungen uber Labmagen-verlagerung (Dislocatio abomasi) bei Milchkuhen in Griecheland. *Mh. Vet.-Med., 47,* 35-40.

LeBlanc, S.J., Leslie, K.E. & Duffield, T.F. (2005). Metabolic predictors of displaced abomasum in dairy cattle. *J. Dairy Sci., 88,* 159–170.

Moore, G.R., Rilley, R.F., Westcott, R.W. & Conner, G.H. (1954). Displacement of the bovine abomasum. *Vet. Med., 19,* 49-51.

Nilsson, L.S. (1962). Etiology of abomasal disolacement. *Mod. Vet. Prac., 43,* 68-70.

Pinsent, R.J., Neal, P.A. & Ritchie, H.E. (1961). Displacement of the bovine abomasum: A review of 80 clinical cases. *Vet. Rec., 73,* 729-735.

Poike, A. & Furll, M. (2000). Zur Epidemiologie der Labmagenverlagerung (dislocatio abomasi) in Mitteldeutschland. In: Furll, M. (Ed.), *Atiologie, Pathogenese, Diagnostik, Prognose, Therapie und Prophylaxe der Dislocatio abomasi. Proceedings Internationaler Workshop, Leipzig 1998* (pp. 29–39). Leipzig, Germany: Leipziger Universitatsverlag.

St Jean, G., Constable, B.L. & Rings, D.M. (1989). Abomasal volvulus in cattle following correction of left displacement by casting and rolling. *Cornell Vet., 79,* 345–351.

Stengarde, L.U. & Pehrson, B.G. (2002). Effects of management, feeding, and treatment on clinical and biochemical variables in cattle with displaced abomasum. *Am. J. Vet. Res., 63,* 137–142.

Stober, M. & Saratsis, P. (1974). Vergleichende Messungen am Rumpf von schwarzbunten Kuhen mit und ohne linksseitige Labmagenverlagerung. *Dtsch. Tierarztl. Wochenschr., 81,* 549–604.

Van Winden, S.L.C. (2002). Displacement of the abomasum in dairy cows – risk factors and pre-clinical alterations. Dissertation Faculty of Veterinary Medicine, Utrecht.

Wolf, V., Hamann, H., Scholz, H. & Distl, O. (2001). Einflusse auf das Auftreten von Labmagenverlagerungen bei Deutschen Holstein Kuhen. *Dtsch. Tierarztl. Wochenschr.,* *108,* 403–408.

Wolf, V., Hamann, H., Scholz, H. & Distl, O. (2001). Einflusse auf das Auftreten von Labmagenverlagerungen bei Deutschen Holstein Kuhen. *Dtsch. Tierarztl. Wochenschr.,* *108,* 403–408.

Chapter 9

ADAPTATIONS OF CATTLE TO STRESSFUL ENVIRONMENTS

Concepta McManus[1], Samuel Paiva[2], Luiza Seixas[3], José Braccini Neto[1], Júlio Otavio Jardim Barcellos[1], Maria Eugênia Andrighetto Canozzi[1], Bruno Stefano Lima Dallago[5], Cristiano Barros de Melo[5] and Michiel Scholtz[6,7]

[1]Departamento de Zootecnia, Universidade Federal de Rio Grande do Sul, Av. Bento Gonçalves, Porto Alegre, Rio Grande do Sul, Brazil
[2]Laboratório de Genética Animal, Embrapa Recursos Genéticos e Biotecnologia, Brasília, DF, Brazil
[3]INCT/CNPq - Informação Genético-Sanitária da Pecuária Brasileira (INCT-Pecuária), Belo Horizonte, MG, Brazil
[4]Escola de Veterinária, Universidade Federal de Goiás, Goiânia,GO, Brazil
[5]Universidade de Brasília, Campus Darcy Ribeiro, Brasília, Brazil
[6]ARC – Animal Production Institute, Private Bag X2, Irene 0062, South Africa
[7]University of the Free State, P O Box 339, Bloemfontein 9301

ABSTRACT

Local cattle breeds in South America originated from cattle that escaped from or were left behind by the colonizers in expeditions through the region in the 16th century. These animals were isolated by rivers and forests and became adapted to specific local conditions such as high temperatures (savannah (cerrado), sertão and Pantanal), as well as extremely low (savannah and sertão) or high (Pantanal) humidity. Disease challenges in these regions are unique and survival has meant that these animals have acquired traits that will be important in the face of future climate challenges with changes in rainfall and temperature patterns. Recent importations of Zebu and European cattle have led to the survival of these animals becoming threatened, but recently, studies have shown that the adaptation to the environment and *Bos taurus* origin have given these animals a unique combination of high heat tolerance and disease resistance combined with high carcass quality. The behaviour of these animals is such that they can walk up to 20km per day in search of water and food, and their social behaviour is more primitive than modern cattle breeds. These breeds are still reared in highly extensive systems and give us an insight into behaviour and adaptation mechanisms needed for survival in highly stressful environments. On the other hand, these changes determine the configuration of new production systems which should be linked to new Technologies, to the economic outcome and consumer demand.

Keywords: Genetic, disease, nutrition, behavior, challenge, production systems

INTRODUCTION

The only animals that are considered domesticated today that were present in Latin America at the time of the Discovery of the Americas in 1454 were camelids (llamas, alpacas, vicuñas, and guanacos), as well as the guinea pig. All other animals came from Europe (Iberian Peninsula) and North Africa and underwent approximately 500 years of natural selection in the diverse environments. From the end of the 19th century there were other cattle imports from mainland Europe for use in more intensive and controlled production systems in the South and South east and Zebu cattle from India for use in more extensive systems in the north, northeast and centerwest (Primo, 2004). In these systems, all animals from the same breed tended to be selected for the same phenotypic characteristics, and reproduction among breeds was seriously reduced (Taberlet et al., 2008). More recently, selection pressures were increased to improve productivity with the use of modern animal breeding techniques and reproductive technologies.

Climate worldwide has also been changing and these changes are predicted to be highly dynamic in the near future (Jones & Thornton, 2009). An increase in the average global surface temperature between 1.8 and 4.0°C by 2100 is predicted (IPCC, 2007), while crop productivity may change with crop yields falling by 10–20% by 2050 in some regions, because of warming and drying (Jones & Thornton, 2003). Changes are expected in southern hemisphere environments and vegetation with decreases in grazing capacity (Scholtz et al., 2010). Romanini et al. (2008) predict that the expected increase of 5 °C in air temperatures in Brazil may lead to a decrease in pasture capacity by up to approximately 50%. Tropical and subtropical climates have both direct (temperature, solar radiation, humidity and wind) and indirect (digestibility of feed, intake, quality and quantity of grazing, pests and diseases, which are themselves directly influenced by climate change) effects on livestock.

A key goal of biology with modern farming practices is to understand phenotypic and genetic relationships between characteristics such as health, disease and evolutionary fitness (Houle et al., 2010). The most important trait of local breeds is their adaptation potential and some, such as the Curraleira Pé-duro, Pantaneiro and Crioula Lageano cattle breeds in Brazil, have shown natural resistance to hostile environments (McManus et al., 2009b; McManus et al., 2011) without interference from man, while others have been exposed to a process of extinction (Primo, 1992). These naturalized breeds are generally smaller than commercial breeds (Bianchini et al., 2006) with high heat tolerance (McManus et al., 2011) and disease resistance (Juliano et al., 2007). The slow growth and small size of these cattle is in harmony with the harsh conditions in the South American ecosystems. This adaptation led to the formation of a potentially important resource for cattle farming in adverse climatic conditions (Britto, 1998).

GENETIC CHALLENGE IN MODERN FARMING SYSTEMS

The twentieth century may be considered a turning point for the way animals are bred and farmed. The human population explosion gave rise to widespread competition with other species for agricultural land, and many of the well adapted species and breeds became extinct or are now threatened with extinction (Flint & Woolliams, 2008). The industrial culture also influenced the environment in which animals are raised with increased intensification of production and the consequences include changes in production systems, the breeds used and eventually climate change. Adequate within-breed genetic diversity needs to be maintained to preserve populations (McManus et al., 2010) and guarantee the long-term sustainable exploitation of livestock, especially in the light of predicted climate changes which include increased mean temperatures and decreased growing days (Romanini et al., 2008; Scholtz et al. 2010).

Breed substitution has been based on the supposition that these breeds are more productive than local breeds but in harsh environments such as the Pantanal in Brazil, it had been shown that while Nellore cattle have a calving interval of almost two years, whereas the naturalized breeds such as Pantaneiro or Curraleiro Pé-Duro calve once a year (McManus et al., 2002).

Modern animal breeding is based on integrating many sciences and technologies, including genetics (both quantitative and molecular), statistics and computing science, information technology, as well as the physiology and endocrinology underlying growth, disease resistance, reproduction and fertility. Apart from desired effects of genetic selection on high economic production efficiency, negative side effects have become apparent. Animals in a population that have been genetically selected for high production efficiency seem to be more at risk for behavioural, physiological and immunological problems (Rauw et al., 1998) as well as increased susceptibility to disease and reduced heat tolerance (McManus et al., 2009a,c), which will be important given predicted environmental changes.

Generally, tropical cattle breeds have low productivity and their roles in traditional societies were multiple and different from the present as society began to act in a market based economy (Mariante et al., 2008). The most important attribute of tropical breeds is better survival under difficult and stressful conditions, occasioned by parasites and diseases and low feed availability and quality (Cunningham & Syrstad, 1987). Studies have shown that naturalized breeds (Scholtz, 1988; Prayaga, 2004; Prayaga & Heanshall, 2005) have the ability to survive, grow and reproduce in the presence of endemic stress factors such as ecto- and endo-parasites, diseases, hot climates (high heat and humidity) and poor seasonal nutrition. For example, McManus et al. (2002) showed that the locally adapted Pantaneiro cattle had approximately double the reproductive rate of Nellore cattle in the harsh environment found in the Brazilian Pantanal.

Mirkena et al. (2010) reviewed adaptation to humans and consequences of domestication on predator aversion, mechanisms of adaptation to available feed and water resources, severe climates and genetic evidence of disease tolerance or resistance, with emphasis on gastrointestinal parasites and bacterial diseases. These authors found that resource allocation by the animal to production and fitness traits has a genetic background under both optimal and sub-optimal conditions. If information on such resource allocation is available, it would help in identifying the most appropriate and adapted genotypes to cope with the environmental challenges posed by the different production systems.

Breeding objectives for ruminants assume that an increase in individual production will be followed by an increase in the economic margin per animal. This is acceptable only if selection for production maintains or increases feed efficiency and product quality, which may not be true. There is evidence that selection for milk yield increases both feed intake and mobilization of body reserves to support milk production (Marie-Etancelin et al., 2002; Veerkamp, 2003). Selection for production also results in poorer female fertility in dairy cattle, probably as a result of more negative energy balance (Veerkamp et al., 2003). Although positive trends for milk production have been seen, several studies show negative results for protein and fat percentages. Breeding for increased milk production has been found to have negative side effects on health and fertility (Pryce et al., 2004; de Jong, 2007), including increases in days to first service, days open, calving interval and decreases in conception and pregnancy rates (Washburn et al., 2002; Rajala-Schultz & Frazer, 2003).

Samoré et al. (2008) found that larger values of somatic cell score were genetically associated with increased production. Few Holsteins cows in the US currently survive beyond their fifth parity and their average lifetime parity number has fallen over the past 20 years from 3.4 to only 2.8 (Tsuruta *et al.,* 2005). A study of the erosion rate of South African Jersey cattle (Du Toit et al., 2004) indicated that their productive herd life had declined from 7.9 lactations in 1970 to a level of 2.3. Rauw et al. (1998) reviewed over 100 studies showing the undesirable (cor)related effects of selection for high production, with metabolic, reproduction and health traits, in broilers, pigs and dairy cattle. Further discussion can be found in Wathes et al. (2008).

Adaptive traits may be rapidly lost by poorly designed crossbreeding leading to dilution of local genetics by exotic germplasm (McManus et al., 2010). Crossbreeding with a breed with higher production levels is widespread and can affect the specific adaption traits of a native or naturalised breed within a few generations. Recovery from such loss can be difficult, requiring many generations of backcrossing. McManus et al. (2009a) showed that local breeds are better adapted to harsh climate conditions, with lower heart and breathing rates as well as lower rectal temperature. Tick counts, fecal worm egg counts (FEC), rectal temperatures and coat scores have been used as indicator traits of adaptability of animals to assess the suitability of particular genotypes to tropical environments (Prayaga & Henshall, 2005; McManus et al., 2009b).

O'Neill et al. (2010), studying four adapted taurine breeds, concluded that these and other breeds that have undergone similar evolutionary trajectories, would possess candidate genes that could contribute to improving the productivity of cattle in challenging environments. However, the physiological antagonism between production potential and adaptation ensures no genotype achieves highest performance in all environments (Blackburn et al., 1998). Several studies on unique aspects of criolla cattle and their crosses have been carried out. A major gene for hair length (slick hair) has been found in the Venezuelan Carora (a two-breed composite of Brown Swiss and local Criollo) (Olson et al. 2003). This gene has been found to contribute to improving the animal's thermoregulatory ability. It is also thought that the Mexican Criollo from the Chihuahuan Desert possesses alleles that allow it to survive with variations in water consumption, fluctuations in ambient temperature, metabolism of a variety of herbaceous plants, and alternating between browsing and grazing (O'Neill et al., 2010). This has implications for other livestock rearing in other semi-arid regions (Masters et al., 2006). In South Africa it was observed that the native Nguni cattle breed was more capable of maintaining its body weight during winter than other breeds and that it had higher blood urea (N) and ruminal NH_3 levels (Linington, 1990).

The results of studies carried out with animals produced by the crossing of resistant with susceptible breeds have demonstrated that the degree of resistance of the hybrids can vary as a function of the breeds evaluated, the age of the animals and whether the evaluations were from natural or artificial infections (Amarante et al., 2009). Depending on the production system used, crossbreds are not necessarily better than purebreds (Rocha et al., 2009). In harsh and undeveloped areas or pastoralist systems, pure breeding with naturalized breeds (such as the Pantaneiro) may be the only production strategy that can be followed. The level of stress factors, management and nutrition may not be sufficient to meet the higher demands of crossbreds (Scholtz et al., 2011). The availability of diverse cattle breed resources with large adaptive and productive differences allow breed types to be matched with the different environments, management capabilities and markets - thereby maximizing the opportunity for sustainable production and profitability.

The impact of changes in adaptation may not be limited to the livestock populations. Increased use of drugs to control emerging diseases on wildlife health was studied by Blanco & Lemus (2010) who found high concentrations of multiple veterinary drugs, primarily fluoroquinolones, in most failed eggs and nestlings of threatened avian scavengers feeding upon medicated livestock carcasses. These deaths were associated with multiple internal organ damage. Livestock pathogens caused disease in these birds, especially septicaemia by swine pathogens and infectious bursal disease.

DISEASE CHALLENGE

One of the potential significant and permanent consequences to changes in the climate is altered patterns of diseases in animals. This may include (a) the emergence of new disease syndromes and (b) a change in the prevalence of existing diseases, particularly those spread by biting insects. A wider geographic distribution of known vectors and/or the recruitment of new strains to the vector pool could result in infections spreading to more and potentially new species of hosts (Summers, 2009). Changes in climate will influence arthropod vectors, their life cycles and life histories, resulting in changes in both vector and pathogen distribution and changes in the ability of arthropods to transmit pathogens (Tabachnick, 2010). Therefore animals will be exposed to different parasites and diseases as indicated from the predicted change in the distribution of, for example, Tsetse in Africa (Herrero et al., 2008); putting an even greater pressure on production and the survival of livestock breeds. There is evidence for host genetic variation in aspects of disease resistance for many diseases, in all major domestic livestock species (Bishop, 2005).

Anomalous climatic conditions caused by El Ninõ Southern Oscillation (ENSO) are recognized to be linked with outbreaks of various human and livestock diseases in various countries (Glantz, 1991). The OIE Scientific Commission has therefore concluded that climatic changes are likely to be a factor in determining the spread of some diseases, especially those that are vector-borne. Economic effects arise due to death and reduced production (Pegram et al., 1989; Cêtre-Sossah et al., 2009) as well as restrictions on animal movement and the trade of animals and animal products (Anyamba et al., 2001; Calistri et al., 2004; Wilson et al., 2009) and opens up the possibility of secondary attacks from other parasites. Some of the most mentioned emerging and re-emerging cattle diseases in a recent OIE survey were Bluetongue and Rift Valley fever (OIE, 2008). Climate also plays a vital part in determining distribution of ticks, which are responsible for diseases such as East Coast Fever, Heartwater, Gallsickness, and Red Water. Prevalence and intensity of tick infestation have been associated with temperature and humidity. In a study in Pakistan, a mean maximum temperature above 26.8 °C and mean humidity ranging from 38.5% to 65% were found favorable for the tick population (Sajid et al., 2009). On the other hand, higher altitude and lower temperatures delay the activity of ticks (Jouda et al., 2004). According to Cassis (1998) one of the consequences of global climate change will be the reduction of biodiversity, which may increase the probability of ticks feeding on cattle (Olwoch et al., 2009).

While the number of animals seropositive for babesosis in a given region is also a consequence of climatic variations, topography and herd management (Osaki et al., 2002; Souza et al., 2002). Juliano et al. (2007) working with native Curraliero Pé-Duro cattle in Brazil found an age effect for the percentage of animals seropositive for *Babesia bovis* and *B. bigemina*. Geleta (2001) found this to be caused by a fall in re-infection due to in part an increase of resistance in host animals while Juliano et al. (2007) correlated this with natural selection due to exposure of these animals to vectors which is common in local breeds (Solorio-Rivera & Rodriguez Vivas, 1997).

Although less important from the clinical view, but essential for livestock production, the diversity and abundance of gastrointestinal (GI) infections could also be influenced by climate. For example, most helminth parasites have free life cycle stages in the environment or in invertebrate intermediate hosts or vectors. The development and survival of these stages are sensitive to climatic conditions, either directly or due to climatic influences on the abundance, behavior and distribution of intermediate hosts and vectors. General predictions for pathogens in a warmer and wetter world are for increased transmissions rates, longer periods for transmission, and shifts in spatial and temporal patterns of pathogen diversity and associated disease (Harvell et al., 2002; Kutz et al., 2005; Polley & Thompson, 2009). For example, the level and type of infective strongylate nematode larvae on pasture in some coastal savanna regions of Ghana was high during the period of and soon after the rains, and very low or none in the absence of rainfall (Agyei, 1997). In addition, the number of infective larvae on pasture was directly related to the pattern of rainfall.

Several studies have been carried out with commercial and native breeds. Indigenous Nguni cattle have been shown to be more resilient to gastrointestinal (GI) nematodes than exotic cattle breeds on semi-arid rangelands in the Eastern Cape (Ndlovu et al., 2008). Crossbreeding can be an important tool where in tropical conditions in Australia and the United States, O'Kelly (1980) and Peña et al. (2000), respectively, observed greater resistance of *Bos taurus* × *Bos indicus* crossbreeds in relation to purebred *B. taurus* animals. Holgado and Cruz (1994), in Argentina, found that Criollo-Nelore were more resistant to GI than Criolla, Hereford and Nelore animals, the latter the most sensitive. Both Zebu and Criolla cattle have undergone less intensive selection for commercial traits such as growth or carcass quality.

Controlling these diseases will be a challenge for future farming systems. This includes both genetic (breeding for tolerance or resistance) and management solutions. The difference between resistance and tolerance is that resistance protects the host at the expense of the parasite, while tolerance saves the host from harm without having any direct negative effects on the parasite (Råberg et al., 2009), therefore the consequences of resistance and tolerance should differ. While resistance should reduce the prevalence of the parasite in the host population, tolerance should have a neutral or positive effect on parasite prevalence (Boots, 2008). Resistance may impose selection on the parasite to overcome host defense, which in turn may impose selection for improved resistance in the host, leading to antagonistic coevolution between host and parasite (Woolhouse *et al.,* 2002). Tolerance, on the other hand, does not have any negative effect on the performance of the parasite, and so there should not be any selection on the parasite to overcome this type of defense (Rausher, 2001; Boots, 2008). Therefore breeding tolerant animals is of interest to the farmer.

BEHAVIORAL AND NUTRITIONAL CHALLENGE

As a result of global warming, livestock in the developing countries of the southern hemisphere, will need to adapt to higher ambient temperatures, lower nutritional value of the grass in some cases, and expansion of diseases, especially ticks and tick borne diseases (Scholtz et al., 2010). Under such challenges balancing genotypes with production environments will become a crucial element requiring the utilization of diverse genetic resources with appropriate genetic potentials for growth, milk production, resistance to disease and prolificacy (Blackburn & Mezzadra, 2006). The question is how to measure adaptation and how to select for it.

Nutrition stress has the largest indirect effect on the grazing animal in the tropics and subtropics. In these environments, natural pasture has both lower nutritional value and lower tiller density than in temperate regions (Linington, 1990). These tropical grasses (C_4) have developed a different photosynthetic pathway to adapt to the climate. The C_4 refers to a 4 carbon compound compared to a 3 carbon compound (C_3) in temperate grasses. C_4 plants have a higher photosynthetic rate, which results in high fibre content, low stem to leaf ratio, reduced digestibility and intake (Leng, 1984). Climate change will thus have the greatest impact on ruminant species (Blackburn & Mezzadra, 2006).

Studies in wild animals or breeds reared in highly extensive systems can give us an insight into behaviour and adaptation mechanisms needed for survival in highly stressful environments and can help in understanding effects on domestic populations. Emergency feeding is typically employed to buffer extreme climatic conditions (Ouellet *et al.,* 2001). This is thought to have an effect on populations because it takes place during the periods with potentially the strongest selection. In wild populations, winter feeding has been shown to reduce natural selection (Schmidt & Hoi, 2002; Lewis & Rongstad, 1998; Bishop *et al.,* 2009). Artificial feeding also limits the animal's range and affects feeding patterns (Sahlsten *et al.,* 2010; van Beest *et al.,* 2010), and might change the mating system and reproductive success (Carranza et al., 1995; Bårdsen *et al.,* 2008). This is thought to change selection pressure and reduce social learning (Rolshausen *et al.,* 2009). Therefore one can presume that domestic animals reared without interference from man should present similar reactions to management policies.

Social interactions between individuals, such as co-operation and competition, are key factors in evolution by natural selection. Biologists have studied theories to attempt to understand the consequences of social interactions for response to natural selection. Current genetic improvement programmes in animal husbandry largely ignore these. Results have shown that including animals with better social skills into breeding programmes may reduce negative social interactions in farm animals and increase positive social interactions (Rodenberg et al., 2010).

Maternal behaviour has been shown to depend on a complex interaction among genetic, physiological factors and maternal experience (Le Neindre, 1989; Buchenauer, 1999). Artificial selection has resulted in changes in production levels and adaptation of cattle breeds. While milk production uses the cows' ability to provide nourishment for her young, selection may be against a strong maternal bond with the offspring. Systems with longer periods of cow–calf contact and strong maternal bond (Grandinson, 2005) are more evident in beef cattle production. When domesticated cattle in extensive conditions rear their young, the behaviors associated with maternal care are similar to those observed in wild ungulates (von Keyserlingk & Weary, 2007). It seems natural that looking at feral or semi-wild cattle, or those that have not undergone specific selection processes could give some insights to the development of maternal-offspring bonds (Bouissou et al., 2001). The degree of domestication depends on (i) the level of human control over breeding, mortality, food supply, space use and thereby selection pressures; (ii) how much these differ from original states; and (iii) how strongly phenotypic traits have been affected relative to the wild counterpart (Mysterud, 2010).

Farmers of local breeds noted several traits they regards as important (Castanheira, 2006). All stated that the dam hides the calf more than other breeds reared by these farmers (Tabapuã, Nelore, Caracu) and abandonment is rare. The famers considered the calf highly insistent in the face of denial by the dam, with each suckling lasting approximately five minutes. Younger calves suckled more often than older ones. A specific trait of this breed was the fact that the cow doesn't stay close to the calf, which she tends to hide alone or with groups of calves while she leaves to find food and water. The hiding behaviour of calves by these cattle is reminiscent of wild ungulates where hiding young is a strategy used to protect the young from predators (Bongi et al., 2008). Some farmers related cases of cows walking distances up to 15 to 20km from their calf looking for water. Curraleiro Pé Duro cattle are generally reared in highly extensive systems on native pastures with little interference from man (Fioravanti et al., 2008). The farmers accounts of the ability of this breed to walk long distances leaving their young with other cows in search of water and food is also seen in other wild and feral species, where large home ranges are seen in wild ungulates (Ciuti et al., 2006).

Allo-suckling was also commented by farmers and observed by Castanheira (2006). While the rate of allo-suckling is low in mammals, mothers have been observed to nurse alien offspring in 68 species (Packer et al., 1992). Roulin (2002) put forward several hypothesis as to why this occurs (misguided parental behavior; reciprocal nursing; nursing related juveniles for inclusive fitness benefits; nursing alien offspring to evacuate milk that their own offspring did not drink; Inexperienced females that lactate spontaneously without reproducing themselves or that have lost their litter nurse alien offspring to improve their maternal skills). Most of these reasons are linked to survival and fitness of the animal group.

Allo-suckling is common in herds of domestic female water buffalo (*Bubalus bubalis*) (Murphey et al., 1991; Murphey et al., 1995), although Andriolo et al. (1994) stated that this approach has never been reported for cattle in nature. Víchová & Barto□ (2005) stated that their observed herd was extensively reared but these were housed in a free stall barn with a single pen and fed hay and corn silage during the observation period. Le Neindre (1989) described this behavior, but the calves are undergoing food deprivation and the cows were restrained, to become adapted to the new calf. Kiley-Worthington & de la Plain (1983) reported that allo-feeding can occur in cattle, when the introduced calf would learn to nurse along with the natural offspring of the cow. There were no descriptions of voluntarily allo-suckling, without the interference of man, in cattle raised extensively as here (Paranhos da Costa et al., 2006).

No measurements of distance between parent / offspring throughout the day were found in the literature. Cows did not stay with their calves in this study which is different from behaviour observed with Nelore and Guzerat cattle (Souza et al., 2009) where 60% to 80% of the time was spent with the calves. Crèche formation with cow guards is common in cattle (Vitale et al., 1986; Sato et al., 1987). Their formation is thought to be related to protection against predators, help in decrease flies and socialization of calves.

An individual is always a consequence of the environment where he lives, the factors of environmental change and at the same time, an environmental factor common to all subjects of his and other species (Silva, 2000). In this context, maternal care must be highlighted as being essential to the survival and development of offspring, for a better adaptation of the animal to the production system and a consequent rational exploration. In cattle, as well as in other mammals, the relationship between mother and offspring begins early.

Enteric fermentation from livestock is responsible for 28% of global methane emissions (IPCC, 2007). The livestock industry should be aware of the effect of livestock on climate change and therefore it is important that mechanisms are put in place to mitigate this effect (Scholtz et al., 2012). Breeding objectives to reduce enteric methane production from beef cattle under extensive production systems can therefore play a significant role in addressing climate change. Wall et al. (2009) reported variations between animals, between breeds, and across time, providing the potential for improvement through selection. Nkrumah et al. (2006) reported that beef cattle with low residual feed intake produced up to 28% less methane than those with high residual feed intake. Residual feed intake is calculated as the difference between actual feed intake and the expected feed requirements for maintenance of body weight and a certain level of production (Hegarty et al., 2007). The lower methane production was attributed to differences in ruminal microbial population and Nkrumah et al. (2006) stated that the differences could be heritable.

PRODUCTION SYSTEMS

The production system represents the synchronized management of elements used to obtain a product derived from animal husbandry. Thus, genetic, environmental, infrastructure, technology and market aspects closely interact in the face of any internal or external change in this system. Environmental changes which lead to breaking the state of equilibrium in animal-environment relationships, may redirect production systems to ensure the level of competitiveness and maintenance of sustainability (Marques et al., 2011).

In the last decade, new drivers configured systems for the production of beef cattle, in particular the high cost of land, competition with agricultural areas, new consumer demands and environmental issues as well as international health policies (Euclides Filho, 2004). These shaped substantial changes in production methods, particularly the need to maintain production levels in stressful environments as well as the appearance of new stressors. These environments require a system whose viability is difficult in both the physical and economic spheres.

Faced with this new scenario, the calf rearing system was the most challenged as the cow had to migrate to new environments with new limiting factors, represented by the presence of endo-and ectoparasites, mineral deficiencies, heat stress and pastures of lower quality, but with the demand to maintain maximum efficiency in these systems. Thus, an extensive system by nature, which depended essentially on process technologies to define productivity when the environment was favorable, now requires the inclusion of technological innovation, particularly technology inputs, to offset these environmental stressors (Barcellos et al., 2011).

Technological innovations to minimize the environmental constraints in systems create barriers that are invariably operational and economical for their use to be more widespread (Lampert et al., 2010). Thus, the search for better adapted genotypes and recovery of strains or biotypes resistant to the environment shape beef cattle production. However, if this is applied to calf rearing, growing and fattening beef cattle (Barcellos & Lobato, 1992) have other types of challenges and these are presented simultaneously with the need to strengthen the systems, because demand for meat is increasing. Therefore, new production systems, even if modified, must maintain the sensory quality of meat as demanded by the market (Pereira et al., 2011). The adaptive adjustments of more intensive systems require the development of new housing, resulting in a more favorable ambience for growing and finishing animals. Parallel to this, adjustments will be required in diets that lead to lower caloric intake, increased use of agro-industrial residues and reduced methane production in South America for finishing cattle.

The regions and countries that will prosper in a climate-changed world (Llewellyn, 2007) will tend to be those that recognize its importance and inexorability; foresee that there may be at least some implications for their industry (including farms); and take appropriate steps well in advance. O'Neill et al. (2010) argue that the knowledge of interactions between genotype, environment and management in the livestock systems will be required to generate genotypes for efficient livestock production that are both economically and environmentally sustainable. They also argue that farmers will have less reliance on infrastructure and veterinary products to alleviate environmental stress and more on the animal's ability to achieve fitness in a given production environment.

Aside from purely biological aspects, the systems that favour the potential for adaptation of animals to environmental stress will require new methods of management and management of production resources. Therefore, the combination of technologies and training of human resources to operationalize these are key factors to minimize the risks involved with new forms of production.

FINAL CONSIDERATIONS

Almost three quarters of world production are in low to medium input agriculture systems, where the environment includes combinations of sources of stress (food, diseases and climate). With the tendency to concentrate production in a few strains and breeds in these systems, it is difficult to reach high production levels, productivity and sustainability in comparison with other production systems. The insistence to use these few breeds can mean modification of properties of systems of production which alternatively could be used on systems with low to medium input (Hammond, 1994).

Animals in temperate regions are generally more productive than those in the tropics and adapt quickly to a new environment, within the temperate regions (Hodges, 1990). Animals from the tropics have relatively low productivity and their use in traditional societies was different from today, as society has come to act in a market economy. The most important aspect in relation to animals adapted to the tropics is to survive in difficult conditions due to disease and lack of or poor quality food. Production levels can vary depending on the breed. Initially the differences were attributed to the action of parasites (Miller & Monge, 1946), however, with increasing control of parasites by drug use, it became increasingly clear that differences in productivity were associated with physiological differences related to the ability to withstand high temperatures. Increased productivity can be achieved through better nutrition, better handling of breeding and physiological studies of adaptation (Galina & Arthur, 1989). Environmental stress causes a decrease in the probability of survival, growth rates and reproductive characteristics (Calow, 1989). Some genotypes are less influenced than others and these will be favored since the stress will act as selection pressure. The adaptation of species to the environment is usually evaluated by physical changes caused by hormonal and physiological conditions under which the animal lives. The establishment of an economically viable production system in a given region requires the choice of breeds or varieties that are suited to local environmental conditions. A common theme for many arguments for conservation genetics is the resistance to disease, because it affects the conservation in several ways. Disease resistance is conceived as one of the future challenges for genetics and animal husbandry with genetic solutions to many current and future problems present in existing populations. Breeds or populations requiring conservation are often those with high variability of disease or adaptation to harsh environments. A second theme linking disease resistance and conservation is the disease risk to the integrity of small or endangered populations, and to improve existing strategies. The size of the population, individually, is a risk, especially when considering diseases to which the population is not resistant. A third issue is the relationship between disease resistance (or environmental adaptation) and productivity. In extreme conditions, associated with endangered populations, there is often a confusion of productivity and disease resistance / environmental challenges.

REFERENCES

Amarante, A. F. T.; Susin, I.; Rocha, R. A.; Silva, M. B.; Mendes, C. Q. & Pires, A. V. (2009). Resistance of Santa Ines and crossbred ewes to naturally acquired gastrointestinal nematode infections. *Veterinary Parasitology, 165 3-4,* 273-280.

Andriolo, A., Paranhos da Costa, M. J., Schmidek, B. (1994). Comportamento de amamentação em búfalo (Bubalus bubalis) In: Proceedings of the 12th Encontro Nacional De Etologia, Sociedade Brasileira de Etologia, pp.1-7.

Anyamba, A.; Linthicum, K. J. & Tucker, C. J. (2001). Climate-disease connections: Rift Valley fever in Kenya. *Cadernos de Saúde Pública, 17 suppl.,* 133–140.

Barcellos, J. O. J. & Lobato, J.F.P. (1992). Efeito da época de nascimento no desenvolvimento de terneiros Hereford e suas cruzas. II. Peso ao desmame, ao ano e sobreano. *Revista da Sociedade Brasileira de Zootecnia,* 21 1, 150-157.

Barcellos, J. O. J.; Queiroz Filho, L. A.; Ceolin, A. C.; Gianezini, M.; McManus, C.; Malafaia, G.C.; Oaigen, R.P. (2011). Technological innovation and entrepreneurship in animal production. *Revista Brasileira de Zootecnia / Brazilian Journal of Animal Science,* 40, 189-200. (supl. especial).

Bårdsen, B. -J.; Fauchald, P.; Tveraa, T.; Langeland, K.; Yoccoz, N. G. & Ims, R. A. *(2008)* Experimental evidence of a risk-sensitive reproductive allocation in a long-lived mammal. *Ecology, 89,* 829–837.

Bianchini, E.; McManus, C.; Lucci, C. M.; Fernandes, M. C. B.; Prescott, E.; Mariante, A. S. & Egito, A. A. (2006). Características corporais associadas com a adaptação ao calor em bovinos naturalizados brasileiros. *Pesquisa Agropecuária Brasileira, 41 9,* 1443-1448.

Bishop, C. J.; White, G. C.; Freddy, D. J.; Watkins, B. E. & Stephenson, T. R. *(2009).* Effect of enhanced nutrition on mule deer population rate of change. *Wildlife Monographs, 172 1,* 1–28.

Bishop, SC. Disease resistance: genetics. In: Pond WG, Bell AW editors. *Encyclopedia of Animal Science.* New York: Marcel Dekker Inc.; 2005; 288–290

Blackburn, H. & Mezzadra, C. (2006). Policies for the management of animal genetic resources. 8th World Congress of Genetics Applied in Livestock Production. 33(2): 1-7. www.wcgalp8.org.br/wcgalp8/articles.

Blackburn, H., Lebbie, S. H. B. & van de Zijpp, A. J. (1998) Animal Genetic Resources and sustainable development. In: World Congress on Genetics Applied To Livestock Production, 6.,1998, Armidale, UNE:6WCGALP/ FAO Symposium, 28, 3-10.

Blanco G. & Lemus J. A (2010). Livestock drugs and disease: the fatal combination behind breeding failure in endangered bearded vultures. *Plosone, 5 1,* e14163.

Bongi, P.; Ciuti, S.; Grignolio, S.; Del Frate, M.; Simi, S.; Gandelli, D. & Apollonio, M. (2008). Anti-predator behaviour, space use and habitat selection in female roe deer during the fawning season in a wolf area. *Journal of Zoology, 276 3,* 242–251.

Boots, M. (2008). Fight or learn to live with the consequences. *Trends in Ecology and Evolution, 23 5,* 248–250.

Bouissou, M-F; Boissy, A; Le Neindre, P & Veissier, I. The social behaviour of cattle. In: KL Keeling & HW Gonyou editors. *Social behaviour in farm animals.* New York: CAB International; 2001; 113-145.

Britto, C. M. C. (1998). *Citogenética do gado Pé–Duro.* Teresina: EDUFPI, 80p.

Buchenauer, D. Genetics of behaviour in cattle. In: R Fries & A Ruvinsky editors. *The genetics of the cattle.* Wallingford: CAB International; 1999; 365–390.

Calistri, P.; Giovannini, A.; Conte, A.; Nannini, D.; Santucci, U.; Patta, C.; Rolesu, S. & Caporale, V. (2004). Bluetongue in Italy: part I. *Veterinaria Italiana, 40 3,* 243–251.

Calow, P. (1989). Proximate and ultimate responses to stress in biological systems. *Biological Jornal of Linnean Society, 37 1-2,* 173-181.

Carranza, J.; Garcia-Munoz, A. J. & Dios Vargas, J. D. *(1995)*. Experimental shifting from harem defence to territoriality in rutting red deer. *Animal Behaviour, 49 2,* 551–554.

Cassis, G. (1998). Biodiversity loss: a human health issue [editorial]. *The Medical Journal of Australia, 169 11-12,* 568–569.

Castanheira, M. (2006). Comportamento materno-filial de bovinos da raça curraleiro: amamentação de bezerros. Master´s dissertation in Animal Science, Universidade Federal de Goias, Brasil.

Cêtre-Sossah, C.; Billecocq, A.; Lancelot, R.; Defernez, C.; Favre, J.; Bouloy, M.; Martinez, D. & Albina, E. (2009). Evaluation of a commercial competitive ELISA for the detection of antibodies to Rift Valley fever virus in sera of domestic ruminants in France. *Preventive Veterinary Medicine, 90 1-2,* 146–149.

Ciuti, S.; Bong, P.; Vassale, S. & Apollonio, M. *(2006).* Influence of fawning on the spatial behaviour and habitat selection of female fallow deer (*Dama dama*) during late pregnancy and early lactation. *Journal of Zoology, 268 1,* 97–107.

Copyright cap livroAgyei, A. D. (1997). Seasonal changes in the level of infective strongylate nematode larvae on pasture in the coastal savanna regions of Ghana. *Veterinary Parasitology, 70 1-3,* 175-82.

Cunningham EP ; Syrstad, O. *Crossbreeding Bos indicus and Bos taurus for milk production in the tropics*. Rome: FAO; 1987.

de Jong, G. Usage of predictors for fertility in the genetic evaluation, application in the Netherlands. 2007. Available from: https://global.crv4all.com/68143/67761/67689/67751.

Du Toit, J., Olivier, J. J., van Wyk, J. B., 2004. An investigation into erosion rate of lactation records in South African Jersey cattle. Proc 2nd Joint Congr. Grassland Soc. and S. Afr. Soc. Anim. Sci., Goudini, South Africa, 118.

Euclides Filho, K. (2004). Supply chain approach to sustainable beef production from a Brazilian perspective Original Research Article. *Livestock Production Science,* 90, 53-61.

Fioravanti, M. C. S.; Juliano, R. S.; Costa, G. L.; Abud, L. J. & Cardoso, W. S. (2008). Características dos criatórios de bovinos da raça Curraleiro nos Estados de Goiás e Tocantins. In: Proceedings of the II Simpósio Internacional de Savanas Tropicais e IX Simpósio Nacional do Cerrado, Brasília: EMBRAPA, 2008. CD.

Flint A. P. F. & Woolliams J. A. (2008). Precision animal breeding. *Philosophical Transactions of the Royal Society of London, Series B, 363,* 573-590

Galina, C. S. & Arthur, G. H. (1989). Review of cattle reproduction in the Tropics. Part 1. Puberty and age at first calving. *Animal Breeding Abstracts, 57,* 583-590.

Geleta, A. R. (2001). Antibody response to Babesia bovis and Babesia bigemina by vaccinated and unvaccinated cattle in an endemic area. Master´s dissertation in Veterinary Science, Faculdade de Ciências Veterinárias da Universidade de Pretoria, Africa do Sul.

Glantz, MH. Introduction. In: MH Glantz, RW Katz & N Nicholls editors. *Teleconnections linking world wide climate anomalies: scientific basis and societal impact*. New York: Cambridge University Press; 1991; 1-12.

Grandinson, K. (2005). Genetic background of maternal behavior and its relation to offspring survival. *Livestock Production Science, 93 1,* 43-50.

     Concepta McManus, Samuel Paiva, Luiza Seixas et al.

Hammond, K. (1994) Conservation of Domestic Animal Diversity: Global Overview. In: Proceedings of the 5th World Congress of Genetics Applied in Livestock Production, Guelph, 21, 423-430.

Harvell, C. D.; Mitchell, C. E.; Ward, J. R.; Altizer, S.; Dobson, A. P.; Ostfeld, R. S. & Samuel, M. D. 2002. Climate warming and disease risks for terrestrial and marine biota. *Science, 296 5576,* 2158-2162.

Hegarty, S. R.; Goopy, J. P.; Herd, R. M. & McCorkell, B. (2007). Cattle selected for lower residual feed intake have reduced daily methane production. *Journal of Animal Science, 85 6,* 1479–1486.

Herrero, M; Hanotte, O; Notenbaert, A; Thornton, PK. Potential of modelling animal genetic resources data in relation to other existing data sets. In: D Pilling, B Rischkowsky & B Scherf. *Report on the FAO/WAAP workshop on production environment descriptors for animal genetic resources report.* Italy: FAO/WAAP; 2008; Annexure 2.9.

Hodges, J. (1990). *Animal Genetic Resources. A Decade of Progress, 1980-1990.* Rome: FAO.

Holgado, F. D. & Cruz, L. (1994). Tolerancia de diferentes biotipos a los parasitos gastrointestinales. *Revista de Investigaciones Agropecuarias, 25 3,* 81–89

Houle D.; Govindaraju D. R. & Omholt, S. (2010). Phenomics: the next challenge. *Nature Reviews Genetics, 11,* 855-866

IPCC. Climate change: impacts, adaptation and vulnerability. Summary for policy makers. 2007. Avaialable from: http://www.ipcc.cg/ SPM13ap07.pdf.

Jones, P. G. & Thornton, P. K. (2003). The potential impacts of climate change in tropical agriculture: the case of maize in Africa and Latin America in 2055. *Global Environmental Change, 13,* 51–59.

Jones, P. G. & Thornton, P. K. (2009). Croppers to livestock keepers: livelihood transitions to 2050 in Africa due to climate change. *Environmental Science & Policy, 12 4,* 427-437.

Jouda, F.; Perret, J. & Gern, L. (2004). Ixodes ricinus density, and distribution and prevalence of Borrelia burgdorferi sensu lato infection along an altitudinal gradient. *Journal of Medical Entomology, 41 2,* 162–169.

Juliano, R. S.; Machado, R. Z.; Fioravanti, M. C. S.; Andrade, G. M. & Jayme, V. A. (2007). Soroepidemiologia da babesiose em rebanho de bovinos da raça Curraleiro. *Ciência Rural, 37 5,* 1387-1392.

Kiley-Worthington, M., & de la Plain, S. (1983). *The behaviour of beef suckler cattle.* Birkhauser: Verlang.

Kutz, S. J.; Hoberg, E. P.; Polley, L. & Jenkins, E. J. (2005). Global warming is changing the dynamics of artic host-parasite systems. *Philosophical Transactions of the Royal Society of London, Series B, 272 1581,* 2571-2576.

Lampert, V. N.; Marques, P. R.; Barcellos, J. O. J. (2010). Sistemas de cria: eficiência bioeconômica e iniciativas de organización de productores. In: Proceedings of the IV Congresso Internacional de La Carne Bovina, Assunção. CD-ROM.

Le Neindre, P. (1989). Influence of cattle rearing conditions and breed on social relationships of mother and young. *Applied Animal Behaviour Science, 23 1,* 117-127.

Leng, RA. Supplementation of tropical and subtropical pastures for ruminant production. In: FMC Gilchrist & RI Macki editors. *Herbivore nutrition in the tropics and subtropics.* Craighall: The Science Press Ltd.; 1984; 129–144.

Lewis, T. L. & Rongstad, O. J. (1998) Effects of supplemental feeding on white-tailed deer, *Odocoileus virginianus*, migration and survival in northern Wisconsin. *Canadian Field-Naturalist, 112*, 75–81.

Linington, M. J. The use of Sanga cattle in beef production. South Africa: Department of Agriculture; 1990; 31–37.

Llewellyn, J. (2007). *The business of climate change: challenges and opportunities.* USA: Lehman Brothers.

Mariante, AS; McManus, C; Mezzadra, C; Rovere, G & Euclides, K. The role of the Southern Cone of Latin America in world beef production. In: A Rosati, A Tewolde & C Moscani editors. *Animal production and animal science worldwide.* Wageningen: Wageningen Academic; 2008; 35-40.

Marie-Etancelin C.; Such X.; Barillet F.; Bocquier F. & Caja G. (2002). Nutrition, alimentation et élevage des brebis laitières: mâýtrise de facteurs de production pour réduire les coûts et améliorer la qualité des produits. *Options Méditerranéennes, 42 B*, 57–71.

Marques, P.R.; Barcellos, J.O.J.; McManus, C.; Oaigen, R.P.; Collares, F.C.; Canozzi, M.E.A. & Lampert, V.N. (2011). Competitiveness of beef farming in Rio Grande do Sul State, Brazil. *Agricultural Systems*, 104 9, 689-693.

Masters, D.; Edwards, N.; Sillence, M.; Avery, A.; Revell, D.; Friend, M.; Sanford, P.; Saul, G.; Beverly, C. & Youg, J. (2006). The role of livestock in the management of dryland salinity. *Australian Journal of Experimental Agriculture, 46 7*, 733-741.

McManus C.; Paiva S. & Araujo R. O. (2010). Genetics and breeding of sheep in Brazil. *Revista Brasileira de Zootecnia, 39 (supl. especial)*, 236-246.

McManus, C..; Abreu, U. G. P.; Lara, M. A. C. & Sereno J. R. B. (2002). Genetic and environmental factors which influence weight and reproduction parameters in Pantaneiro cattle in Brazil. *Archivos de Zootecnia, 51 194*, 91-97.

McManus, C.; Louvandini, H.; Paiva, S. R.; Oliveira, A. A.; Azevedo, H. C. & Melo, C. B. (2009b). Genetic factors of sheep affecting gastrointestinal parasite infections in the Distrito Federal, Brazil. *Veterinary Parasitology, 166 3-4*, 308-313.

McManus, C.; Paludo, G. R.; Louvandini, H.; Gugel, R.; Sasaki, L. S. B. & Paiva, S.R. (2009c). *Heat tolerance in Brazilian sheep: physiological and blood parameters. Tropical Animal Health and Production, 41 1*, 95-101.

McManus, C.; Prescott, E.; Paludo, G. R.; Bianchini, E.; Louvandini, H. & Mariante, A. S. (2009a). Heat tolerance in naturalized Brazilian cattle breeds. *Livestock Science, 120 3*, 256–264.

McManus, C.; Castanheira, M.; Paiva, S. R.; Louvandini, H.; Fioravanti, M.C.; Paludo, G. R.; Bianchini, E. & Corrêa, P. S. (2011). Use of multivariate analyses for determining heat tolerance in Brazilian cattle. *Tropical Animal Health and Production, 43 3*, 623-630.

Miller, J. C. & Monge, L. (1946). Body temperature and respiration rate and their relation to adaptability in sheep. *Journal of Animal Science, 5 2*, 147-153.

Mirkena, T.; Duguma, G.; Haile, A.; Tibbo, M.; Okeyo, A. M.; Wurzinger, M. & Sölkner J. (2010). Genetics of adaptation in domestic farm animals: a review. *Livestock Science, 132 1-3*, 1-12.

Murphey, R. M.; Paranhos da Costa, M. J. R.; Lima, L. O. S. & Duarte, F. A. M. (1991). Communal suckling in water buffalo (Bubalus bubalis). *Applied Animimal Behaviour Science, 28 4*, 341–352.

Murphey, R. M.; Paranhos da Costa, M. J. R.; Silva, R. G. & Souza, R. C. (1995). Allonursing in river buffalo, Bubalus bubalis: nepotism, incompetence or thievery? *Animal Behaviour, 49 6,* 1611–1616.

Mysterud, A. (2010). Still walking on the wild side? Management actions as steps towards 'semi-domestication' of hunted ungulates. *Journal of Applied Ecology, 47 4,* 920–925.

Ndlovu, T.; Chimonyo, M. & Muchenje, V. (2008). Monthly changes in body condition scores and internal parasite prevalence in Nguni, Bonsmara and Angus steers raised on sweetveld. *Tropical Animal Health and Production,* 41 7, 1169–1177.

Nkrumah, J. D.; Okine, E. K.; Mathison, G. W.; Schmid, K.; Li, C.; Basarab, J. A.; Price, M. A.; Wang, Z. & Moore, S. S. (2006). Relationships of feedlot efficiency, performance and feeding behaviour with metabolic rate, methane production, and energy partitioning in beef cattle. *Journal of Animal Science, 84 1,* 145–153.

O′Neill, C. J; Swain, D. L & Kadarmideen, H. N. (2010). Evolutionary process of *Bos taurus* cattle in favourable versus unfavourable environments and its implications for genetic selection. *Evolutionary Applications, 3 5-6,* 422-433.

O'Kelly, J.C. (1980). Parasitism and blood composition in genetically different types of cattle grazing in a tropical *environment. Veterinary Parasitology, 6 4,* 381–390

OIE. Report of the Meeting of the OIE Scientific. Commission for Animal Diseases. 2008. Available from: http://www.oie.int/downld/SC/ 2008/A_SCAD_feb2008.pdf.

Olson, T. A.; Lucena, C.; Chase Jr, C. C. & Hammond, A. C. (2003). Evidence of a major gene influencing hair length and heat tolerance in Bos taurus cattle. *Journal of Animal Science, 81 1,* 80-90.

Olwoch, J. M.; Reyersb, B. & van Jaarsveldt, A. S. (2009). Host–parasite distribution patterns under simulated climate: implications for tick-borne diseases. *International Journal of Climatology, 29 7,* 993–1000.

Osaki, S. C.; Vidotto, O.; Marana, E. R. M.; Vidotto, M. C.; Yoshihara, E.; Pacheco, R. C.; Igarashi, M. & Minho, A. P. (2002). Ocorrência de anticorpos anti-*Babesia bovis* e estudo sobre a infecção natural em bovinos da raça Nelore, na região de Umuarama, Paraná, Brasil. *Revista Brasileira de Parasitologia Veterinária, 11 2,*77-83.

Ouellet, J. -P.; Crête, M.; Maltais, J.; Pelletier, C. & Huot, J. *(*2001*).* Emergency feeding of white-tailed deer: test of three feeds. *Journal of Wildlife Management, 65 1,* 129–136.

Packer C.; Lewis S. & Pusey A. (1992). A comparative analysis of non-offspring nursing. *Animal Behaviour, 43 2,* 265-281

Paranhos da Costa, M. J. R.; Albuquerque, L. G.; Eler, J. P.; Silva, J. A. II. V., 2006, Suckling behaviour of Nelore, Gir and Caracu calves and their crosses. *Applied Animal Behaviour Science, 101 3,* 276–287.

Pegram, R. G.; Lemche, J. & Chizyuka, H. G. B. (1989). Effect of tick control on live weight gain of cattle in central Zambia. *Medical and Veterinary Entomology, 3 3,* 313–320.

Peña, M. T.; Miller, J. E.; Wyatt, W. & Kearney, M. T. (2000). Differences in susceptibility to gastrointestinal nematode infection between Angus and Brangus cattle in South Louisiana. *Veterinary Parasitology, 89 1-2,* 51–61

Pereira, P. R.; Barcellos, J. O. J.; Federizzi, L. C.; Lampert, V. N.; Canozzi, M.E.A.; Marques, P. R. (2011). Advantages and challenges for Brazilian export of frozen beef. *Revista Brasileira de Zootecnia / Brazilian Journal of Animal Science,* 40, 200-209.

Polley, L. & Thompson, R. C. A. (2009). Parasite zoonoses and climate change: molecular tools for tracking shifting boundaries. *Trends in Parasitology, 25 6,* 285-291.

Prayaga, K. C. & Henshall, J. M. (2005). Adaptability in tropical beef cattle: genetic parameters of growth, adaptive and temperament traits in a crossbred population. *Australian Journal of Experimental Agriculture, 45 8,* 971-983.

Prayaga, K. C. (2004). Evaluation of beef cattle genotypes and estimation of direct and maternal genetic effects in a tropical environment. 3. Fertility and calf survival traits. *Australian Journal of Agricultural Research, 55 8,* 811–824.

Primo, A. T. (1992). El ganado bovino ibérico en las américas 500 anõs despues. *Archivos de Zootecnia, 41 154,* 421-432.

Primo, A. T. (2004). *América: conquista e colonização: a fantástica história dos conquistadores ibéricos e seus animais na era dos descobrimentos.* Porto Alegre: Movimento.

Pryce, J. E; Royalb, M. D; Garnsworthy, P. C & Mao, I. L (2004). Fertility in the high-producing dairy cow. *Livestock Production Science, 86 1-3,* 125–135.

Råberg, L.; Graham, A. L. & Read, A. F. (2009). Decomposing health: tolerance and resistance to parasites in animals. *Philosophical Transactions of the Royal Society of London, Series B, 12 364,* 37-49.

Rajala-Schultz P. J & Frazer G. S. (2003). Reproductive performance in Ohio dairy herds in the 1990s. *Animal Reproduction Science, 76 3-4,* 127-142.

Rausher M. D. (2001). Co-evolution and plant resistance to natural enemies. *Nature, 411,* 857–864.

Rauw W. M.; Kanis E.; Noordhuizen-Stassen, E. N. & Grommers F. J. (1998). Undesirable side effects of selection for high production efficiency in farm animals: a review. *Livestock Production Science, 56 1,* 15-33.

Rocha, L. P.; Fraga, A. B.; Araújo Filho, J. T.; Figueira, R. F.; Pacheco, K. M. G.; Silva, F. L. & Rodrigues, D. S. (2009). Desempenho de cordeiros cruzados em Alagoas, Brasil. *Archivos de Zootecnia, 58 221,* 145-148.

Rodenburg, T. B.; Bijma, P.; Ellen, E. D; Bergsma, R.; de Vries, S.; Bolhuis, J. E.; Kemp, B. & van Arendonk J. A. M (2010). Breeding amiable animals? Improving farm animal welfare by including social effects in breeding programmes. *Animal Welfare, 19 suppl. 1,* 77–82

Rolshausen, G.; Segelbacher, G.; Hobson, K. A. & Schaefer, H. M. *(2009).* Contemporary evolution of reproductive isolation and phenotypic divergence in sympatry along a migratory divide. *Current Biology, 19 24,* 2097-2101.

Romanini, C. .B., Nääs, I.D.A., D'Alessandro Salgado, D. Lima, K.A.O., do Valle, M.M., Labigalini, M.R., de Souza, S.R.L., Menezes, A.G., de Moura D.J. (2008) Impact of Global Warming on Brazilian Beef Production, Livestock Environment VIII, Iguassu Falls, Brazil 701P0408

Roulin, A. (2002). Why do lactating females nurse alien offspring? A review of hypotheses and empirical evidence. *Animal Behaviour, 63 2,* 201-208.

Sahlsten, J.; Bunnefeld, N.; Månsson, J.; Ericsson, G.; Bergström, R. & Dettki, H. *(2010).* Can supplementary feeding be used to redistribute moose? *Wildlife Biology, 16 1,* 85–92.

Sajid, S. M.; Iqbal, Z.; Khan, M. N.; Muhammad, G. & Khan, M. K. (2009). Prevalence and associated risk factors for bovine tick infestation in two districts of lower Punjab, Pakistan. *Preeventive Veterinary Medicine, 92 4,* 386–391.

Samoré A. B.; Groen A. F.; Boettcher P. J.; Jamrozik J.; Canavesi F. & Bagnato A. (2008). Genetic correlation patterns between somatic cell score and protein yield in the Italian Holstein Friesian population. *Journal of Dairy Science, 91 4*, 4013-4021.

Sato, S.; Woodgush, D. G. M. & Wetherill, G. (1987). Observations on creche behavior in suckler calves. *Behavioural Processes,* 15, 333-343.

Schmidt, K. T. & Hoi, H. *(2002)* Supplemental feeding reduces natural selection in juvenile red deer. *Ecography, 25 3,* 265–272.

Scholtz, M.M. (1988) Selection possibilities for hardy beef breeds in Africa: The Nguni example. In: Proceedings of 3rd World Congress on Sheep and Beef Cattle Breeding, 2, 303-319.

Scholtz, M. M.; Furstenburg, D.; Maiwashe, A.; Makgahlela, M. L.; Theron, H. E. & van der Westhuizen, J. (2010). Environmental-genotype responses in livestock to global warming: A Southern African perspective. *South African Journal of Animal Science, 40 5,* 408-413.

Scholtz, M. M.; McManus, C., Okeyo, A. M.& Theunissen, A. (2011). Opportunities for beef production in developing countries of the southern hemisphere. *Livestock Science,* 142: 195 - 201.

Scholtz, M. M., Steyn, Y., Van Marle-Koster, E. & Theron, H. E. (2012). Improved production efficiency in cattle to reduce their carbon footprint for beef production. *South African Journal of Animal Science, 42 5, 450 – 453.*

Silva, R. G. (2000). Introdução a bioclimatologia animal. São Paulo: FAPESP/Nobel.

Solorio-Rivera, J. L. & Rodriguez-Vivas, R. I. (1997). Epidemiologia de la babesiosis bovina. I. Componentes epidemiológicos. *Revista Biomédica, 8 1,* 37-47.

Souza, A. P.; Surkamp, V.; Bellato, V.; Sartor, A. A. & Farias, L. M. (2002). Prevalência de anticorpos anti-Babesia em bovinos no planalto Norte de Santa Catarina. *Revista Ciência Agroveterinária,1 1,* 21-23.

Souza, E. A.; Andrea, M. V.; Santos, C. S.; Paranhos da Costa, M. J. R.; Bittencourt, T. C. B. S. C. & Marcondes, C. R. (2009). Relações materno-filiais e sua influência no peso pré-desmama de animais Nelore da Bahia. *Archivos de Zootecnia, 58 224,* 729-732.

Summers, B. A. (2009). Climate change and animal disease. *Veterinary Pathology, 46 6,* 1185–1186.

Tabachnick, W. J. (2010). Challenges in predicting climate and environmental effects on vector-borne disease episystems in a changing world. The *Journal of Experimental Biology, 213 6,* 946-954.

Taberlet, P.; Valentini, A.; Rezaei, H. R.; Naderi, S.; Pompanon, F.; Negrini, R. & Ajmone-Marsan, P. (2008). Are cattle, sheep, and goats endangered species? *Molecular Ecology, 17 1,* 275–284, 2008.

Tsuruta S.; Misztal, I. & Lawlor T. J. (2005). Changing the definition of productive life in US Holsteins: effect on genetic correlations. *Journal of Dairy Science, 88 3,* 1156–1165.

van Beest, F.; Loe, L. E.; Mysterud, A. & Milner, J. M. *(2010).* Comparative space use and habitat selection of moose around feeding stations. *Journal of Wildlife Management, 74 2,* 219–227.

Veerkamp R. F.; Beerda B. & van der Lende T. (2003). Effects of genetic selection for milk yield on energy balance, levels of hormones, and metabolites in lactating cattle, and possible links to reduced fertility. *Livestock Production Science, 83 2,* 257–275

Víchová, J. & Barto□, L. (2005). Allosuckling in cattle: gain or compensation? *Applied Animal Behaviour Science, 94 3,* 223–235.

Vitale, A. F.; Tenucci, M.; Papini, M. & Lovari, S. (1986). Social behaviour of the calves of semi-wild Maremma cattle, *Bos primigenius Taurus. Applied Animal Behaviour Science, 16 3,* 217-231.

von Keyserlingk, M. A. G.; Weary, D. M. (2007). Maternal behavior in cattle. *Hormones amd Behavior, 52 1,* 106-113.

Wall, E.; Simm, G. & Moran, D. (2009). Developing breeding schemes to assist mitigation of greenhouse gas emissions. *Animal, 4 3,* 366-376.

Washburn S. P.; Silvia W. J.; Brown C. H.; McDaniel B. T. & McAllister, A. J. (2002). Trends in reproductive performance in Southeastern Holstein and Jersey DHI herds. *Journal of Dairy Science, 85 1,* 244-251.

Wathes D. C.; Brickell, J. S.; Bourne, N. E.; Swali, A. & Cheng, Z. (2008). Factors influencing heifer survival and fertility on commercial dairy farms. *Animal, 2 8,* 1135-1143.

Wilson, W. C.; Mecham, J. O.; Schmidtmann, E.; Jimenezsanchez, C.; Herrero M. & Lager, I. Current status of bluetongue virus in the Americas. 2009. Available from: http://ddr.nal.usda.gov/dspace/bitstream/10113/ 23231/1/IND44152599.pdf.

Woolhouse M. E. J.; Webster J. P.; Domingo E.; Charlesworth, B. & Levin, B. R. (2002). Biological and biomedical implications of the co-evolution of pathogens and their hosts. *Nature Genetics, 32,* 569–577.

In: Cattle: Domestication, Diseases and the Environment   ISBN: 978-1-62417-820-7
Editor: George Liu   © 2013 Nova Science Publishers, Inc.

Chapter 10

NATIVE CATTLE GENETIC RESOURCES IN CHINA

Dongxiao Sun[1], Yali Hou[2]*, Qin Chu[3], Yi Zhang[1] and Yuan Zhang[1]*

[1]College of Animal Science and Technology, China Agricultural University
[2]Beijing Institute of Genomics, Chinese Academy of Sciences
[3]Institute of Animal Husbandry and Veterinary Medicine,
Beijing Academy of Agriculture and Forestry Sciences

ABSTRACT

China has abundant cattle breed resources, including 92 local breeds, 9 developed and 13 introduced breeds. The local breeds are comprised of Chinese Yellow cattle, water buffalo, Yak, as well as Gayal. Chinese Yellow cattle are the major breeds with high genetic divergence, and can be categorized into Northern group (*Bos taurus* like Yanbian), Southern group (*Bos indicus* like Zhaotong) and Central group (*Bos taurus* and *indicus*, like Qinchuan, Nanyang, Jinnan, Luxi) with the Yellow River, the Qinling mountain and Yangtze River as boundaries. Water buffalo in China are mostly swamp rather than river type, consisted of two clades from *Yangtze Valley* and the *South of China* respectively, present three divergent mitochondrial DNA lineages (A, B1 and B2). There are also multiple introduced breeds mainly for the breed improvement purpose. Chinese Holstein is the most dominant dairy cattle (approximately 80%), which has the most complete genetic improvement system for the last 30 years, including breed registration, dairy herd improvement, progeny testing, genetic evaluation, and recently genomic selection.

Keywords: Chinese, cattle, buffalo, genetic resource, Chinese Holstein, genetic improvement

---

* Corresponding authors: Dongxiao Sun, Yali Hou.

1. GENERAL INTRODUCTION ON CATTLE BREEDS IN CHINA

China has abundant cattle breed resources. According to the survey results in 2010 (Genetic resources of cattle in China, 2011), there are 114 cattle breeds in China, composed of 92 local breeds, 9 developed and 13 introduced breeds. 92 local breeds were grouped into 53 Chinese Yellow cattle breeds, 26 water buffalo breeds, 12 Yak breeds, as well as Gayal. Developed breeds include 8 *Bos taurus* and one Yak breeds. Introduced breeds have 10 *Bos taurus*, 2 water buffalo and one *Bos indicus* breeds. According to their usages, Chinese cattle are categorized into beef cattle, dairy cattle, and dual-purpose cattle. Chinese Yellow cattle are the major resources of beef cattle, out of which, there are five famous breeds named as Qinchuan, Nanyang, Luxi, Jinnan and Yanbian. Chinese Holstein was developed from cross-breeding between Chinese Yellow cattle and European Holstein over the past 100 years. It is the most dominant dairy cattle (approximately 80%), which has the most complete genetic improvement system for the last 30 years, including key procedures such as breed registering, dairy herd improvement, progeny testing, and genetic evaluation, and achieved substantial progresses. Furthermore, Chinese Simmental, Xinjiang Brown, Chinese Grassland Red, Mongolian Sanhe constitute the majority of dual-purpose cattle. Majority of Chinese buffalo are draft and beef purpose and few of them are dairy type. Yaks (*Bos grunniens* or *Bos mutus*) are produced in the high frigid region above the altitude of over 3000 m in the Qinghai-Tibetan Plateau and have the features of multi-purpose of milk, meat and hair production, and pack transportation. Gayal or mithun (*Bos frontalis*) in China is the domesticated form of the gaur. It is a very rare semi-wild and semi-domestic bovine species. There still exist debates on Gayal's origin and taxonomic status. Besides them, there is a certain degree of introduced breeds, including Simmental originated from German and France respectively, Jersey, Shorthorn, Hereford, Charolais, Piemontese, South Devon, Limousin, Angus, German Yellow, Belgian Blue-White, Brahman, Murray Grey. Until 2010, there are 12.60 million heads of dairy cattle registered, 80 million heads of beef cattle, 22.75 million heads of buffalo, as well as 14 million heads of Yak. This Chapter will focus on Chinese native Yellow cattle, Chinese Swamp water buffalo and Chinese Holstein, summarizing the aspects of genetic resources and existing genetic improvement programs.

2. GENETIC RESOURCES OF CHINESE YELLOW CATTLE

Chinese Yellow cattle is the major Chinese native cattle breed, which is famous for its advantageous characteristics of high meat quality, great ability of roughage-resistance and stress resistance, constituting one of the precious cattle resources worldwide. Compared to Chinese Holstein, genetic origination and divergence of Chinese Yellow cattle still remains elusive. Several groups have analyzed the genetic structure and relationship of Chinese Yellow cattle based on the summary data from skull classification, coat color, blood protein polymorphisms, body stature, ecological characters, chromosome group, microsatellite, mtDNA, and archaeological discoveries. For example, Chen et al. (2001) found that Chinese cattle breeds derive from two major origins. One was *Bos taurus*, including turino mongolian in the regions outside of the Great Wall and draft taurine on the Qinghai Tibet plateau. The other origin was *Bos indicus*, of which there were three influences. The first was the

Africander type from West Asia, like Nanyang cattle; the second was an indicus origin, influencing Yunnan humped cattle; and the third was Southeast Asian in origin, which was supposedly the result of crosses between *Bibos banteng* and local high hump cattle. Geographically, Chinese Yellow cattle can be roughly classified into three groups (Chen et al, 2001): Northern group (Mongolian group, such as Yanbian, Mongolian et al), Central group (Huanghe and Huaihai group, like Qinchuan, Jinnan, Luxi, Nanyang, Jiaxian et al) and Southern group (Changjiang and Zhujiang group, including Xizhen, Xuanhan, Ebian, Wenling, Wenshan, Hainan et al.) (Figure 1).

It is showed that there is controversy in the breed geographical category, like Nanyang and Luxi, which were recommended to be grouped into Southern group by Lei et al (2000). In our chapter, we treat them still as Central group as tradition. It is remarkable to note that breed morphologies closely correlate with geographical locations in this three-group classification system. Interestingly, two ecological systems (the Yangzte River and Qinling Mountains along the Yellow River) separate three groups. For example, humpless cattle are mainly from Northern group, including the Mongolian breed and their derived breeds, and Tibetan draft cattle. The Nanyang breed, a low humped cattle in Central group, is obviously influenced by the Africander type. When this form breeds with others, the resulting forms have a well developed chest dewlap and folds. High humped cattle breeds in Southern group especially in Southeast region have chest dewlaps with poorly developed fold and without an abdominal dewlap.

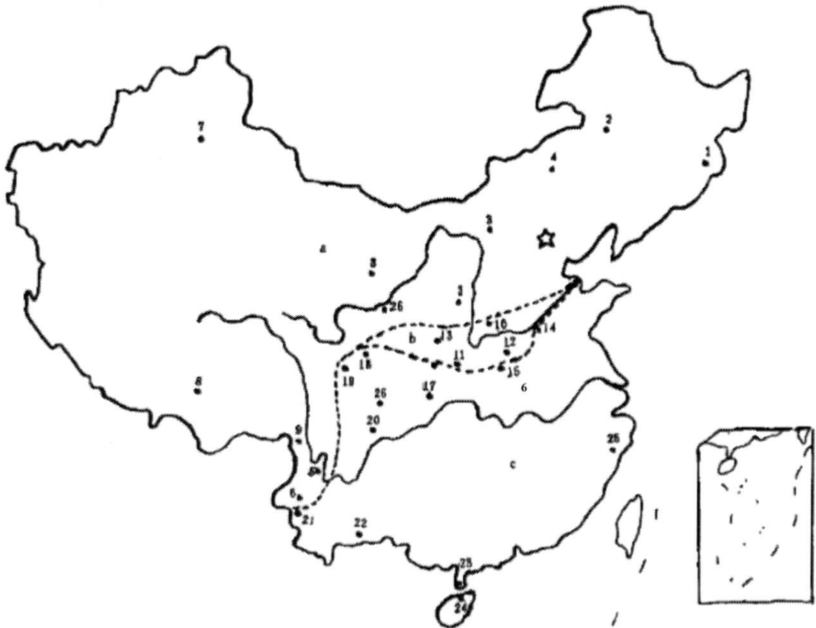

Figure 1. Distribution map of 26 yellow cattle breeds in China (cited from Lei et al., 2000). a. Northern group; b. Central group; c. Southern group. a, b, c were separated by Y chromosomes morphologies by Lei et al (2000). 1. Yanbian cattle; 2. Horqin cattle; 3. Mongolian cattle; 4. Wuzhumuqin cattle; 5. Diqing cattle; 6. Lijiang cattle; 7. Xinjiang brown; 8. Tibetan cattle; 9. Gayal; 10. Jinnan cattle; 11. Lingnan cattle; 12. Jiaxian red cattle; 13. Qinchuan cattle; 14. Luxi Cattle; 15. Nanyang cattle; 16. Xizhen cattle; 17. Xuanhan cattle; 18. Pingwu cattle; 19. Sanjiang cattle; 20. Ebian cattle; 21. Yunnan hump cattle; 22. Wenshan cattle; 23. Xuwen cattle; 24. Hainan cattle; 25. Wenling hump cattle; 26. Chinese Black-and-White cattle.

Normally, higher heterogeneity was detected in Central group than in both Northern and Southern groups. Chen et al also illustrated some obvious distinctions between Chinese Zebu and Indian Zebu breeds (Chen et al, 2001). However, with the introduction of foreign advanced cattle breeds in the forms of frozen semen and embryo, as well as the gradually decreases of profit of native cattle industry, there is accelerating the loss of local cattle genotypes. A few Chinese indigenous Yellow cattle breeds are becoming extinct, such as Zhoushan, Fuzhou, Pinglu, and other breeds while several breeds including Dengchuan, Tangjiao and Jinan breeds have already been extinguished (Chen et al, 2001). Facing such a severe situation, it is urgent to investigate and conserve Chinese Yellow cattle genetic resources. Interestingly, different Y chromosome morphologies exist between *Bos taurus* and *Bos Indicus*. *Bos taurus* usually has metacentric Y chromosomes while *Bos indicus* has acrocentric Y chromosomes. By using chromosome G-, C-, RBA-banding analyses, Yu et al. (1993) surveyed the Y chromosome polymorphisms using 119 individuals of nine local breeds of Chinese Yellow cattle, concluded that Y chromosome polymorphism was related to the classification and origin of Chinese Yellow cattle to some extent.

The Northern humpless taurus breeds like Mongolia and Yunbian, have submetacentric and metacentric Y chromosomes. The humped breeds such as Xizhen, Luxi, Nanyang and Wenling, have telocentric (Xizhen) and acrocentric Y chromosomes. Out of them, Nanyang and Luxi are located in the central region but on its southeast edge, while Xizhen and Wenling belonged to Southern group. Within Central groups, three types of Y chromosomes (metacentric, submetacentric, and acrocentric) were identified in cattle like Qinchuan, Jinnan, and Jiaxian. These results supported the hypothesis that besides Mongolia breed which had submetacentric Y chromosome, there was probably another ancestral humpless cattle breed which possessed metacentric Y chromosome, later on, this ancestor was pointed out as draft taurine on the Qinghai Tibet plateau by Chen et al (2001). The Northern Chinese Yellow cattle were originated from *Bos taurus*; the Southern cattle were influenced by *Bos indicus*; and the Central cattle were formed as the consequence of both *Bos taurus* and *indicus*. In addition, the differentiation of humped cattle had already occurred in the wild ancestors of Chinese Zebu living in ancient China. Later, Lei et al (2000) extended this technique to a larger group including 26 Chinese local breeds, reached a similar conclusion with a few exceptions. Furthermore, based on counting a genetic marker (AgNORs, Silver-staining in nucleolar organizer regions), Chen et al (1994) analyzed 40 individuals from 4 local cattle breeds (Mongolia, Qingchuan, Lingnan and Xizhen), obtained the same conclusion as those derived by Y chromosome morphologies.

3. GENETIC DIVERSITY OF CHINESE YELLOW CATTLE BASED ON MICROSATELLITE MARKERS

Microsatellite markers are a valuable tool to investigate the genetic structure in different populations due to their large polymorphisms. By using 12 microsatellite DNA markers (BM1824, HEL5, SPS115, TGLA122, TGLA126, TGLA53, BM1818, ETH185, HEL13, ILSTS054, MM12, TGLA227; http://www.fao.org) recommended by the Food and Agriculture Organization of the United Nations (FAO) and the International Society of Animal Genetics (ISAG), Li et al. (2007) investigated the genetic diversity of 9 Chinese native cattle breeds (Yanbian, Changbai, Enshi, Liping, Jiaxian, Zaosheng, Zhaotong, Pinglu, Chuannan) and 3 introduced breeds (Simmental, Charolais and Germany Yellow). For each breed, approximately 60 typical unrelated individuals were sampled. After generating the PCR products, they detected all the products by using ABI3100-Avant auto gene sequenator, and genotyped them using GeneMapper Version3.2. They further calculated the allele frequencies and heterozygosity (H) for each breed at the 12 microsatellite locus by using GENEPOP, inferred polymorphism information content (PIC) according to the algorithm derived by Botstein et al (1980), as well as Nei's standard genetic distance (D_S) and Nei's genetic distances (D_A) by using DISPAN. They found Chinese local breeds had more allele numbers (8.42~10.58), higher H (0.712~0.827) and PIC (0.67~0.80) than introduced breeds (allele number: 7.00~7.75, H: 0.661~0.696, PIC: 0.61~0.66).

The Northern breeds like Yanbian and Changbai possess relatively lower allele number, H and PIC, while the Central breeds have the highest H and PIC, especially the Jiaxian breed. These results indicate Chinese Yellow cattle has abundant genetic diversity and higher heterogeneity compared to introduced breeds. Although the Northern breeds like Yanbian and Changbai went through certain extent of selection and inbreed, the Central breeds show highest heterogeneity, consistent with the fact that the Central breeds are impacted by both *Bos taurus* and *Bos indicus*. Based on the calculated D_A between each breed, cluster analysis was performed by using UPGMA method. They clustered the 12 breeds into four groups (Figure 2). The first group includes the Southern cattle breeds such as Enshi, Liping, Zhaotong and Chuannan; the second group embraces the Central cattle breeds like Jiaxian and Zaosheng, Pinglu; the third group covers the Northern cattle breeds including Yanbian and Changbai, which presents the lowest D_A; and the fourth group consists of foreign breeds including Germany Yellow, Simmental and Charolais. In addition, the Central breeds were clustered firstly with the Southern breeds and then both of them were clustered with the Northern breeds, suggesting that the Central breeds are more influenced by *Bos indicus* than by *Bos taurus*. These results clearly support the conclusions derived in the previous studies as described above.

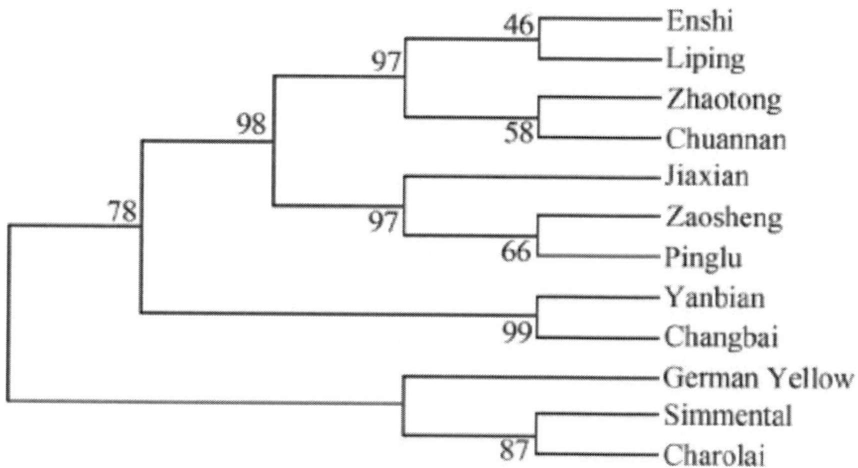

Figure 2. UPGMA/D_A dendrogram of 12 cattle breeds.

4. GENETIC DIVERSITY OF CHINESE YELLOW CATTLE BASED ON MITOCHONDRIAL DNA

Mitochondrial DNA (mtDNA) can be used to study cattle's maternal origin, evolution and genetic diversity. In mtDNA, the D-loop region is 5~10 times more variable than the other regions, making it an ideal marker. Jia et al (2007) sequenced the 910bp PCR-products of the mtDNA D-loop regions from 123 individuals in 12 Chinese cattle breeds (Enshi from Hubei, Wenling from Zhejiang, Dabieshan from Anhui, Guangfeng from Jiangxi, Longlin, Nandan, Weizhou from Guangxi, Yanjiang from Liaoning, Altay White Head from Xinjiang, Zhaotong from Yunnan, Xigaze Humped, Apeijiaza from Tibet) and two individuals in Germany Yellow cattle breed respectively. After sequences alignment and editing by using Mega3.1 and DnaSP4.0, they detected 93 variations and 57 haplotypes, derived average number of nucleotide difference as 22.708, nucleotide diversity (π) as 0.0251 ± 0.00479, and haplotype diversity (H_d) as 0.888 ± 0.026, indicating large genetic diversity in Chinese cattle breeds. Based on the estimated Kimura-2-parameter genetic distances (0~0.049) between these 13 breeds, Neighbor-Joining (NJ) tree was constructed, showing two main clades, corresponding to *Bos taurus* and *Bos indicus*, as well as one specific clade occupied by the Apeijiaza cattle in Tibet, which could represent some introgression of yak. They identified a specific haplotype which was ubiquitous in almost all Chinese Indicus with the exception of Weining in Guizhou Province, Gaofeng in Yunnan Province, and Tibetan Zebu, which suggests most Chinese Zebu come from only certain number of individuals having this haplotype, and Zebu in Tibet, Guizhou, and Yunnan are distinct from the Chinese Zebu. They also inferred that Yunnan may be the entrance of Indian Zebu into China because Yunnan breeds (Zhaotong and Gaofeng) expressed abundant haplotypes. They emphasized the importance of Tibetan Zebu in the distribution and origin of Chinese Zebu, based on the fact that both Tibetan Zebu (Xigaze Humped cattle and Apeijiaza cattle) accommodated *Bos indicus* haplotypes (35.7% and 50% respectively). This was inconsistent with the conclusion derived by Chen et al (2001) that Tibetan cattle breed was one of Taurine breeds. This discrepancy could be due to the fact that they sampled distinct breeds from Tibet. They further investigated the origin of Tibetan Zebu, and came up with the hypothesis that these two Tibetan Zebu breeds may be affected by Yunnan and Indian Zebu, however, the relationship remained uncertain.

Using the sequences of mtDNA D-loop from European cattle (GenBank Accession No, V00654), Brahman (DQ887761), and Nellore (AY126697) as standards, Zhang et al (2009) studied the same mtDNA D-loop regions as did by Jia et al (2007) in 206 individuals from 16 different Chinese Yellow breeds (Guanling, Wuchuan Black, Weining from Guizhou Province, Diqing and Zhaotong from Yunnan province, Wannan from Anhui province, Ji'an from Jiangxi province, Pinglu from Shanxi province, Sanjiang, Xuanhan, Pingwu, Liangshan, and Chuannan from Sichuan province, Tibetan, Xigaze Humped, and Apeijiaza from Tibet). They corrected and identified the complete D-loop sequencing by using DNAMAN, aligned homologous sequences by using CLUSTALX, determined haplotype number and polymorphisms, constructed the NJ phylogeny tree by using MEGA2.0, calculated H_d, π by DnaSP 4.10.7, clustered haplotypes by using Network 4.2. They identified 101 variations and 99 haplotypes (73 *Bos taurus* haplotype, 26 *Bos indicus* haplotype), calculated the similar values of the average number of nucleotide differences and nucleotide diversity (22.6920 and

0.0227) to Jia et al (2007), and slightly higher haplotype diversity (0.9320), again indicating high genetic diversity in this group of Chinese indigenous cattle. Within them, Guanling, Weining, Zhaotong, Tibetan and Xigaze Humped cattle had the most number of haplotypes of 12, while Ji'an had the least number of 3; Guanling, Xuanhan and Wannan showed the highest genetic variation, while Sanjiang had the least. They proved that Tibetan breed belonged to *Bos taurus* because it did not have the Indicus Haplotype, and it also accommodated large genetic divergences, which supported that Tibetan breed could be the most ancient in China, and has not been impacted by the other breeds. When they defined the mtDNA D-loop sequence of Nellore as H3 haplotype, only 50 out of the 206 individuals had H3 haplotype and only 16% were highly similar to the sequence of Nellore, which supported that Chinese Indicus cattle had their own specific characteristics. For example, Ji'an and Wuchuan Black had the top high proportion of H3 (83.3% and 73.3%). Although Diqing, Xigaze Humped, and Apeijiaza were similar to Indicus, they did not have H3 haplotype. By constructing NJ tree and network of haplotypes, it was illustrated that the *Bos indicus* haplotypes identified in this study overlap with Indian Indicus haplotype (H3) more or less. These haplotypes were categorized into additional 4 groups (H3A, H3D, H3B, and H3K): H3A in Ji'an, Pingwu, Sanjiang, Xuanhan, Chuannan, Wuchuan, Guanling, Zhaotong, Pinglushan, H3D in Wannan, Chuannan, Liangshan, Weining, H3B in Guanling, Wuchuan, Zhaotong, Xuanhan, Ji'an, and H3K in Pingwu and Sanjiang. It was further inferred that *Bos indicus* in China had experienced at least 4 population expansions during their immigrations.

5. GENETIC DIVERSITY OF CHINESE DOMESTIC BUFFALO BASED ON MICROSATELLITE MARKERS

Domestic Asian buffalo (*Bubalus bubalis*) are classified into the swamp type (2n = 48) found in China and Southeast Asia, and river type (2n = 50) in the Indian subcontinent and further west. Archaeological data suggest that swamp buffalo was domesticated in China about 7000 years ago (Chen & Li, 1989). As a draft animal, domestic buffalo are extremely important historically and closely related to agricultural civilization in the Southern China. To study their degree of genetic diversity and differentiation, Zhang et al (2007) examined 30 microsatellite loci in 18 Chinese indigenous swamp buffalo populations: Dehong (DH),Guizhou (GZ), Guizhoubai (GB), Yanjin (YJ), Fuling (FL), Enshi (ES), Jianghan (JH), Haizi (HZ), Shanqu (SQ), Dongliu (DL), Xiajiang (XJ), Fuzhong (FZ), Fu'an (FA), Xinfeng (XF), Xinglong (XG), Xilin (XL), Diandongnan (DD), Dechang (DC) and two introduced river buffalo breeds: Nili-Lavi (NL) and Murrah (MR) (Figure 3). These 30 microsatellite markers were recommended by FAO and ISAG for domestic buffalo diversity studies (Hoffmann et al. 2004). A total of 394 alleles were detected across the 30 microsatellite loci. Total number of allele (TNA) observed at each locus varied from 1 (HMH1R) to 17 (DRB3). Both ILSTS008 and RM099 were polymorphic in swamp but not river buffalo. The locus with the largest mean number of alleles (MNA) was CSSM019 for the swamp (10.3) and CSSM047 for the river (11.0) buffalo, respectively. In total, 37 private alleles (i.e. found in only one population) were identified. They were distributed in 14 populations across 22 loci. The population with the maximum number of private alleles was DH (10), followed by NL (5), MR (3), GB (3), HZ (3), and XF (3).

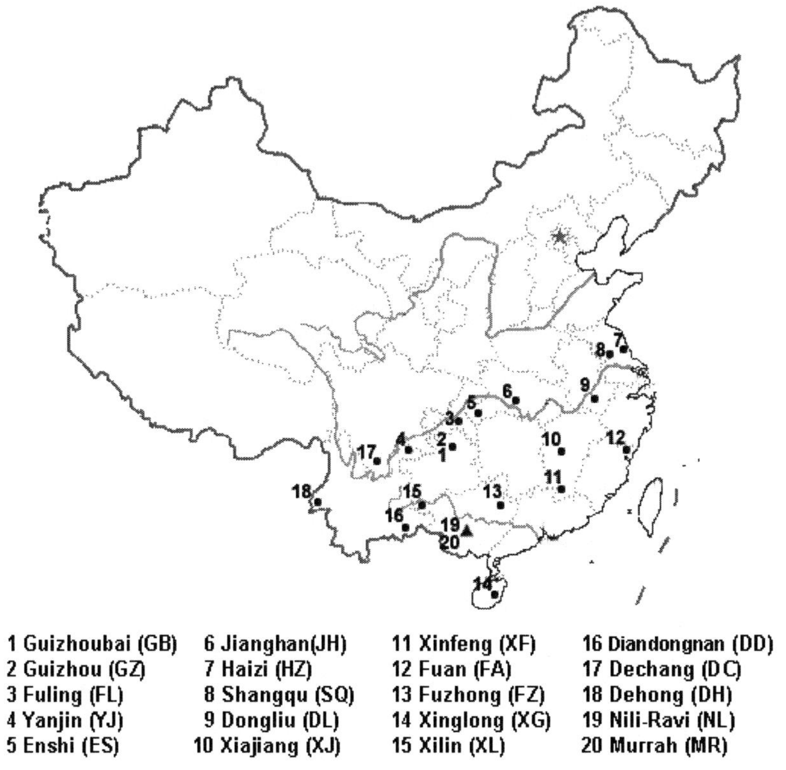

Figure 3. Geographical location of 20 domestic buffalo populations sampled. Abbreviations of populations are given in parentheses (cited from Zhang et al, 2007).

Significant deviations from Hardy-Weinberg Equilibrium (HWE) were observed for 58 population-locus combinations from 600 tests. For all loci examined, the number of deviations ranged from zero (XJ) to six (DH and MR). Among the 30 microsatellites examined, CSSM022 showed the maximum number of 12 populations in disequilibrium due to heterozygote deficiency, which might be attributable to the presence of null alleles. The remained twenty-nine loci gave zero (CSSM041, BRN, CSSM008, ILSTS005) to six (DRB3) significant results for HWE test. The MNA varied from 4.17 in the YJ to 6.40 in the DH.

The expected heterozygosity ranged from 0.517 (YJ) to 0.609 (DH). Wilcoxon signed rank tests were conducted to examine the significant differences in the number of alleles and gene diversity between each pair of populations. Of all populations examined, DH had the significant higher genetic variability. DD also had large genetic variability while YJ and FL had low genetic variability. F_{ST} estimates were significantly different from zero for all loci in Chinese buffalos. Values were relatively low and ranged from 0.017 (CSSM036) to 0.039 (CSSM046). There was considerable differentiation (30.24%) between but not within (2.03%) buffalo type. When DH was considered as a unique group from other Chinese local populations, more than the twice genetic variation existed between groups (Dehong / other Chinese buffalo populations) compared to within group; 5.29% vs. 2.10%. All F_{ST} values were significantly different from zero except the three pairs of GZ-GB, JH-GZ, JH-GB. Amongst Chinese local populations, DH had a larger differentiation from the other populations, ranging from 0.046 to 0.086. For river-swamp population pairs, genetic differentiation varied from 0.254 to 0.352.

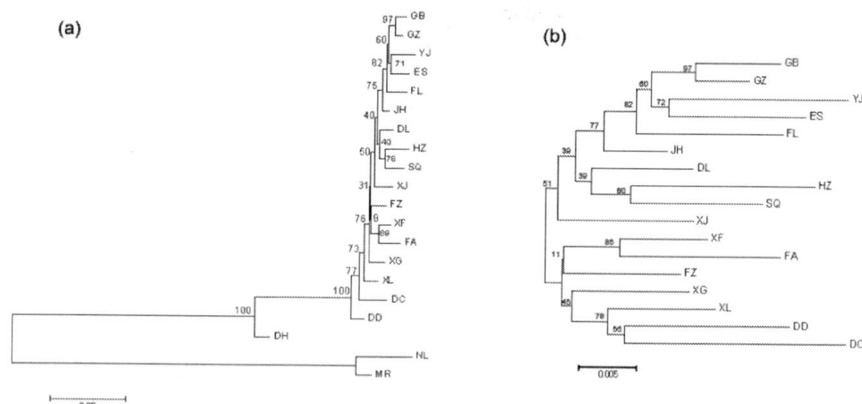

Figure 4. Neighbor-joining (NJ) trees (a) of 18 Chinese indigenous buffalo populations and two introduced river buffalo breeds and (b) of 17 Chinese indigenous buffalo populations without DH.

Correlations between geographical distances and genetic distances were significant regardless if DH was included ($r = 0.572$; $P < 0.0001$) or excluded ($r = 0.545$; $P < 0.0001$). The analysis with DH suffered a large error sum of squares than without it (0.039 vs. 0.011). Due to its genetic admixture nature, DH tended to show relatively higher genetic distance than the other populations when the geographical distances were similar. When DH was excluded, a linear relationship between the geographical and genetic distances emerged for all population pairs except the DC-YJ. A neighbor-joining tree (Figure 4a) was constructed using a D_A genetic distance matrix. The obtained topology was supported by relative high bootstrap values. As expected, the 20 populations are divided into two distinct groups, i.e. swamp and river. Among the 18 Chinese buffalo populations, DH was most divergent from the other 17 populations, which were clustered closely. When two river breeds and DH were excluded from the distances matrix, there was a new clustering tree (Figure 4b) which consisted of two large clusters, the *Yangtze Valley* and the *South of China*. In the *Yangtze Valley* cluster, aside of XJ, there were two sub-clusters, i.e. the *Upper and Middle Reaches of Yangtze* (GZ, GB, YJ, FL, ES, and JH) and the *Lower Reaches of Yangtze* (HZ, SQ, and DL). The *Southern China* cluster was also further divided into two sub-clusters, the *South-China* (FA, XF, FZ) and the *Southwest* (XG, XL, DD, DC). The topology was generally consistent with their geographical distribution.

5. MOLECULAR PHYLOGENY OF CHINESE BUFFALO INFERRED FROM MITOCHONDRIAL CONTROL REGION SEQUENCES

Zhang (2006) also inferred the molecular phylogeny of Chinese buffalo by analyzing the mitochondrial control region sequences (includes the D-loop along with adjacent transcription promoter regions). PCR primers for amplification and sequencing of mtDNA control region (CR) were designed from the published mitochondrial DNA sequence of domestic buffalo (GenBank accession no. AF488491). A total of 100 samples from 18 Chinese indigenous swamp buffalo populations: Dehong (DH),Guizhou (GZ), Yanjin (YJ), Enshi (ES), Jianghan (JH), Haizi (HZ), Shannan (SN), Shanqu (SQ), Dongliu (DL), Xiajiang (XJ), Fuzhong (FZ),

Fu'an (FA), Xinfeng (XF), Xinglong (XG), Xilin (XL), Diandongnan (DD), Dechang (DC), Binhu (BH) and two introduced river buffalo breeds Nili-Lavi (NL) and Murrah (MR), out of which, 18 of them are mentioned above. Five animals in each population were randomly selected for sequencing. Complete mitochondrial CR sequences were determined for 90 Chinese swamp buffalo and 10 river buffalo (GenBank accession no. EF597573-EF597599; EF597600-EF597672). In agreement with Kierstein *et al.* (2004), three single nucleotide repeat regions, displaying length polymorphisms, were observed. One is a poly-G motif located in the left hypervariable segment (HVSI), the others are two adjacent poly-C stretches in the right hypervariable segment (HVSII). Most significantly, the observed G-stretch showed distinct variation patterns for different lineages. Excluding all gaps, comparisons of these sequences revealed 68 polymorphic sites that defined 50 haplotypes, with 45 in swamp buffalo and 5 in river buffalo, respectively. Hap1 exhibited the highest frequency with 28% and was present in all swamp buffalo populations but BH. The haplotype and nucleotide diversity of Chinese buffaloes were 0.898 and 0.016, respectively, slightly higher than those found by Lei *et al.* (2007).

The sequence alignment and the neighbor-joining tree reflected the similar phylogenetic relationship among Chinese mtDNA haplotypes as reported by Lei *et al.* (2007). As expected, strong differentiation was confirmed between Chinese swamp and river buffalo and two divergent mtDNA lineages (A and B) were observed in swamp buffalo, with A predominant (77%). Moreover, lineage B could be subdivided into B1 (11%) and B2 (12%). Results of PCR-RFLP analysis also indicated that the two lineages (A and B) occurred at a similar frequency in all swamp buffalo populations (frequencies of B = 16% ± 7%). The estimated divergence times between observed lineages were as follows: B1 versus B2, 240,000 year ago (YA); A versus B1/B2, 650,000 YA; River versus A/B1/B2, 1,780,000-1,860,000 YA. In order to perform a more complete meta-analysis, we pooled 209 available mtDNA CR sequences of Chinese swamp buffalo, including the sequences determined in this study and those reported by Lei *et al.* (2007) (DQ364160-DQ364189, DQ658051-DQ658139). A total of 79 haplotypes were identified. In the media-joining network (Figure 5), there were 30 mutation steps between A and B, indicating their substantial divergence, and B1 was separated from B2 by 8 mutation steps. Lineage A showed a typical star-like phylogenetic pattern with derived variants surrounding the ancestor. Likewise, both B1 and B2 were characterized as a starburst network in spite of fewer haplotypes included. This kind of evolutionary relationship implies a history of population expansion that is indicative of domestication events (Troy *et al.*, 2001). Additionally, the significantly large negative Fst values support recent demographic growth. Using an estimated mutation rate of approximately one substitution per 11,000 years for the 240bp sequence of mtDNA HVSI in cattle (Troy *et al.*, 2001), we estimated the expansion times for A (6,133 ± 2,086 years), B1 (5,958 ± 2,633 years) and B2 (7,333 ± 3,116 years).

These estimates are in good agreement with the possible domestication time revealed by archeological evidence (7,000 YA) (Chen & Li, 1989). To explore the phylogenetic relationships among domestic buffalo populations in three main geographical regions in Asia, i.e. China, Indian subcontinent and Southeast Asia, an integrated evolutionary network was constructed based on the150-bp sequence of the mtDNA D-loop hypervariable region. In the network (Figure 6), two major kinds of mtDNA haplotypes, which were identified in Chinese swamp buffalo and Indian subcontinent river buffalo respectively, constituted the backbone of the network with marked divergence.

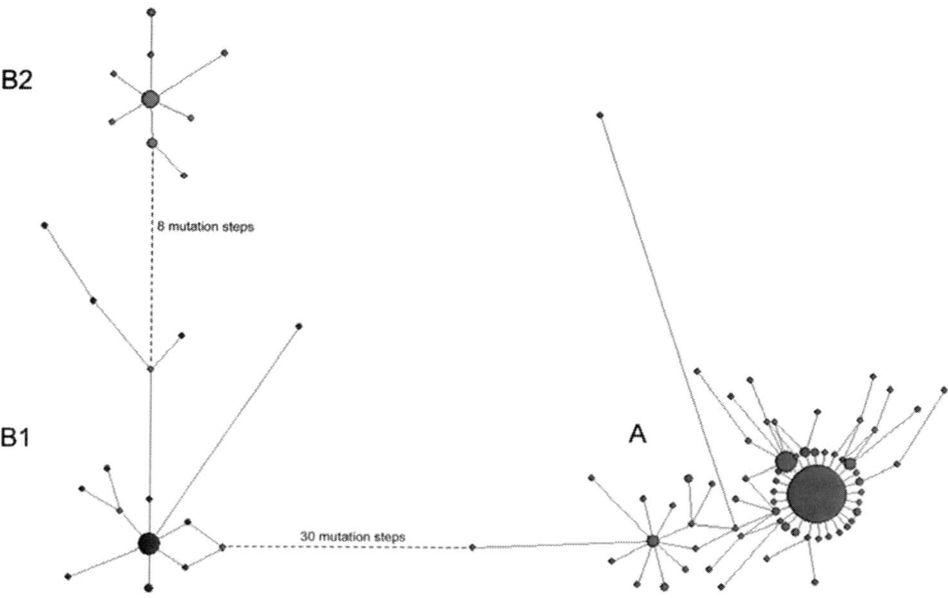

Figure 5. Media-joining network of mtDNA CR sequences in Chinese swamp buffalo. Three mtDNA haplotype groups are A, B1 and B2, respectively. Circle areas are proportional to haplotype frequencies and branch lengths correspond to the number of mutation steps. There are 30 mutation steps between A and B1, and 8 mutation steps between B1 and B2.

Notably, both swamp buffalo from China and river buffalo from the Indian subcontinent show the star-like patterns of haplotypes without much sequence shared between them. The haplotypes from Southeast Asian buffalo were scattered around the network, suggesting all eight swamp populations of Southeast Asia had both maternal ancestries. It is noted that in this pooled data the proportions of swamp and river samples were nearly equal (29:28) and the ratio of A against B (23:6, i.e. 20% of B) was similar to that in Chinese water buffalo (16% ± 7% of B) reported by Zhang et al (2007).

6. Genetic Improvement Program of Chinese Holstein

6.1. Background

Chinese Holstein was developed from cross-breeding between Chinese Yellow cattle and European Holstein over the past 100 years since 1870. Foreign Holstein bulls, embryos and frozen semen have been continuously imported, mainly from USA and a few from Canada and Europe (Sun et al., 2009) , which were directly used in AI or crosses with Chinese Holstein cows through planned mating to generate breeding bulls. It was first recognized as a breed in 1986. Chinese Holstein was used to be called as Chinese Black-and-White cattle and it is now the major breed of dairy cattle in China. Although it is mainly distributed in Northern China, Chinese Holstein cattle are the backbone of dairy cattle herds, accounting for 80% of the total dairy cattle inventory in the nation. Cow milk production makes up over 90% of the gross production of milk in China. The current selection direction of the breeding programs for Chinese Holstein is aimed at higher milk yield and protein percentage while retaining fat percentage.

6.2. Overview of Dairy Bull Progeny Testing in China

For the traditional genetic evaluation based on progeny testing system, most of the developed countries for dairy industry have been using the animal BLUP (best linear unbiased prediction) model to genetically evaluate breeding value of bulls. For example, Canada uses test day model to estimate breeding value since 2004. Similarly in China, multiple traits test-day model has been used to estimate breeding value of milk performance traits and SCS (somatic cell score) of bulls and animal model BLUP for type traits of bulls since 2006. Dairy Association of China (DAC) was founded in 1982.

It had organized several registrations and published 8 Chinese Holstein herd books. In 1992, the association by law, "Regulation of Chinese Holstein Registration", was drafted and approved by Ministry of Agriculture. In 2007, the national breed standard of Chinese Holstein was established. To facilitate progeny test and genetic evaluation, DAC established the data processing center and formally initiated the implementation of breed registration for dairy cattle in China in 2006.

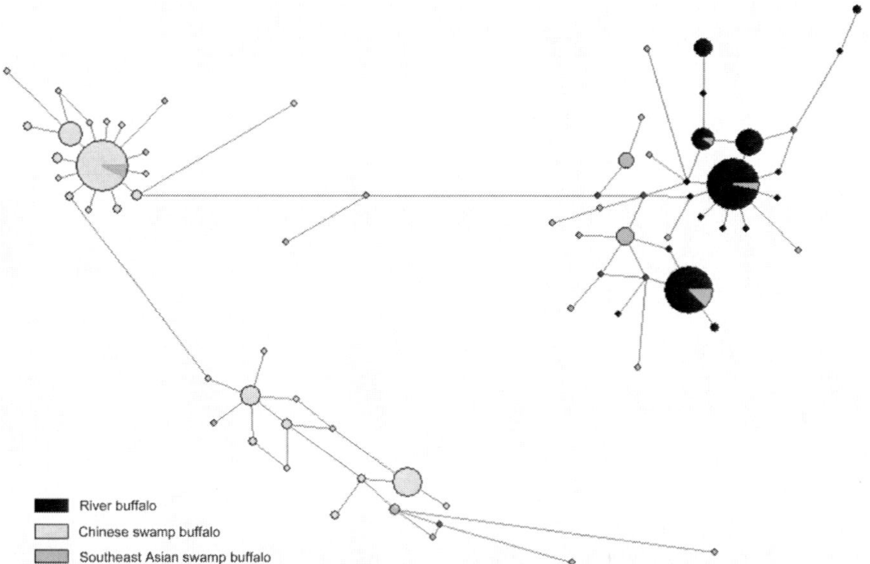

Figure 6. Media-joining network showing genetic relationships among mtDNA control region haplotypes of Chinese swamp buffalo, Southeast Asian swamp buffalo and river buffalo. It was constructed using a 150 bp fragment of the hypervariable region within mtDNA control region (Lau *et al.*, 1998). Circle areas are proportional to haplotype frequencies and branch lengths correspond to the numbers of mutation steps. Color coding indicates to which regional populations the haplotypes belong. Median vectors, representing missing or not sampled haplotypes, are illustrated by red dots. The whole data set included sequences from Chinese buffalo reported by Zhang et al (2007) and Lei *et al.* (2007) (DQ364160-DQ364189, DQ658051-DQ658139), 80 Southeast Asian/Australian buffalo (Lau *et al.*, 1998) (AF016397), 80 Brazilian/Italian river buffalo (Kierstein *et al.*, 2004) (AF197196-AF197223; AY195589-AY195599) and 120 Indian buffalo (AF475159 - AF475278).

In China, the progeny test of dairy bulls, organized by Dairy Association of China (DAC), started at 1983, with two batches were tested annually after 1994. As of December 2011, totally 46 batches of bull (1400 heads) were tested. The numbers of young sires tested annually in the developed dairy countries usually are ~1500 heads in US, 1100 head in France, 600 heads in Canada, 350 head in Netherlands, and 310 head in Italy. Since 1983, DAC started to organize national bull progeny test, and totally 46 batches (1400 bulls) were tested as of 2010.

The total amount of bull tested for the past 28 years in China was similar to those in developed countries for dairy industry in one year. Average number of tested bulls per year was about 120 since 2008. Currently total number of bull held in AI stations was about 2000 in China.

6.3. Overview of Developing Status of Dairy Herd Improvement (DHI) in China

Dairy Herd Improvement (DHI) test started from Shanghai in 1995, supported by Canada-China Integrated Dairy Cattle Breeding Project. Before 2005, only limited amount of performance data was available. There were only few herds of dairy cattle that can participate in progeny test. However, the current performance data has been greatly improved through the continuous effort of DAC. Based on the results of the last tests, the total number of cattle joined DHI test was about 410,000 heads in China at the end of 2010. The system carrying data collection and genetic evaluation has been well established. Multiple trait test day model for milk production traits and multiple trait animal model for type trait was used for sire evaluation.

Also, a defined selection index, i.e. China Performance Index (CPI), has been set up in 2004 and used for sire ranking. In 2009, CPI has been further developed and used in China till now, which includes milk production traits, type, mammary system, foot and leg, SCS. DHI tests and genetic level of bull participating progeny tests needs to be improved. Due to the rapid development of bull population in every AI station, the total amount of bulls participating progeny test was increased. However, due to disease and other reason, importation of elite genetics and live bulls were extremely limited. The pedigree genetic level of bulls that AI station selected for test was therefore affected. This situation decreased the overall genetic level of bulls under tests. In the recent year, with the increase of international exchange and cooperation, dairy breeding system had been improved in some areas in China. With the establishment of the Data processing center of DAC, data collection had been more systematic and efficient (see below). With the Animal Husbandry Act was put into action on July, 1, 2006, AI stations in China paid more attention to and put more emphasize on progeny test.

Currently, there are DHI testing labs located in Beijing, Shanghai, Tianjin, Xi'an, Hangzhou, and etc. The establishment of these testing labs facilitates the development of national DHI testing system, and benefits the national dairy genetic improvement at the same time. Currently with more serious requirement of the milk quality and better integration of the price system in China, more farms are requesting to join the DHI program.

6.4. Identification System and Registration Software System of Chinese Dairy Cattle

The data processing center of DAC is responsible for the breed registration of Chinese Holstein. Internationally most of the developed dairy countries are using a coding system of 12 digits. To facilitate the breed registration, the data processing center of DAC imported the IRIS dairy information management system from Netherlands, and developed its own "Breed Registration System of Chinese Holstein" which can be independently used on farms. This on farm system can easily input and output cattle information. According to the rules for numbering cow from Dairy Association of China, it takes 12 digits, consists of 2 digits codes for the province/city/autonomous region, 4 digits codes for the farm, 2 digits codes for birth year of the animal, and 4 digits codes for the sequential birth order of the animal. By adopting the unified numbering system, it is easier to accurately record and establish the regional central databases. Currently, the data processing center of DAC is focusing on choosing data collection unit in each province, and will soon initiate data collection and assist training local technicians. There are more than 10 million dairy cattle in China according to a recent formal statistics. The establishment of the new ID system and the importation of the IRIS system created the platform of genetic improvement of Chinese dairy cattle. It will improve feed and management of dairy farm and provide reliable evidence, which can assist decision-making of local animal husbandry division. With the application and development of the registration system, the dairy breeding system in China will step into its maturity and brings improvement to the cattle population.

6.5. Genomic Selection Program in China

With two cattle genome assemblies available (Btau_4 and UMD3), the cattle research community has been focusing on single nucleotide polymorphisms (SNPs) as the main source of genetic variation in cattle. This effort led to the multiple SNP genotyping arrays like the Illumina Bovine SNP50, BovineHD, and Affymatrix Bos1 platforms. Based on SNP genotyping assays, Decker et al. (2009) reported resolving the evolution of extant and extinct ruminants with high-throughput phylogenomics. Evaluations of genetic merit based on SNPs became a reality in early 2009 leading to an acceleration of improvements to dairy and beef breed stocks (VanRaden et al., 2009; Wiggans et al., 2009; Hayes et al., 2009). Genomic selection (GS) is a promising marker-assisted selection method, in which high density markers covering the whole genome are selected simultaneously. GS can increase the accuracy of estimated breeding values, decrease the generation interval by selecting individuals at the early stage of life and accelerate genetic progress. With the availability of high density whole genome SNP chips for many species, GS is reshaping the conventional livestock animals, plant and aquaculture genetic evaluation systems.

Study on genomic selection of dairy cattle in China has been conducted by the research team in China Agricultural University (Zhang et al, 2010, 2011), so for, genomic selection technology platform for Chinese Holstein cattle has been successfully established. In this study, a novel GS method was developed, which was named as best linear unbiased prediction with a trait-specific marker-derived relationship matrix (TABLUP). Comparison analysis results showed that, compared with GBLUP method, TABLUP increased the predicting ability. Also, the reference population including 5000 cows from 52 sire families for genomic selection of Chinese Holstein has been established, in which each individual was genotyped with Illumina 50K chip. A preliminary application of GS in Chinese Holstein cattle population was carried out. The marker effects profile and genomic estimated breeding values (GEBV) of five milk performance traits in Chinese Holstein was plotted and predicted, respectively. Results showed that the accuracy of GEBV of three yield traits ranged from 0.6~0.75. By the end of 2011, the technology platform of genomic selection in Chinese Holstein has been well established by China Agricultural University. Base on such platform, genetic evaluation using genomic data (Illumina 50 K chip) for Holstein bulls was first applied to the national genetic improvement program of dairy cattle in China organize by DAC and Ministry of Agriculture, in which a novel selection index, GCPI (Genomic China Performance Index), was set up to combine the traditional EBV and GEBV with different weight.

ACKNOWLEDGMENT

Funding: Natural Science Foundation of China (30901015, 31072016), "948"Project (2006-G48) and National Key Technologies R & D Program (2002BA518A01). We appreciate Dr. George Liu's English editing which significantly improved this chapter.

REFERENCES

Botstein D, White RL, Skolnick M, Davis RW. Construction of a genetic linkage map in man using restriction fragment length polymorphisms. *Am. J. Hum. Genet.*, 1980, 32: 314–331.

Chen H, Qiu H, Zhan T. Studies on genetic relationship between cattle breeds by Ag-NORs. *Journal of Chinese Yellow Cattle*, 1994, 20 (3): 3-11.

Chen Y, Li X. New evidence of the origin and domestication of the Chinese swamp buffalo (*Bubalus bubalis*). *Buffalo J.*, 1989, 1: 51-55.

Chen YC, Cao HH. Diversity of Chinese Yellow cattle breeds and their conservation. *Biondiversity Science*, 2001, 9(3): 275–283.

China Dairy Statistical Summary 2011, *Dairy Association of China.*

China Dairy Yearbook 2006, *China Agriculture Press.*

Decker JE, Pires JC, Conant GC, McKay SD, et al. Resolving the evolution of extant and extinct ruminants with high-throughput phylogenomics. *PNAS*, 2009, 106 (44) : 18644-18649.

Genetic resources of cattle in China, 2011, China Agriculture Press.

Hayes BJ, Bowman PJ, Chamberlain AJ, Goddard ME. Invited review: Genomic selection in dairy cattle: progress and challenges. *J. Dairy Sci.*, 2009, 92:,433–443.

Hoffmann I, Marsan PA, Barker JSF, Cothran EG, Hanotte O, Lenstra JA, Milan D, Weigend S, Simianer H. (2004). New MoDAD marker sets to be used in diversity studies for the major farm animal species: recommendations of a joint ISAG/FAO working group. In: Proc. 29th *International Conference on Animal Genetics*. Tokyo, Japan.

Jia S, Chen H, Zhang G, Wang Z, Lei C, Yao R, Han X. Genetic variation of mitochondrial D-loop region and evolution analysis in some Chinese cattle breeds. *Journal of Genetics and Genomics*, 2007, 34(6): 510-518.

Kierstein G, Vallinoto M, Silva A, Schneider MP, Iannuzzi L, Brenig B. Analysis of mitochondrial D-loop region casts new light on domestic water buffalo (*Bubalus bubalis*) phylogeny. *Molecular Phylogenetics and Evolution*, 2004, 30: 308-24.

Lau CH, Drinkwater RD, Yusoff K, Tan SG, Hetzel DJS, Barker JSF. Genetic diversity of Asian water buffalo (*Bubalus bubalis*): mitochondrial DNA D-loop and cytochrome b sequence variation. *Animal Genetics*, 1998, 29: 253-64.

Lei C, Chen H, Hu S. Studies on Y chromosome polymorphism and the origin and classification of Chinese Yellow cattle. *Acta Agriculturae Boreali-occidentalis Sinica*, 2000, 9(4): 43−47.

Lei C, Zhang W, Chen H, Lu F, Liu R, Yang X, Zhang H, Liu Z, Yao L, Lu Z, Zhao Z. Independent maternal origin of Chinese swamp buffalo (*Bubalus bubalis*). *Animal Genetics*, 2007, 38(2): 97-102.

Li R, Zhang G, Wang Z, Wang H, Han X, Wang D, Wang J. Analysis of the genetic structure of 12 Chinese and foreign cattle breeds using DNA microsatellite markers. *Hereditas,* 2007, 29 (12): 1463-1470.

Sun DX, Jia J, Ma Y, Zhang Y, Wang YC, Yu Y, Zhang Y. Effects of DGAT1 and GHR on milk yield and milk composition in the Chinese dairy population. *Animal Genetics*, 2009, 12: 997-1000.

Troy CS, MacHugh DE, Bailey, JF, Magee DA, Loftus RT, Cunningham P, Chamberlain AT, Sykes BC, Bradley DG. Genetic evidence for Near-Eastern origins of European cattle. *Nature*, 2001, 410: 1088-1091.

VanRaden PM, Van Tassell CP, Wiggans GR, Sonstegard TS, Schnabel RD, Taylor JF. et al. Invited review: reliability of genomic predictions for North American Holstein bulls. *J. Dairy Sci.*, 2009, 92: 16–24.

Wiggans GR, Sonstegard TS, VanRaden PM, Matukumalli LK, Schnabel RD, Taylor JF. et al. Selection of single-nucleotide polymorphisms and quality of genotypes used in genomic evaluation of dairy cattle in the United States and Canada. *J. Dairy Sci.*, 2009, 92: 3431–3436.

Yu R, Xin C, Chen L. Studies on Y chromosome polymorphism and the origin of Chinese Yellow cattle. *Agricultural Sciences in China*, 1993, 26(5): 61-70.

Zhang G, Zheng Y, Wang Z, Han X, Jia S, Chen H. Genetic diversity and origin of mitochondria DNA D-loop region of some Chinese indigenous cattle breeds. *Hereditas*, 2009, 31(2): 160-168.

Zhang Y, Sun D, Yu Y, Zhang Y. Genetic diversity and differentiation of Chinese domestic buffalo based on 30 microsatellite markers. *Animal Genetics*, 2007, 38: 569-575.

Zhang Y. Studies on genetic diversity of Chinese domestic buffalo. PhD thesis. *China Agricultural University*, 2006.

Zhang Z, Liu J, Ding X, Bijma P, Koning D, Zhang Q. Best linear unbiased prediction of genomic breeding values using a trait-specific marker-derived relationship matrix. PLoS ONE, 2010, 5(9): e12648. Zhang Z, Zhang Q, Ding X. Advance in genomic selection in domestic animals. *Chinese Science Bulletin*, 2011, 56 (25): 2655-2663.

In: Cattle: Domestication, Diseases and the Environment
Editor: George Liu

ISBN: 978-1-62417-820-7
© 2013 Nova Science Publishers, Inc.

Chapter 11

ECONOMIC EVALUATION OF PERFORMANCE AND FUNCTIONAL TRAITS IN DUAL-PURPOSE HUNGARIAN FLECKVIEH CATTLE

I. Komlósi[1] and B. Húth[2]
[1]University of Debrecen, Hungary
[2]Hungarian Fleckvieh Association, Hungary

ABSTRACT

A bio-economic model was used to estimate economic values of 14 milk production, functional, growth and carcass traits for Hungarian Fleckvieh (Simmental). The highest relative economic importance was obtained for milk yield (29%), followed by productive lifetime of cows (20%) and daily gain in the rearing period (11%). Other functional traits (calving difficulty score, still birth, total conception rate of heifers, cows and calf mortality) reached a relative economic importance of 15%. Based on these results, the inclusion of productive lifetime and cow fertility in the breeding program for Hungarian Fleckvieh is advisable.

Keywords: Hungarian Fleckvieh, cattle, economic weight, bio-economic model

INTRODUCTION

The cattle sector needs to breed animals that convert the available resources effectively and profitably and bears in mind economic and environmental factors to enhance market-competitiveness. The introduction of the quota system attracted attention on functional traits (Reinsch and Dempfle, 1998; Veerkamp et al., 2002; Vargas et al., 2002; Kulak et al., 2004; Wolfová et al., 2007). Functional traits are the ones associated with both product increase and cost decrease (Groen et al., 1997). Disregarding factors affecting the cow's life performance, such as fertility and health, can result in income decrease. Moreover, it also increases the burden on the environment as well as consumer disapproval of breeding and production conditions (Olesen et al., 2000; Stott et al., 2005). It has become evident that cost reduction and effective farming should be based not only upon continuous production increase (of milk and beef) but also upon healthy cow herds of long productive life (Miesenberger and Fürst, 2003).

As a member of the Mountain Fleckvieh group, the Hungarian Fleckvieh is a dual-purpose breed with good fitness attributes and high milk yield. In 2010, there were 312,000 cows registered in Hungary, out of which 14,800 heads were dual-purpose Hungarian Fleckvieh cows. The members of the group adapt well to extreme environments, ensuring good beef and milk production even during the peak periods. During the past decades the milk production of the Mountain Fleckvieh breed variants increased, while, in the absence of direct selection − fitness traits such as productive life, vitality, and fertility showed slightly unfavourable changes (Füller, 2010).

The first breeding value estimation and selection for functional traits were started in Austria in 1995 for productive life of breeding bulls, which was followed by the other traits in the subsequent years (1998) (Fürst, 2001). As a result, milk yielding traits had a share of 88.2%, beef yielding traits 4.2%, fitness traits 7.6% progress in economic value (Miesenberger and Fürst, 2006).

German and Austrian Mountain Fleckvieh breeders targeted their breeding goals at improving milk protein, fitness and animal health, life performance, while maintaining beef yielding traits. They aimed at functional productive life with 30,000 kg of milk yield. Tischler (2002) highlights that the importance of production traits (milk and beef) and fitness traits in Mountain Fleckvieh breeding programs varies between countries in Europe and overseas, which can be explained by the differences in market and socio-political requirements resulting from the role of the sector. Countries aiming at maximum profit stress the importance of production oriented traits (USA, New Zealand, Canada), while in European countries where agriculture is a multifunctional branch (Germany, Austria, France, Italy), production and fitness traits weigh in almost equal proportions in their breeding programs (Füller, 2010).

Breeding goals identified by the Hungarian Fleckvieh Association in 2009 are high milk and beef yielding capacity, high feed intake necessary for high performance, fertility, good growth rate and adaptability. The adaptability is expressed in productive life. Traits such as firm, easily milking udder of appropriate shape; limbs with flawless, strong, dry foot; muscularity and optimal frame are prioritized.

As breeding goals for dual-purpose herds they translate into 6500 kg milk, 4.1% fat, 3.6% protein, 2.0 kg/s average milking speed. Heifers are to be mated between 16-18 months of age, with 380-400 kg of body weight, productive life covers 5-7 calvings and lactations on the average. Adult cows are not to surpass 700 kg of body weight. The cow herds recorded produced 5416 kg of milk, 3.86% fat, and 3.8% protein on average (based on yearly performance of 2008). To achieve these goals, performance and selection indices were applied to the following traits: amount of milk (kg), milk fat (kg; %), milk protein (kg; %), somatic cell count, productive life and conformation traits.

Groen (1990) claimed that proper economic consideration of traits is imperative for the improvement of profitability. The present chapter aims at calculating the economic value of the traits which affect profitability, thus facilitate their proper weighing in selection.

MATERIAL AND METHODS

Description of Model

To calculate the economic value of indices we used the ECOWEIGHT program package (Wolf et al., 2007). The bio-economic model of the package was described in detail by Wolfová et al. (2005). The basis of the program is constituted by a bio-economic model containing deterministic and stochastic elements.

Revenues and costs were calculated per animal of each group of cattle. To take into account the time when a trait influences revenues and costs during an animal's lifetime, all revenues and costs were discounted to the date of calving (birth of progeny). We expressed these production values and costs on a yearly basis per cow, and multiplied it with the number of individuals in a given age group. The criterion for the economic efficiency of the production system is the present value of profit calculated as the difference of discounted revenues and costs per cow per year. State subsidy increased income. The marginal economic value of the trait is the partial derivative of the trait's profit function. With continuously changing traits, the marginal economic value was calculated from the difference of the average increase of the trait multiplied by 0.5% and average decrease multiplied by 0.5%. If and describe the increase and decrease of trait l, while and for increase and decrease, respectively, the marginal economic value can be described with the equation below:

$$ev_l = \frac{profit_h - profit_l}{TV_l^h - TV_l^l} \cdot \qquad (1)$$

The marginal economic values of discrete variable (categorical) traits (e.g. calving ease) were calculated following the procedures given in Wolfová et al. (1995). The calculation is based on a threshold model in which the normal (average) distribution was shifted to the right and to the left by 0.05 standard deviation. The difference in distribution was calculated as an average difference in score, then the above equation was applied. Some traits (mature weight, carcass traits) can be expressed only once in the lifetime of an animal, while others (milk yield, conception rate) several times. The former ones are the so-called direct traits; the latter are the maternal traits, for example. Some of the traits belong to both groups, such as calving ease, which is a direct trait for the calf, but a maternal trait for the cow.

To take into account the different number of expressions for both trait components transferred by a certain group of selected parents, the economic weights for direct and maternal trait components for this selection group were calculated by multiplying the marginal economic value of each trait by the number of discounted expressions (NDEs) for direct and maternal effects of this trait. The gene-flow method developed by Hill (1974) and Elsen and Mocquot (1974) is applied for this calculation, which was a part of the program ECOWEIGHT (Wolf et al. 2007). The equations for the calculation of the NDEs are given in Nitter et al. (1994). The economic weight (ew_{lj}) for trait l within the jth group of traits (direct or maternal) for the particular selection group of animals was calculated as

$$ew_{lj} = ev_l \times NDE_j \qquad (2)$$

where is the marginal economic value of trait and is the number of discounted expressions for maternal or direct effects of trait l, discounted either to the year of birth or of selection of the animal group with a given discount rate and summed over a defined investment period. The discount rate was set to 6% for a 25-year investment period.

To express the relative importance of different traits, relative standardized economic weights for direct and maternal traits or trait components were calculated as follows:

$$ewr_{lj} = 100\left|ew_{lj} \times s_l\right| \bigg/ \sum_l \sum_j \left|ew_{lj} \times s_l\right| \tag{3}$$

where is the economic weight for component of trait l, is the genetic standard deviation of trait l. The product is the standardized economic weight for component of trait l. The relative economic weight for component of trait expresses therefore the standardized economic weight for component of trait as percentage of the sum over all traits and trait components of the absolute values of the standardized economic weights. Since no separate genetic standard deviation was available for the direct and maternal traits, the genetic standard deviations for the Austrian Fleckvieh published by Miesenberger et al. (1998) were applied. We calculated with the same standard deviation of the given trait.

Input Parameters Used for Calculation

Various sources of information were used to identify the herd structure, including characteristics of breeding, management, and production values and costs. Data were collected by the Performance Recording Ltd and by the Hungarian Fleckvieh Association between 2000 and 2007. Data regarding maintenance costs and profitability derived from the average of those provided by farms with herds of over 100 cows. We presupposed maximum five pure-bred artificial inseminations for cows, and three for heifers. Non-fertile cows were culled after lactation. Due to health problems resulting from dystocia, 10% of the cows were culled at 30 days after calving. Cows performed maximum of 8 lactations. Non-pregnant heifers were culled at 24 months of age. Male calves were marketed at 180 days of age, while 0.5 percent was sold to artificial insemination centres as replacement breeding bulls at the age of 300 days. We calculated with the rearing of female calves on the farms where they were born, and with the marketing of surplus pregnant heifers at the age of 22 months.

Table 1 displays the basic statistics of traits related to calving for Hungarian Fleckvieh heifers and cows based on national data. Heifers are more likely to have a higher abortion rate and calving difficulties. Cows' conception rate is lower than that of heifers. During each lactation 9-16% of cows were culled due to health issues, and 16-18 % due to low milk production. The mortality rate for cows was between 2-4%. The basic characteristics of traits regarding milk, fat, and protein yield, body weight, and the offspring's vitality are shown in Table 2. Our calculations considered labour costs, feeding, housing, breeding, and health care costs. Additional costs (interest rate, energy, transport, insurance, overhead) were calculated as fixed costs per age groups per day. Feeding costs were calculated on the basis of daily net energy and protein requirements of animals for maintenance, growth and milk production based on the market price of purchased feed for the given age group as well as the production costs for self produced feed. Costs for water – used for drinking and otherwise – were also added. Feeding costs calculated for the various age groups can be seen in Table 3.

Table 1. Basic statistics of traits related to calving for Hungarian Fleckvieh heifers and cows (expressed in %)

Name	1st calving	2nd and further calvings
Abortion rate	3	2
Relative frequency of calving score 3 out of the total no. of calvings when female/male calf is born	11/14	3.6/7.2
Relative frequency of calving score 4 out of the total no. of calvings when female/male calf is born	1/2	0.08/1.1
Cows' conception rate from 1st to 5th inseminations	50, 51, 51, 55, 55	
Heifers' conception rate from 1st to 3rd inseminations	65, 62, 63	
Decrease of conception rate after dystocia (calving difficulties)	15	
Cows' culling rate after dystocia[a]	10	
Cows' culling rate due to calving difficulties in 1st to 8th lactations[b]	9, 9, 9, 12, 14, 14, 15, 16	
Cows' culling rate due to low milk yield in 1st to 8th lactations	19, 19, 17, 16, 18, 18, 19, 19	
Cows' mortality rate in 1st to 8th lactations	2, 2, 3, 2, 3, 3, 4, 4,	

[a] Easy calving includes calving scores 1 and 2, dystocia includes calving scores 3 and 4; [b]except for calving difficulty

Detailed calculations were published by Wolfová et al. (2007). Housing costs were those for bedding (cost for straw minus revenue for manure). Breeding costs included ones related to insemination, such as price of semen, inseminator's wage per fertilization. Health care costs included dystocia cost expressed per calving, cost for medication, and those of removing and rendering dead animals. Major costs other than those for feeding can be seen in Table 4.

Revenues are mainly derived from milk, male calves marketed, breeding bulls, marketing surplus pregnant heifers, culled cows and heifers, and from manure.

Milk price was calculated as the average of those provided by five major milk processing firms that purchase 76% of the entire amount of milk. The standard price for milk was 0.29 EUR per liter if somatic cell count/ml was below 400,000, and 0.12 EUR if exceeding it.

Table 2. Some characteristics of important traits for Hungarian Fleckvieh cow and progeny

Trait (Unit)	Means
Average milk yield/year (kg)	5950
Milk fat (%)	3.96
Milk protein (%)	3.45
Insemination after calving (day)	85
Slaughter % heifers/cows	58/54
Rate of still birth after easy/difficult calving[a]	
in 1st calving (%)	6/16
2nd and subsequent calvings (%)	5/17
Calf mortality within 48 hours after easy/difficult calving	

Table 2. (Continued)

Trait (Unit)	Means
in 1st calving (%)	2/20
in 2nd and subsequent calvings (%)	1/15
Rate of calf mortality from 2nd day to end of rearing period (193 days) (%)	3.0
Birth weight for female/male calves (kg)	45/50
Body weight gain during rearing period for female/male calves (kg/day)	0.8/0.9
Heifers' body weight gain until 1st insemination (kg/day)	0.8
Heifers' body weight gain from 1st insemination until calving (kg/day)	0.7
Heifers' body weight at 1st insemination (kg)	400

Table 3. Content and price of fodder for different age groups

Age group	Dry matter content (DM) kg DM/kg feed	Net energy content MJ NE/kg DM	Raw protein content[a] PDI/kg DM	Price of fodder portion EUR/100 kg feed
Cows	0.54	7.08	140	8.85
Calves up to 3 months of age	0.35	7.85	170	29.63
Calves from 3 to 6 months of age	0.73	7.20	140	7.78
Breeding heifers	0.65	6.0	130	8.81

[a]For the raw protein requirement, the French system was applied and the amount of protein is given in grams of PDI (protéines vraies réellement digestibles dans l'intestin grêle).

The standard price was paid for milk with 3.7% fat and 3.3% protein. Bonus was granted for higher - or penalty for lower - fat percentage (1.27 EUR/kg) for protein percentage, (3.10 EUR/kg). Non-pregnant Hungarian Fleckvieh heifers were sold at 2.15 EUR/kg, and pregnant heifers at 3.45 EUR/kg, respectively. A Hungarian Fleckvieh cow culled was sold at 1.38 EUR/kg. We used 0.029 EUR/L as government subsidies to milk.

Table 4. Main parameters for the calculation of non-feed costs

Variable (unit)	Cost (EUR)
Fixed cost (EUR/animal per day) for	
cows	1.81
reared calves up to 6 months of age	0.48
breeding heifers from 6 months until calving	0.41
breeding bulls from 6 months	0.41
Cost for veterinary treatment for	
cows (EUR/animal per lactation)	41.37
reared calves until 6 months of age	8.27
breeding heifers from 6 months until calving	17.38
breeding bulls until selling to AI stations)	6.96
Veterinary cost connected with dystocia	
calving score 3	10.34
calving score 4	17.24

Variable (unit)	Cost (EUR)
Cost for removing and rendering dead animals	
mature animals	155.17
young animals	38.79
Price of semen	13.79
Price for water (EUR/100 L)	0.068
Price for bedding straw (EUR/100 kg)	3.44

Traits Evaluated

Milk Production Traits

This group of traits included milk yield during a 305-day lactation with constant average fat and protein content as well as fat and protein content at constant milk yield.

In other words, we assumed that fat and protein increase was achieved at constant milk yield. The increase of milk yield, however, was assumed under constant lactation curve.

Currently a quota system is operated in Hungary and EU countries, but the South-East Asian market is expected to open in 2015. Since the national quota is not fully exploited at the moment, we assumed unrestricted milk production as did by Pärna et al. (2007) and Wolfová et al. (2007).

Functional Traits

This group of traits included calving difficulty score, total conception rate for heifers and cows, calf mortality, length of productive life, somatic cell count, tendency to mastitis. The economic value of conception rate (%) was calculated as the difference between the 0.5% score increase and decrease of the trait. Calf mortality at birth included abortions, still birth, calves dying within 48 hours after birth, while cases between the 2nd day to weaning (90 days) and from weaning to the end of rearing (180 days) were considered separately. Time in production covered the period from the first calving to culling or death. The somatic cell score (SCS) was calculated from the somatic cell count (SCC) (ml/l) according to Da et al. (1992) equation:

$$SCS = \log_2\left(\frac{SCC}{100\ 000}\right) + 3$$

(4)

The approach described above for categorical traits was applied for calculation of the economic value of somatic cell score assuming a normal distribution. Incidences of clinical mastitis were calculated as case/year/cow.

Growth and Carcass Traits

This group of traits included birth weight, growth rate of calves until weaning and in the rearing period, from month 6 until first calving, weight increase during the fattening period, mature weight of cows, dressing percentage. Both sexes were considered when calculating the economic value of birth weight and weight increase, but it was expressed for females only. The economic value of growth traits depended on the price of feeding matter covering the nutritional requirements because neither feed intake nor feed conversion were included as separate traits.

RESULTS

The stationary age structure of the herd is shown in Table 5. The average lactation number for the Hungarian Fleckvieh was 2.83 with an interval of 408 days between two calvings. After insemination 94.6% of the heifers and 95.2% of the cows were conceived. The general calving difficulty score was 1.70 and 1.77 for female and male calves born, respectively.

Table 5. Structure of the herd in the stationary state

Variable	Proportion (%) of cows in a given lactation and means
Lactation	
1	30.3
2	22.1
3	16.7
4	12.3
5	8.4
6	5.3
7	2.9
8	2.0
Interval between two calvings (day)	408
Number of female calves reared/100 calvings	42.24

Table 6. Mean, genetic standard deviation (s_I) and marginal economic values (ev_I) in EUR per unit of the trait and per Hungarian Fleckvieh cow per year

Trait (Unit)	Mean	s_I [d]	ev_I
305-day milk yield[a] (kg)	5950	350	0.15
305-day fat yield (kg)	236	15.0	0.71
305-day protein yield (kg)	205	11.0	1.57
Somatic cell score (score)	4.38	0.23	-11.66
Calving difficulty score (score)[b]	1.79	0.08	-42.70
Calf mortality at birth (%)	6.8	1.0	-0.61
Calf mortality in rearing (%)	5.4	1.0	-1.92
Conception rate of heifers (%)	95	1.5	0.47
Conception rate of cows (%)	97.5	5.0	1.33
Length of productive life of cows (years)	2.73	0.49	77.39
Birth weight of calves[b] (kg)	40	1.6	0.45
Mature weight (kg)	700	20.5	-0.66
Daily gain in the rearing period of calves[b] (g/day)	700	47	0.37
Dressing percentage[c] (%)	56.7	1.14	1.67

[a]Milk with average fat and protein percentages averages over all lactations. [b]Mean is given for females, economic values include both sexes. [c]Means of these traits are given for heifers, economic weights include heifers and cows. [d]The genetic standard deviations are those of the Austrian Fleckvieh (Miesenberger et al., 1998)

Table 7. Economic weights[a] for direct and maternal trait components (ew_{lj}, in EUR per unit of the trait and per cow per year), absolute values of standardized economic weights[b] (ews_{lj}, in HUF per genetic standard deviation) and relative standardized economic weights (ewr_{lj} in %, see equation [3])

Trait and trait components	ew_{lj}	ews_{lj}	ewr_{lj}
305-day milk yield	0.14	48.42	28.6
305-day fat yield	0.63	9.51	5.6
305-day protein yield	1.40	15.41	9.1
Somatic cell score	-10.41	-2.39	1.4
Calving difficulty score - direct	-47.08	-3.77	2.2
- maternal	-38.11	-3.05	1.8
Calf mortality at birth - direct	-0.68	-0.68	0.4
- maternal	-0.55	-0.55	0.3
Calf mortality in rearing	-2.11	-2.11	1.3
Conception rate of heifers - direct	0.52	0.78	0.5
- maternal	0.42	0.63	0.4
Conception rate of cows - direct	1.47	7.36	4.4
- maternal	1.19	5.96	3.5
Length of productive life of cows	69.06	33.84	20.0
Birth weight of female calves- direct	0.49	0.79	0.5
- maternal	0.40	0.64	0.4
Mature weight of cows	-0.59	12.07	7.2
Daily gain in the rearing period of calves	0.40	18.97	11.2
Trait and trait components	ew_{lj}	ews_{lj}	ewr_{lj}
Dressing percentage	1.84	2.10	1.2
Total		168.39	100.0

[a]Marginal economic values multiplied by the number of discounted expression of the trait during 25-year interval. [b]Calculated as where is the genetic standard deviation of the trait (the same genetic standard deviation was used for direct and maternal trait components).

For the modelled production system, income was 179.45 EUR/cow/year with 130.94 EUR production value including 155.18 EUR government subsidies. Table 6 shows the marginal economic weights and the corresponding genetic standard deviation calculated for each trait. The negative economic values of somatic cell score, calving difficulty, and calf mortality indicate that the increase of a trait by one unit to the mean value will result in economic loss. The negative values for mature weight also show that increased weight resulted in increased feed costs for maintenance, which were not offset by higher revenues deriving from cows' higher slaughter weight. Daily gain in the rearing period, however, resulted in positive economic value which indicates that the faster weight gain heifers reach mature age for breeding, and the better heifers sell when pregnant.

The economic weights, standardized and relative economic weights of direct and maternal components of different traits were calculated from equations [2] and [3]; the results are shown in Table 7.

Of the traits evaluated for the Hungarian Fleckvieh, milk yield proved to be the most important (28.6%), followed by the length of productive life (20.0%). Calves daily weight gain (11.2%), however, has higher relative economic value than milk protein yield (9.1%). Cows' mature weight causes substantial economic loss (7.2%). The importance of milk fat

(5.6%) is higher than the conception rate of cows (3.5-4.4%), while that of calving difficulty is about 2%. The importance of the other traits failed to reach 2%. The three trait groups affected the profitability of the breed: milk production by 43.3%, functional traits by 36.2%, and beef production by 20.5%.

DISCUSSION

In the present chapter the economic value of various traits for the Hungarian Fleckvieh were calculated. The marginal economic value can be applied to design a selection index, or to calculate the profitability of a breeding program when genetic progress is available for individual traits. The relative economic weight reveals the significance of individual traits to the breeder, while the correlation between the heritability value and the traits are also to be considered.

In most countries it is only the amount or percentage of milk fat and milk protein that are included in the index. The economic values for these traits are determined by the pricing policy for the milk components and the feeding costs (Gibson et al., 1992). Although we express the economic values of fat and protein per kg, what we examine is the relationship expressed in percentage between the two traits. The price of protein and fat is 2:1 in Hungary, which can explain the relative economic weight ratio between them of 1.64:1. This value was estimated as 1.41 alongside to the price ratio of 1.25:1 by Reinsch and Dempfle (1998). If purchase price for milk was independent of milk components, then it would result in negative economic value (Pärna et al., 2007, St-Onge et al., 2002). Milk protein has recently gained significance, which is expressed in the indices of the major Holstein breeding countries (Canada, Germany, Italy and the Netherlands). The economic weight of milk protein is 2-4.8 times larger than that of milk fat (Miglior et al., 2005). The marginal economic value of mature weight is negative. In a paper surveying 12 studies, Koenen et al. (2000) published the economic values of mature weight for cows between -1.28 and +0.02 EUR/kg/cow. The economic value of -0.61 EUR/kg calculated in the present work corresponds to this interval. Van Raden claimed (2002) that not only does bigger body weight require more feed, but it results in higher housing costs too. Moreover, cattle of larger body weight reach mature weight later, thus rearing smaller heifers may be more profitable (Owens et al., 1993; Püski et al., 1999). Should we consider all these factors, the economic value of mature weight would be even more negative. In the light of these results, monitoring the mature weight of cows seems justified. The positive economic value for growth rate indicates that this value needs attention in the rearing phase. Building fitness traits into the index has been attracting growing attention for the past years, partly due to the quota system, and partly to such low fertility that endangers even the replacement of breeding stock (Miglior et al., 2005). Our calculations show that productive life is the second most important factor contributing to the profitability of a farm. Its marginal economic value (0.21 EUR/day) falls into the top third of data published in the literature. For dairy farms in Germany the value of this trait is 0.09 – 0.16 EUR/day (Reinsch, 1993; Wünsch and Bergfeld, 2001), in Italian herds 0.46 – 0.56 EUR/day (Brandts et al., 1996), in the UK 1 EUR/day (Pryce et al., 1999), and in Finland 1.12 EUR/day (Toivakka et al., 2005). The economic value for calving difficulty and stillbirth with the Hungarian Fleckvieh was smaller than that of the length of productive life, which is similar to the results obtained for the Austrian Feckvieh (Miesenberger et al., 1998). Mack (1996) and Miesenberger et al. (1998), however, found the economic value of still birth higher (3%) than that of calving difficulty (1.3%). Our current values are 0.7 and 4.0, respectively, for the Hungarian Fleckvieh. The economic significance of calving difficulty was 4.0%, which is derived from the relatively high rate of dystocia in the Hungarian herds. Berry et al. (2007b) claimed that cows experiencing dystocia have lower milk fat and milk protein concentration, but higher somatic cell count, thus the indirect economic value surpasses the direct one. Instances of infertility and culling due to biological reproductive reasons increase following dystocia. With the Hungarian Fleckvieh the frequency of calving difficulty is higher at the first calving (14.4%) than that in the Austrian Fleckvieh (5.0%) (Fürst and Egger-Danner, 2003). The Italian Simmental index weighs milk yielding traits in 44%, beef yielding traits in 24%, conformation traits in 19.5%, and fitness traits in 12.5% (INTERBULL, http://www-interbull.slu.se, accessed:13/06/2011). Conformation traits are not included in the selection index for Hungarian Flecvieh. For the selection of elite cows and for mating plans, selection is carried out by independent culling levels for conformation traits. If conformation is considered as a trait in correlation with the length of productive life, then our results calculated for milk, functional, and beef traits in a ratio of 44:36:20, respectively, show results close to the Italian index. The length of productive life is the second most important trait in the dual-purpose type, and in beef type it is the most important or second most important trait depending on market conditions (Krupa et al., 2005). Despite the fact that the economic value for the functional traits is high, only a slow selection response can be expected in these traits due to the low heritability. Having reviewed papers by several authors, Keller et al. (2008) concluded that the most important traits in the various cattle breeds are the proportion of lean meat, protein and solid content of milk, as well as the length of productive life. From economic aspects Keller et al (2009) found fertility, weaning weight, and length of productive life the most important in national herds depending on the production system.

A solid index is highly accepted by the breeders. Seventy percent of the Austrian breeders apply the total merit index for breeding stock selection (Miesenberg and Fürst, 2006). In the Austrian index milk traits represent 38% and the ratio of milk protein and milk fat is close to 8:1. In the Hungarian index it is close to 2:1, and this latter result was also supported by our calculations. Miesenberger and Fürst (2006) claimed that the total merit index for the Austrian Fleckvieh, which included beef and fitness traits together with milk yield, resulted in 11% higher economic growth as compared to the index considering merely milk yielding traits. The beef traits included in selection index currently include killing out percent, net body weight gain, and the EUROP carcass conformation class. Since 2012, selection has been carried out by a combined index, including fitness, milk and beef traits based on our calculations.

REFERENCES

Berry D. P., Lee J. M., Macdonald, K. A., Roche, J. R. (2007). Body condition score and body weight effects on dystocia and stillbirths and consequent effects on post-calving performance. *J. Dairy Sci., 90*, 4201-4211.

Brandts, A., Canavesi, F., Cassandro, M. (1996). Economic weights for longevity in the Italian Holstein breed. *Interbull Bulletin, 14*, 76-80.

Da, Y., Grossman, M., Misztal, I., Wiggans, G. R. (1992). Estimation of genetic parameters for somatic cell score in Holsteins. *J. Dairy Sci., 75*, 2265-2271.

Elsen, J. M., Mocquot, J. C. (1974). Méthode de prévision de l'evolution du niveau génétique d'une population soumise à une opération de sélection et dont les génerations se chevauchent. INRA *Bull. Tech. Dépt. Génét. Anim., 17,* 30-54.

Fürst, C. (2001). Zucht auf Fitness und Gesundheit beim Fleckvieh-Nutzungsdauer und Langlebigkeit. 24. Kongress der Europäischen Vereinigung der Fleckviehzüchter. 10-14. 10. 2001. Romania, Brasov.

Fuerst, C., Egger-Danner, C. (2003). Multivariate evaluation for calving ease and stillbirth in Austria and Germany. *Interbull Bulletin, 31,* 47-51.

Füller, I. (2010). Hústermelő képesség javítására irányuló szelekció továbbfejlesztése a magyartarka fajtában. Ph.D Dissertation. Kaposvár University.

Gibson, J. P., Graham, N., Burnside, E. B. (1992). Selection indexes for production traits of Canadian dairy sires. *Can. J. Anim. Sci., 72*, 477-491.

Groen, A. F. (1990). Influences of production circumstances in situations with output limitations. *Livest. Prod. Sci., 22,* 1-16.

Groen, A. F., T. Steine, J. J. Colleau, J. Pedersen, J. Pribyl, Reinsch, N. (1997). Economic values in dairy cattle breeding, with special reference to functional traits. Report of an EAAP-working group. *Livest. Prod. Sci., 49*, 1-21.

Hill, W. G. (1974). Prediction and evaluation of response to selection with overlapping generations. *Anim. Prod., 18*, 117-139.

Hungarian Fleckvieh Association (2009). A magyartarka fajta tenyésztési programja. In http.//www.magyartarka.hu date of access: 06.13. 2011.

Keller, K., Fördős, A., Szabó, F. (2008). Értékmérők ökonómiai súlyozása a szarvasmarha-tenyésztésben. *Állattenyésztés és Takarmányozás, 57,* 1, 23-37.

Keller, K., Wolfová, M., Wolf, J., Fefete, Zs., Komlósi, I., Szabó, F. (2009). Der Einfluss des Kuhgewichts auf die Betriebsrentabilität und auf die ökonomischen Gewichte der Fleischrindmerkmale. *Arch. Tierz., 52*, 3, 255-264.

Koenen, E. P. C., Berentsen, P. B. M., Groen, A. F. (2000). Economic values of live weight and feed-intake capacity of dairy cattle under Duch production circumstances. *Livest. Prod. Sci., 66*, 235-250.

Krupa, E., Wolfová, M., Peskovicá, D., Huba, J., Krupová, Z. (2005). Economic values of traits for Slovakian Pied cattle in different marketing stratgies. *Czech J. Anim. Sci., 50*, 10, 483-492.

Kulak, K., Nielsen, H. M., Strandberg, E. (2004). Economic values for production and non-production traits in Nordic dairy cattle populations calculated by stochastic simulation. *Acta Agric. Scand. Sect. A. Anim. Sci., 54*, 127-138.

Mack, G. (1996). Wirtschaftlichkeit des züchterischen Fortschritts in Milchviehherden, Gesamtbetriebliche Analyse mit Hilfe eines simultan-dynamischen Linearen Planungsansatzes. Dissertation, Universität Hohenheim.

Miesenberger, J., Sölkner J., Essl, A. (1998). Economic weights for fertility and reproduction traits relative to other traits and effects of including functional traits into a total merit index. *Interbull Bulletin, 18*, 78-84.

Miesenberger, J., Fürst, C. (2003). Was bringt die Zucht nach dem Ökonomischen gesamtzuchtwert? 25. Kongress der Europäischen Vereinigung der Fleckviehzüchter. 6-12. 9. 2003. Serbien. *cit. in Füller, I.* (2010). Hústermelőképesség-javítására irányuló szelekció továbbfejlesztése a magyartarka fajtában. Ph.D. Dissertation. Kaposvár University.

Miesenberger, J., Fürst, C. (2006). Experiences in selecting total merit index in the Austrian Fleckvieh breed. *Biotechnology in Animal Husbandry, 22,* 1-2, 17-27.

Miglior, F., Muir, B. L. Van Doormaal, B. J. (2005). Selection indices in Holstein cattle of various countries. *J. Dairy Sci., 88,* 1255-1263.

Nitter G., Graser, H.U., Barwick, S.A. (1994). Evaluation of advanced industry breeding schemes for Australian beef cattle. 1. Method of evaluation and analysis for an example population structure. *Aust. J. Agric. Res., 45,* 1041–1656.

Olesen, I., Groen, A. F., Gjerde, B. (2000). Definition of animal breeding goals for sustainable production systems. *J. Anim. Sci., 78,* 570-582.

Owens, F. N., Dubenski, P., Hanson, C. F. (1993). Factors that alter the growth and development of ruminants. *J. Anim. Sci., 71,* 3138-3150.

Pärna, E., Kiiman, H., Vallas, M., Viinalass, H., Saveli, O. (2007). Development of a breeding objective for Estonian Holstein cattle. *Agric. and Food Sci., 16,* 212-221.

Pryce, J., Simm, G., Amer, P., Coffey, M., Stott, A. (1999). Returns from genetic improvement on indices that include production, longevity, mastitis and fertility in UK circumstances. *Interbull Bulletin,* No. 23, 55-61.

Püski, J., Tran, A. H., Gáspárdy, A., Bozó, S., Szücs, E. (1999). A típus hatása a holstein tehenek tejtermelésének a hatékonyságára az első laktációban. *Állattenyésztés és Takarmányozás, 48,* 323-337.

Reinsch, N. (1993). Berechnung wirtschaftlicher Gewichtungsfaktoren für sekundäre Leistungsmerkmale beim Fleckvieh. Dissertation. München-Weihenstephan, Technische Universität.

Reinsch, N., Dempfle, L. (1998). Investigations on functional traits in Simmental. 3. Economic weights at the stationary state of a Markov chain. *Arch. Tierz., 41,* 211-224.

St-Onge, A., Hayes, J. F., Cue, R. I. (2002). Economic values of traits for dairy cattle improvement estimated using field-recorded data. *Can. J. Anim. Sci., 82,* 29-39.

Stott, A. W., Coffey, M. P., Brotherstone, S. (2005). Including lameness and mastitis in a profit index for dairy cattle. *Anim. Sci., 80,* 41-52.

Tischler, J. (2002). Fleckviehzucht im Wettbewerb mit speziellen Milchrassen. 4. Fleckviehseminar der AGÖF, 2002. April 5. Strass/Zillertal, Tirol.

Toivakka, M., Nousiainen, J. I., Mäntysaari, E. A. (2005). Estimation of economic values of longevity and other functional traits in Finnish dairy cattle. In *56th Annual Meeting of the EAAP* (paper CG2.25.).

Van Raden, P. M. (2002). Selection of dairy cattle for lifetime profit. In *Proceedings of the 7th World Congress on Genetics Applied to Livestock Production* (CD-ROM, No. 01-21.), Montpellier, France.

Vargas, B., Groen, A. F., Herrero, M., Van Arendonk, J. A. M. (2002). Economic values for production and functional traits in Holstein cattle of Costa Rica. *Livest. Prod. Sci., 75,* 101-116.

Veerkamp, R. F., Dillon, P., Kelly, E., Cromie, A. R., Groen, A. F. (2002). Dairy cattle breeding objectives combining yield, survival and calving interval for pasture-based systems in Ireland under different milk quota scenarios. *Livest. Prod. Sci., 76,* 137-151.

Wolfová, M., Wolf, J., Hyánek, J. (1995). Economic weights for beef production traits in the Czech Republic. *Livest. Prod. Sci., 43,* 63-73.

Wolfová, M., Wolf, J., Přibyl, J., Zahrádková, R., Kica J. (2005). Breeding objectives for beef cattle used in different production systems. 1. Model development. *Livest. Prod. Sci., 95,* 201-215.

Wolf, J., Wolfová, M., Krupa, E. (2007). User's Manual for the Program ECOWEIGHT (C Programs for Calculating Economic Weights in Livestock), Version 3.0.2. Programs for Cattle. Institute of Animal Science, Prague Uhříněves, Czech Republic, and Slovak Center of Agricultural Research, Nitra, Slovak Republic.

Wolfová, M., Wolf, J., Kvapilík, J., Kica J. (2007). Selection for profit in cattle. I. Economic weights for purebred dairy cattle in the Czech Republic. *J. Dairy Sci., 90,* 2442-2455.

Wünsch, U., Bergfeld, U. (2001). Berechnung wirtschaftlicher Gewichte für ökonomisch wichtige Leistungsmerkmale in der Milchrinderzucht. *Züchtungskunde, 73,* 3-11.

INDEX

A

access, 72, 186
acclimatization, 47
accounting, 169
acetylation, 61, 62, 63, 65, 66, 68, 69, 70, 72, 74, 79, 82
acid, 29, 40, 54, 70, 77, 80, 97, 124, 134
acidic, viii, 25, 36, 116, 119
acidosis, 116, 119
acquired immunity, vii
acrosome, 85
active site, 28
adaptability, 142, 153, 176
adaptation, vii, x, 41, 139, 140, 141, 142, 143, 145, 146, 147, 148, 149, 152, 153
adaptive immunity, 2, 30
additives, 116
adenocarcinoma, 79
adenovirus, 30
adhesion, vii, 1, 9, 14, 22
adipocyte, 47, 49
adipose, viii, 39, 40, 44, 45, 46, 47, 49, 51, 53, 54, 55, 56, 87
adipose tissue, 40, 45, 49, 51, 54, 55, 56, 87
adiposity, viii, 40, 45, 47, 51
adrenal gland(s), 90
adsorption, ix, 115, 116
adulthood, 94, 100
adverse effects, 94, 95, 121
aetiology, 136
Africa, 143, 151, 152, 156
age, 6, 42, 43, 44, 45, 46, 47, 48, 51, 53, 56, 84, 95, 98, 102, 105, 132, 143, 144, 151, 176, 177, 178, 180, 182, 183
agonist, 87, 102
agriculture, 75, 99, 123, 124, 125, 149, 152, 176
AIDS, 37

air temperature, 140
airway epithelial cells, 37
albumin, 4, 17
alfalfa, 132
algorithm, 163
alimentation, 153
alkaloids, 93
alkalosis, 133, 135
allele, 22, 163, 165
allelic exclusion, 8
alters, 78, 119
aluminium, 116, 124
amenorrhea, 106
amino acid(s), vii, 1, 8, 9, 12, 13, 15, 16, 22, 26, 27, 34, 35, 38, 72, 87
ammonia, 117, 121
ammonium, 117
amphibians, 2
amylase, 119
ancestors, 162
androgen, 73, 91, 93, 94
animal disease(s), 124, 156
animal husbandry, 124, 146, 147, 149, 172
animal welfare, 155
anorexia, 133
antagonism, 142
antibiotic, 110, 112
antibody, vii, 1, 4, 6, 7, 8, 10, 11, 12, 13, 14, 15, 16, 17, 19, 22, 23, 62, 116, 120, 121, 123
anti-cancer, 71
anticancer drug, 81
antigen, vii, 1, 2, 3, 4, 9, 12, 13, 14, 15, 30, 36, 71, 81
antigen exposure, vii, 1, 13, 14, 15
antigen-presenting cell(s), 71, 81
APCs, 30
apoptosis, 18, 61, 63, 71, 72, 77, 78, 79, 97, 98, 102, 103, 104, 105, 106
apoptotic pathways, 98

appetite, 132
aquaculture, 123, 124, 125, 172
aqueous solutions, 119
Argentina, 144
Aristotle, 115, 124, 127
arrest, 61, 65, 66, 67, 69, 77
arrhythmias, 133
ARS, 25, 35, 59
artery(s), ix, 96, 102, 109
arthropods, 143
Asia, 161, 168, 169
astrocytes, 78
ATF, 82
ATP, 49, 54, 73
auscultation, 132, 133
Austria, 176, 186
autoantibodies, 20
autoimmunity, 81
aversion, 141
avian, 143

B

babesiosis, 156
backfat thickness (BFT), viii, 39, 40
bacteria, 29, 71, 75, 76
bacteriophage, 19
barriers, 26, 148
base, 13, 21, 85, 98, 134
base pair, 9
Bayesian estimation, 34
bedding, 95, 179, 181
beef, 15, 47, 56, 100, 101, 103, 123, 124, 146, 147,
    148, 151, 152, 153, 154, 155, 156, 160, 172, 176,
    184, 185, 187, 188
behaviors, 146
Beijing, 159, 171
beneficial effect, 71, 116, 121, 122
benefits, 35, 99, 146, 171
bicarbonate, 120
bile, 121
bile acids, 121
binding globulin, 94
bioavailability, 118, 121
biodiversity, vii, 144
biological processes, 60
biological systems, 150
biosynthesis, 27, 72, 73, 82
biotechnology, 78, 82
birds, 143
birth weight, 181
bisphenol, 93, 104, 105

blood, viii, 4, 15, 19, 30, 39, 41, 42, 45, 49, 51, 54,
    61, 85, 87, 88, 91, 94, 96, 100, 103, 117, 120,
    121, 123, 124, 125, 143, 153, 154, 160
blood flow, 100
blood plasma, 91
blood urea nitrogen, 121
body composition, 56
body fat, viii, 39, 40, 42, 43, 45, 47, 49, 51, 54, 55,
    57, 95
body fluid, 18, 93
body mass index (BMI), 94
body weight, viii, 39, 40, 41, 42, 45, 51, 56, 120,
    121, 143, 147, 176, 178, 180, 184, 185
bonds, 146
bone(s), 3, 5, 49, 53, 89
bone marrow, 3, 5
bradycardia, 132
brain, 73, 81, 84, 88, 90
Brazil, vii, 139, 140, 141, 144, 153, 155
breakdown, 47
breathing, 142
breathing rate, 142
breeding, ix, xi, 83, 95, 100, 106, 140, 141, 143, 145,
    146, 149, 150, 151, 153, 155, 157, 160, 169, 170,
    171, 172, 173, 174, 175, 176, 178, 179, 180, 183,
    184, 185, 186, 187, 188
breeding goal, 176, 187
bronchial epithelial cells, 27, 38
browsing, 143
buffalo, xi, 147, 153, 154, 159, 160, 165, 166, 167,
    168, 169, 170, 173, 174
bursa, 16
by-products, 93, 132

C

calcium, 97, 110, 118, 121, 123, 124, 125
calibration, 41
caloric intake, 148
cancer, 35, 61, 71, 77, 79, 80, 81, 82, 86, 101
cancer cells, 79
carbon, 75, 85, 145, 156
carbon dioxide, 75, 85
carboxyl, 72
carcinogenesis, 60
carnivores, 5, 6
carotene, 121
cartilaginous, 2
casting, 133, 134, 136
castration, 103
catalytic activity, 69
category a, 63
cathepsin G, 28

catheter, 42

cation, 116

causation, 117

cDNA, 21, 31

CEC, 116

cell biology, 78, 80, 81

cell cycle, 61, 63, 65, 67, 69, 71, 77, 78

cell death, 69, 71, 97, 98, 102

cell differentiation, 61, 94

cell division, 65, 69, 78

cell fate, 69

cell line(s), 61, 63, 64, 67, 78, 79

cell surface, 6, 29

cellular homeostasis, 71

cerebrospinal fluid, 53, 56

challenges, x, 78, 99, 139, 142, 145, 148, 149, 153, 154, 173

chaperones, 71

chemical(s), 60, 79, 89, 93, 94, 102, 116, 123

chemical properties, 116

chicken, vii, 1, 4, 5, 8, 17, 21, 22, 31

chimpanzee, 31

China, vi, vii, xi, 159, 160, 161, 162, 164, 165, 167, 168, 169, 170, 171, 172, 173, 174

chitin, 2

chlorine, 110

cholesterol, 47, 89, 101

chromosome, 7, 8, 11, 12, 21, 32, 36, 61, 84, 160, 162

chronic obstructive pulmonary disease, 35

chymotrypsin, 28

circadian rhythm, 40

circulation, 6

CIS, 99

City, 39

civilization, 75, 165

classes, 4, 93

classification, 100, 160, 161, 162, 174

cleavage, 8, 26, 29

climate(s), vii, x, 139, 140, 141, 142, 143, 144, 145, 147, 148, 149, 151, 152, 153, 154, 156

climate change, vii, 140, 141, 147, 152, 153, 154

clinical application, 80

clinical trials, 35

clone, 9

cloning, 31, 40, 54

cluster analysis, 163

clustering, 70, 167

clusters, 62, 167

coding, 9, 31, 33, 69, 70, 80, 170, 172

cognition, 93

colic, 133

colitis, 35

collaboration, 76

colon, 70, 80

colon cancer, 70, 80

color, 160

colorectal cancer, 77, 78

colostrum, x, 4, 5, 6, 18, 115, 120, 121, 123, 124

combinatorial diversity, vii, 1, 3, 10, 12, 13, 14

commercial, 35, 41, 77, 120, 140, 144, 151, 157

communication, 26

community, 172

compaction, 72

comparative analysis, 154

compensation, 157

competition, 69, 141, 146, 148

competitiveness, 148, 175

complement, 7, 9

complementarity, 16, 17, 23

complexity, 2, 12, 19, 23, 68, 98

composition, 26, 41, 42, 75, 136, 154, 174

compounds, 61, 75, 93, 119

computing, 141

conception, xi, 84, 110, 122, 142, 175, 177, 178, 179, 181, 184

condensation, 72, 97

conditioning, 72

conduction, 117

configuration, xi, 140

conformity, 42

Congress, 150, 152, 156, 187

consensus, 67, 74

conservation, 15, 33, 71, 74, 149, 173

constituents, 76

construction, 128

consumers, 116

consumption, 47, 75, 125, 143

contamination, 134

control group, 63, 117, 118, 119

controversial, 44

cooling, 96

cooperation, 171

coordination, 63

COPD, 35

copper, 121

copulation, 84

corpus luteum, 111

correlation(s), 48, 49, 92, 156, 184, 185

correlation coefficient, 49

corticosteroids, 106

cost, 120, 148, 175, 179, 180

Costa Rica, 187

covering, 172, 181

CPI, 171

critical period, 72, 119

Croatia, vii, 109, 114
crop, 140
cross-sectional study, 40
cryptorchidism, 86, 89, 93, 101
crystalline, ix, 115, 116
CSREES, 35
culture, 5, 141
cure, 134
cycles, 63, 100
cycling, 66
cyclins, 63, 65
cysteine, 13, 14, 20
cystic fibrosis, 35
cytochrome, 174
cytokines, 3, 27, 30, 37
cytometry, 62
cytoplasm, 85
cytosine, 69, 79
Czech Republic, 188

D

dairy cattle, x, xi, 15, 81, 113, 115, 116, 119, 120,
    121, 127, 128, 130, 132, 136, 142, 159, 160, 169,
    170, 171, 172, 173, 174, 186, 187, 188
dairy industry, 128, 170, 171
data collection, 41, 171, 172
data gathering, 41
data processing, 170, 172
data set, 74, 152, 170
database, 21
DDT, 93
deacetylation, 70, 73, 80
deaths, 143
decomposition, 117
deduction, 98
defects, 88, 93, 95, 96, 97, 105
defence, 151
defense mechanisms, 26
deficiency(s), 92, 104, 105, 148, 166
deformation, 41
degradation, vii, 4, 30, 35, 37, 65, 69, 72, 97, 121
dendritic cell, 30, 37
dendrogram, 163
denial, 146
deoxyribonucleic acid, 103
Department of Agriculture, 35, 77, 153
deposition, 51
depression, viii, 40, 49, 51, 52, 53, 54
deprivation, 147
depth, 75
detectable, 5, 6, 68, 110
detection, 21, 76, 151

developed countries, 170, 171
developing countries, 145, 156
developmental disorder, 93
deviation, 178, 183
diarrhea, x, 115, 116, 120, 121, 124
diet, 40, 42, 44, 45, 46, 47, 75, 94, 100, 117, 118,
    119, 123, 124, 125, 134, 135
dietary fiber, 61
dietary supplementation, 116, 124
digestibility, 125, 140, 145
digestion, 51, 76, 119, 122, 124, 125
discrete variable, 177
diseases, vii, x, 15, 76, 115, 116, 122, 127, 129, 133,
    134, 135, 140, 141, 142, 143, 145, 149
disequilibrium, 166
disorder, 87
displacement, vii, x, 127, 128, 129, 130, 131, 132,
    133, 134, 135, 136
distilled water, 120
distribution, 5, 12, 17, 18, 20, 35, 55, 74, 100, 130,
    132, 143, 144, 152, 154, 164, 167, 177
divergence, vii, xi, 1, 3, 8, 12, 14, 33, 155, 159, 160,
    168
diversification, vii, 1, 2, 4, 5, 6, 10, 12, 14, 16, 17,
    19, 22, 23
diversity, vii, 1, 2, 3, 6, 10, 12, 13, 14, 16, 17, 19, 20,
    21, 23, 144, 164, 165, 166, 168, 173, 174
DNA, 8, 9, 16, 20, 59, 60, 61, 62, 63, 65, 66, 67, 68,
    69, 71, 72, 73, 74, 77, 78, 79, 81, 82, 85, 94, 96,
    97, 98, 99, 100, 101, 103, 104, 105, 106, 162,
    164, 174
DNA damage, 63, 94, 97, 98, 99, 100, 101, 103, 104,
    106
DNA repair, 69
DNA sequencing, 78
dogs, 32
domain structure, 26, 31
domestication, viii, 25, 26, 141, 146, 154, 168, 173
dopamine, 91, 103
dopaminergic, 91, 99, 103
down-regulation, 6, 60
draft, 160, 161, 162, 165
Drosophila, 66, 69, 73, 82
drugs, 35, 71, 73, 79, 93, 143, 150
dry matter, 61, 116, 120, 135
drying, 140
duodenum, 128, 129, 135

E

East Asia, vii, 181
ecological systems, 161
economic efficiency, 177

economic growth, 185
economic losses, 71, 110
economic values, xi, 175, 177, 182, 183, 184, 187
ecosystem, 75, 76
editors, 55, 150, 151, 152, 153
egg, 142
ejaculation, 84
elafin, 25, 26, 27, 28, 29, 30, 35, 36, 37, 38
elastin, 37
electron, 97, 102
ELISA, 43, 151
elongation, 70
embryogenesis, ix, 83
embryonic stem cells, 79
emission, 75
encoding, vii, 1, 8, 12, 14
endangered, 149, 150, 156
endangered species, 156
endocrine, ix, 83, 84, 93, 98, 99
endocrine system, 93
endocrinology, 141
endometritis, ix, 109, 110, 111, 112, 113, 114
endothelial cells, 36
energy, 44, 61, 75, 84, 101, 119, 120, 122, 132, 142, 154, 156, 178, 180
energy supply, 61
engineering, 21
England, 105, 113
entrepreneurship, 150
environment(s), ix, x, 30, 57, 60, 72, 75, 83, 85, 111, 116, 123, 134, 139, 140, 141, 142, 143, 144, 145, 147, 148, 149, 152, 154, 155, 175, 176
environmental change, 60, 75, 141, 147
environmental conditions, 103, 149
environmental effects, 81, 156
environmental factors, ix, 75, 83, 95, 96, 98, 102, 153, 175
environmental impact, viii, 59, 75, 82
environmental influences, 72
environmental issues, 148
environmental stimuli, 73
environmental stress(es), ix, 59, 60, 71, 73, 94, 148
environmental temperatures, 96
enzyme(s), 3, 37, 68, 73, 85, 117, 119
epidemiology, 132
epidermis, 29, 35, 38
epididymis, 84, 85, 92, 93, 101
epigenetic modification, 73
epigenetics, vii, viii, 59, 60, 72, 75, 76, 77, 80, 82
epistasis, ix, 83
epithelial cells, 5, 27, 36, 37, 61, 63, 71, 77, 78, 121
equal opportunity, 35, 77
equilibrium, 147

erosion, 142, 151
ESI, 26, 37
estrogen, 73, 92, 98, 100, 103, 105
ethanol, 40, 54
ethers, 93
etiology, 94, 109, 127
EU, 181
eukaryotic, 65, 72, 73, 78
eukaryotic cell, 65
Europe, vii, 128, 129, 140, 169, 176
evidence, 2, 9, 12, 20, 22, 40, 41, 61, 63, 65, 69, 73, 99, 100, 105, 141, 142, 143, 150, 155, 168, 172, 173, 174
evolution, viii, 2, 5, 7, 9, 12, 16, 19, 21, 25, 26, 33, 34, 38, 71, 73, 82, 146, 155, 157, 164, 172, 173, 174, 186
exercise, 96, 103
exons, 8, 9, 26, 31, 33
experimental design, viii, 39, 43
exploitation, 141
exposure, vii, 1, 3, 9, 12, 13, 14, 15, 71, 93, 94, 96, 100, 102, 103, 106, 144
expulsion, 110
external environment, 26, 60, 99
extinction, 140, 141
extracellular matrix, 26
extracts, 54, 82

F

families, 8, 10, 11, 12, 19, 20, 33, 73, 99, 173
family members, 38
farmers, 146, 148
farms, 113, 120, 128, 129, 148, 157, 171, 172, 178, 184
fasting, 56, 57
fat, 40, 44, 45, 46, 51, 54, 55, 94, 95, 96, 121, 124, 129, 135, 142, 170, 176, 178, 179, 180, 181, 182, 183, 184, 185
fatty acids, 43, 47, 57, 61, 71, 75, 77, 129
FDR, 63
FEC, 142
feed additives, ix, 115, 116, 121, 124
feed intake reduction, viii, 40, 41, 49, 52, 54
feedstuffs, 118
female rat, 93
fermentation, 51, 61, 75, 76, 117, 122, 123, 124, 125, 128, 129, 147
fertility, vii, ix, xi, 83, 86, 87, 88, 89, 91, 92, 94, 95, 96, 98, 99, 100, 101, 102, 103, 109, 110, 112, 141, 142, 151, 156, 157, 175, 176, 184, 185, 186, 187
fertility rate, 98

fertilization, ix, 83, 85, 86, 94, 96, 111, 179
fetal development, 88
fetus, 5, 6, 7, 14, 17, 18
fever, x, 103, 111, 112, 115, 116, 118, 123, 129, 131,
    132, 144, 150, 151
fiber, 75, 76
fibrinogen, 2
fibroblasts, 35
fidelity, 65
filiform, 84
financial, 99, 120, 128
Finland, 184
fish, 2, 3, 31
fistulas, 117
fitness, 140, 142, 146, 148, 176, 184, 185
fixation, 136
fixed costs, 178
flagellum, 85
flank, 134
flexibility, 4, 10, 13, 14
flora, 82
fluctuations, 143
fluid, 26, 84, 85, 92, 121, 133, 134
fluid balance, 92
fluoroquinolones, 143
FMC, 152
follicle(s), 5, 16, 18, 87, 99, 101, 102, 104, 106
follicle stimulating hormone, 87, 99, 104, 106
follicular fluid, 103
food, x, 40, 54, 55, 56, 57, 61, 140, 146, 147, 149
food intake, 54, 55, 56, 57
Ford, 17
formation, viii, 3, 5, 25, 60, 74, 88, 90, 141, 147
fragments, 15
France, 151, 160, 171, 176, 187
frostbite, 95
functional analysis, 64
fungi, 38, 75, 93
fungus, 93
fusion, 10, 29

G

gamete, 88
gametogenesis, 91
gastrointestinal tract, 27, 61, 77, 117, 118, 129
gene amplification, 69
gene expression, ix, 16, 22, 37, 59, 60, 61, 63, 65,
    66, 69, 70, 71, 72, 73, 76, 77, 79, 80, 81, 82, 93,
    105
gene mapping, 21
gene regulation, 59, 60, 65, 69, 73
gene silencing, 60, 69

genes, viii, 2, 3, 5, 7, 8, 9, 11, 12, 13, 14, 15, 16, 19,
    20, 21, 22, 23, 25, 26, 31, 32, 33, 34, 35, 36, 37,
    59, 60, 63, 64, 65, 66, 67, 68, 69, 70, 71, 72, 73,
    74, 78, 79, 80, 82, 89, 94, 102, 142
genetic background, 142
genetic diversity, 141, 162, 163, 164, 165, 174
genetic information, 65, 72
genetic linkage, 173
genetic marker, 162
genetics, ix, 59, 75, 76, 83, 98, 141, 142, 149, 150,
    171
genome, vii, 7, 9, 11, 12, 14, 19, 23, 31, 59, 60, 61,
    63, 65, 69, 73, 74, 76, 82, 93, 172
genomics, 59, 79, 82
genotype(ing), 49, 54, 142, 148, 156, 172
germ cells, 84, 89, 97, 98
germ line, 85, 93
Germany, 113, 136, 163, 164, 176, 184, 186
germline sequence divergence, vii, 1, 3, 14
gestation, 4, 5, 6, 7, 13, 84, 130
gland, 4, 5, 18, 84
global climate change, 144
global warming, 75, 145, 156
glucagon, 57
glucocorticoid receptor, 73
glucose, viii, 39, 40, 41, 43, 47, 49, 50, 51, 53, 54,
    55, 57, 121, 123
glycol, 93
glycolysis, 94
glycosylation, 9
gonadotropin-releasing hormone (GnRH), 105
gonads, 87, 88, 91
grants, 35
grass(s), 122, 145
grazing, 57, 140, 143, 145, 154
Greece, vii, 115, 124, 127, 128, 132, 136
greenhouse gas, 75, 157
greenhouse gas emissions, 157
growth, ix, xi, 49, 51, 53, 54, 55, 56, 57, 59, 63, 65,
    66, 67, 70, 71, 76, 77, 78, 87, 89, 91, 99, 100,
    101, 102, 103, 104, 107, 140, 141, 144, 145, 149,
    155, 168, 175, 176, 178, 181, 184, 187
growth arrest, 63, 67, 71
growth factor, 77, 78
growth hormone, 54, 88, 99, 100, 101, 102, 103, 104,
    107
growth rate, 149, 176, 181, 184
guidance, 99
guidelines, 41

H

habitat, 150, 151, 156

hair, 41, 89, 134, 142, 154, 160
half-life, 4, 17
haplotypes, 5, 18, 20, 164, 168, 169, 170
harmony, 140
HDAC, 61, 68, 70, 71, 74, 80, 81
health, ix, 26, 109, 110, 112, 115, 116, 121, 122, 124, 140, 142, 143, 148, 155, 175, 176, 178
health care, 178
health care costs, 178
health problems, 178
health status, 116, 121, 124
heat shock protein, 71, 78
hemisphere, 140, 145, 156
heritability, 184, 185
heterochromatin, 66, 74
heterogeneity, 13, 19, 20, 21, 162, 163
heterozygote, 166
high carcass quality, x, 140
histone(s), ix, 59, 60, 61, 62, 63, 65, 66, 67, 68, 69, 70, 71, 72, 73, 74, 76, 77, 78, 79, 80, 81, 82, 97
histone deacetylase, 61, 63, 71, 77, 79, 80
history, 168
HIV, 28, 29, 35, 37
HIV-1, 28, 37
HM, 17, 18, 103
homeostasis, 4, 88, 93, 98, 101, 125
hormonal control, ix, 83
hormone(s), vii, viii, ix, 39, 47, 48, 55, 73, 82, 83, 86, 87, 88, 89, 90, 91, 92, 93, 97, 98, 99, 100, 101, 102, 103, 104, 106, 107, 111, 156
hormone levels, 100, 106
horses, ix, 84
host, vii, 2, 25, 26, 35, 60, 70, 75, 110, 111, 112, 143, 144, 145, 152
host population, 145
hot spots, 96
housing, 132, 148, 178, 184
human genome, 21
human health, 35, 151
human resources, 148
human skin, 37, 38
human subjects, 55
humidity, x, 95, 139, 140, 141, 144
humoral immunity, 15
Hungarian Fleckvieh, vi, xi, 175, 176, 178, 179, 180, 182, 183, 184, 186
Hungary, vii, 175, 176, 181, 184
hydrated aluminosilicates, ix, 115
hydrogen, 75
hyperinsulinemia, 47, 55, 56, 57
hyperplasia, 103
hyperprolactinemia, 103
hypoglycemia, 40

hypogonadism, 87, 89, 91, 100, 105
hypothalamus, 72, 73, 87, 88, 89, 91, 92, 97, 105
hypothermia, 133
hypothesis, 31, 46, 146, 162, 164

I

ideal, 94, 164
identification, 21
identity, 8, 12
idiopathic, 97, 104, 105
IFN, 30
Ig heavy chains, 19
ileum, 18
images, 41
imbalances, 134
immune function, 30, 114
immune response, x, 17, 18, 30, 71, 80, 115, 120
immune system, 2, 3, 7, 14, 15, 16, 19, 26, 30, 71, 80, 85
immunity, vii, viii, 2, 4, 5, 6, 16, 25, 28, 29, 37, 75, 110, 111, 120
immunization, 15
immunogenetics, 15
immunoglobulin(s), x, 2, 3, 5, 6, 15, 16, 17, 18, 19, 20, 21, 22, 23, 115, 120, 121, 123
immunoglobulin superfamily, 2
immunomodulatory, 6, 28
imports, 140
imprinting, 60
improvements, 61, 98, 172
in situ hybridization, 21
in vitro, 27, 29, 38, 40, 47, 61, 68, 78, 117
in vivo, 29, 47, 117
incidence, x, 89, 93, 102, 110, 111, 115, 118, 119, 121, 124, 127, 128, 129, 132, 135
income, 175, 177, 183
independent variable, 43
India, 140
indirect effect, 145
individuals, 146, 162, 163, 164, 172, 177
inducer, 74, 80
induction, 36, 38, 45, 61, 67, 73
industry, 76, 93, 124, 147, 148, 162, 187
infancy, 61, 100
infants, 99
infection, 26, 29, 30, 37, 121, 144, 152, 154
infectious agents, 15
infertility, 86, 87, 88, 89, 90, 91, 93, 94, 96, 97, 98, 99, 100, 103, 104, 106, 185
inflammation, viii, 25, 29, 30, 35, 38, 69, 95, 111
inflammatory bowel disease, 77
inflammatory cells, 27, 30

inflammatory disease, 35
inflammatory responses, 30, 36
information technology, 141
infrastructure, 147, 148
ingest, 57
ingredients, 135
inguinal, 84
inheritance, 73, 82
inhibition, 29, 40, 48, 65, 68, 70, 74, 78, 92, 94
inhibitor, 26, 28, 30, 36, 37, 38, 54, 61, 65, 79
initiation, 52, 63, 65, 70, 73, 81
injections, 42, 49
injury, 134
innate immunity, 2
insects, 2, 31, 143
insertion, vii, 1, 9, 13, 14
institutions, vii
insulation, 105
insulin, viii, 39, 40, 41, 42, 43, 47, 48, 49, 50, 51, 52,
    53, 54, 55, 56, 57, 77, 78, 101
insulin resistance, 47, 57
integration, 171
integrin, 9, 22
integrity, 26, 96, 97, 100, 104, 149
interface, 26
interference, 140, 146, 147
interferon, 30
intervention, 133
intestinal tract, 116
intestine, 6, 121
intron(s), 9, 31, 33, 74
invertebrates, 2
investment(s), ix, 83, 178
iodine, 110
ion-exchange, ix, 115, 118
ions, 26, 84, 117
Ireland, 188
iron, 121
irradiation, 37
isoflavone, 94
isolation, 155
Israel, 38
issues, ix, 109, 178
Italy, 150, 152, 171, 176, 184

J

Japan, 39, 41, 43, 173
jaundice, 133
juveniles, 146

K

Kenya, 150
keratinocyte(s), 27, 30, 37
kidney, 63, 77, 78
kinase activity, 63
Korea, 39

L

labeling, 62
lactation, x, 18, 99, 118, 119, 122, 127, 129, 151,
    178, 180, 181, 182
landscape(s), 74, 75, 76, 77, 81
laparotomy, 134
large intestine, 28, 35, 61
larvae, 144, 151
larval development, 69
Latin America, 140, 152, 153
laws, 79
lead, 49, 61, 69, 86, 87, 88, 89, 91, 140, 147, 148
leakage, 134
learning, 100
leptin, viii, 39, 40, 41, 42, 43, 44, 45, 46, 47, 48, 49,
    51, 52, 53, 54, 55, 56, 57, 87, 106
leucine, 2, 3, 28
leucocyte, 26
libido, 91
life cycle, 143, 144
lifetime, xi, 142, 175, 177, 187
ligand, 97
light, vii, 1, 2, 3, 6, 10, 11, 12, 13, 14, 15, 16, 17, 20,
    22, 23, 35, 141, 174, 184
liver, x, 3, 49, 54, 121, 124, 127, 133, 134
livestock, 17, 45, 82, 93, 140, 141, 143, 144, 145,
    147, 148, 152, 153, 156, 172
local anesthesia, 134
local conditions, x, 139
localization, 17, 18, 38, 103, 104
loci, 12, 32, 165, 166
locus, 2, 7, 8, 9, 11, 12, 20, 21, 23, 32, 33, 36, 163,
    165, 166
longevity, 85, 186, 187
Louisiana, 154
LTA, 29
luciferase, 70
lumen, 4, 96, 117, 121, 128, 134
lung disease, 35
lupus, 20
luteinizing hormone, 54, 55, 85, 87, 88, 99, 100, 101,
    102, 103, 104, 107
lymph, 7, 18

lymph node, 7, 18
lymphocytes, 2, 6, 7, 11, 16, 18, 19, 21
lymphocytosis, 22
lymphoid, 4, 5, 6, 14, 18, 19
lymphoid organs, 4, 5
lymphoid tissue, 5, 6, 18, 19
lysine, 68, 72, 73, 74, 81, 82
lysosome, 85
lysozyme, 110

M

machinery, 15, 70, 72, 80
macromolecules, 4
macrophage inflammatory protein, 30
macrophages, 36
magnesium, 121, 124, 125
magnitude, 54
major histocompatibility complex (MHC), 2, 18
majority, 12, 63, 71, 110, 160
malignancy, 67
mammal(s), ix, 2, 3, 4, 7, 12, 31, 34, 37, 66, 73, 82, 84, 90, 93, 98, 146, 147, 150
mammalian cells, 65, 79, 81
mammalian reproduction, ix, 83
man, 99, 105, 140, 146, 147, 173
management, 94, 95, 113, 129, 134, 135, 136, 143, 144, 145, 146, 147, 148, 150, 153, 172, 178
manipulation, 76
manure, 179
mapping, 19, 20, 21, 74, 75, 79, 82
market economy, 149
marketing, 178, 179, 186
Markov chain, 187
marrow, 3, 7
masking, 73
mass, 28, 94, 100, 102
mastitis, x, 114, 127, 129, 181, 187
materials, ix, 45, 72, 115, 117, 118, 119, 122, 125
maternal care, 146, 147
matrix, 26, 167, 172, 174
matter, 180, 181
measurement(s), 41, 45, 46, 52, 56, 99, 133, 147
meat, ix, 49, 75, 109, 111, 148, 160, 185
media, 168
mediation, 66
medication, 179
medicine, 17, 110
meiosis, 85, 89
melatonin, 84
mellitus, 57
membranes, 29, 62, 110, 112, 113, 129
memory, 82

messenger ribonucleic acid, 101
messenger RNA, 69
meta-analysis, 168
Metabolic, x, 55, 56, 127, 136
metabolic acidosis, 121
metabolic disorder(s), 123
metabolism, 4, 17, 40, 44, 47, 49, 51, 55, 56, 61, 63, 72, 110, 116, 123, 124, 143
metabolites, viii, 39, 47, 55, 82, 123, 156
metabolized, 84
metaphase, 65
methodology, 45
methylation, 60, 61, 68, 69, 70, 73, 78, 79, 81, 94
mice, 3, 5, 11, 12, 13, 16, 23, 30, 37, 40, 54, 91, 92, 93, 94, 100, 103, 105, 106
microbiota, 75, 76, 82
microorganisms, 75, 76, 110
microRNA, ix, 59, 69, 79, 80
microsatellites, 166
migration, vii, 1, 9, 14, 153
milk quality, 171
mineralocorticoid, 73
MIP, 30
mitochondria, 97, 174
mitochondrial DNA, xi, 159, 167, 174
mitogen, 27
mitosis, 65, 78, 85
model system, 81
modelling, 152
models, 35
modifications, ix, 60, 61, 68, 72, 73, 78, 81, 109
modules, 2
molecular biology, 79, 80
molecules, ix, 2, 21, 70, 75, 97, 115
Mongolia, 162
monocyte chemoattractant protein, 30
Moon, 56
morbidity, 35
morphological abnormalities, 95
morphology, ix, 62, 83, 88, 92, 100, 102, 105, 106
mortality, xi, 146, 175, 178, 179, 180, 181, 182, 183
mortality rate, 178, 179
mosaic, 31
Moscow, 122
motif, 38, 168
MR, 17, 19, 55, 56, 100, 106, 165, 166, 168
mRNA(s), 8, 22, 27, 30, 40, 55, 56, 68, 69, 73
mtDNA, 160, 164, 167, 168, 169, 170
mucosa, 111
mucus, 26, 28, 37, 110
mutation(s), 13, 15, 87, 89, 100, 104, 105, 168, 169, 170
mutation rate, 168

mycotoxins, 116

N

Na$^+$, 117
NaCl, 43, 123
NADH, 75
National Academy of Sciences, 79
native species, vii
natural enemies, 155
natural gas, 110
natural selection, 140, 144, 145, 146, 156
necrosis, 38
negative effects, 145
negative relation, 44
nematode, 144, 149, 151, 154
neonates, 14
nerve, 118, 132
Netherlands, 151, 171, 172, 184
neurons, 72, 78, 81, 87, 91, 92, 99, 103
neuropeptides, 87
neurotransmitter, 92
neutral, 145
neutrophils, 30
New Zealand, 176
next generation, 73, 74
nitrogen, 117, 125
nodes, 3
non-insulin dependent diabetes, 57
normal distribution, 181
North Africa, 140
North America, 128, 129, 174
nuclear receptors, 73
nuclei, 78
nucleotide sequence, vii, 1, 9, 10, 13, 14, 20, 22, 60
nucleotides, 3, 13, 14, 69
nucleus, 69, 72
null, 31, 166
nursing, 146, 154
nutrient(s), 51, 60, 61, 74, 75, 121, 125
nutrition, vii, 46, 56, 60, 75, 77, 132, 140, 141, 143, 149, 150, 152
nutritional imbalance, 121
nutritional status, 57, 87

O

obesity, 40, 47, 56, 94, 96, 101
OIE, 143, 154
oil, 41
oligomerization, 67
omentum, 128, 134

oocyte, ix, 83, 84, 85
opportunities, 15, 78, 153
organ(s), 5, 7, 14, 27, 35, 46, 53, 56, 84, 128, 133, 134, 143
organelles, 62
organism, 26, 60, 65, 90
organize, 171, 173
osmotic pressure, 57, 121
osmotic stress, 74
ovaries, 111
overlap, 165
oxidation, 49, 54, 57, 110
oxidative stress, 97, 98, 100
oxygen, 97, 100, 110
oxytocin analogues, ix, 109
ozone, vii, ix, 109, 110, 111, 112, 114

P

p53, 67, 68, 79
pairing, 13, 14
Pakistan, 144, 155
palpation, 133
pancreas, 43
parallel, 43
parallelism, 43
parasite(s), 71, 141, 142, 143, 144, 145, 149, 152, 153, 154, 155
parasitic diseases, 81
parenchyma, 96
parents, 177
paresis, 118, 124, 125
parity, 132, 142
pasture(s), 140, 144, 145, 146, 148, 151, 152, 188
pathogenesis, 129
pathogens, viii, 4, 25, 30, 35, 38, 75, 120, 143, 144, 157
pathology, 79
pathophysiology, 103, 123
pathways, 5, 27, 63, 64, 65, 69, 77, 79, 87, 89, 94
PCR, 31, 163, 164, 167, 168
pedigree, 171
penicillin, 110
penis, 84, 89
peptide(s), vii, 25, 26, 27, 29, 30, 35, 36, 40
perinatal, 5
peripheral blood, 5, 6, 7, 11, 30, 81
peripheral blood mononuclear cell, 81
peritoneal cavity, 84, 134
peritonitis, 134
permeability, 5
permit, 14
pests, 140

pH, x, 85, 115, 116, 119, 123, 124, 133
phage, 9
pharmaceutical, 15
phenotype(s), ix, 59, 60, 61, 73, 75, 83
Philippines, 39, 55
phosphate, 124
phosphorus, 116, 121, 123, 124, 125
phosphorylation, 29, 49, 68, 74
phylogenetic tree, 12
Physiological, 55, 99, 102, 123, 124
physiological factors, x, 127, 146
physiology, 75, 84, 89, 141
pigs, ix, 32, 40, 55, 84, 142
pilot study, 104
pineal gland, 84
pituitary gland, 85
placebo, 102
placenta, ix, x, 4, 17, 18, 109, 110, 112, 113, 114, 127, 131
placental barrier, 4
plants, 143, 145
plasma cells, 22
plasma membrane, 29, 37, 97, 103
plasticity, 60
plastics, 93
platform, 14, 172
plexus, 96, 102
PM, 78, 104, 106, 174
pneumonia, 29
policy, 152, 184
policy makers, 152
pollutants, 93
polycomb repressive complex, 79
polymerase, 72
polymorphism(s), 8, 9, 12, 19, 49, 54, 160, 162, 163, 164, 168, 172, 174
polysaccharides, 26
polyunsaturated fatty acids, 97, 103
population, 6, 30, 62, 71, 102, 128, 141, 144, 147, 149, 150, 155, 156, 165, 166, 167, 168, 171, 172, 173, 174, 186, 187
population structure, 187
position effect, 60
positive relationship, viii, 39, 49, 54
potassium, 121, 124
predators, 146, 147
pre-elafin, 36, 38
pregnancy, 110, 112, 114, 142, 151
prepuce, 84
present value, 177
preservation, 121
prevention, ix, x, 15, 77, 78, 115, 116, 118, 119, 120, 122, 123, 124, 127, 128

primate, 32, 36
priming, 30
prions, 60
probability, 114, 144, 149
probe, 41
probiotic, 76
process control, 76
producers, 27, 95
production costs, 179
profit, 162, 176, 177, 187, 188
profitability, 143, 176, 178, 184
progesterone, 90
prognosis, 133
pro-inflammatory, 28
project, 7
prolactin, 99, 100, 105
proliferation, 6, 18, 61, 79, 91, 92, 104
proline, 9, 14
promoter, 57, 68, 71, 73, 74, 78, 81, 167
propagation, 41, 65
prophylaxis, 136
propositus, 100
prostaglandin(s), ix, 109, 110, 111, 112
prostate gland, 84
protease inhibitors, 26
proteasome, 29, 36, 77
protection, 5, 15, 18, 27, 29, 35, 36, 37, 84, 147
protective role, 97
protein family, 26
protein kinases, 65
protein structure, 26
proteinase, 28, 37
proteins, 2, 4, 17, 19, 26, 29, 38, 63, 65, 68, 72, 74, 75, 77, 81, 92, 97, 100, 121, 135
proteolysis, 4, 17
pseudogene, 33
Pseudomonas aeruginosa, 29, 30
psoriasis, 30
puberty, 84, 87, 90, 92, 94, 100
puerperium, x, 127
purity, 116
pyloric stenosis, 130
pylorus, 134
pyrimidine, 63

R

radiation, 75, 140
rainfall, x, 139, 144
rate of change, 150
RE, 19, 56, 81
reactions, 146
reactive oxygen, 97

reactivity, 23, 43
reality, 172
receptors, 2, 5, 17, 37, 73, 85, 87, 88, 91, 92, 98, 100, 107, 121
recognition, 14, 16, 35, 37, 60, 65, 68, 78, 79
recombination, 2, 3, 5, 7, 8, 10, 11, 12, 13, 16, 20, 22
recommendations, 173
recovery, 43, 110, 133, 134, 148
rectal temperature, 142
reflexes, 95
regression, 43
regression analysis, 43
regulations, 68, 86
relevance, 17, 68, 103
reliability, 174
remodelling, 109
repair, viii, 25, 28, 72
replication, 61, 63, 65, 66, 78
repression, 63, 67, 69, 80
reproduction, ix, 83, 87, 88, 89, 91, 92, 94, 97, 99, 100, 103, 106, 110, 113, 140, 141, 142, 151, 153, 186
requirements, 61, 93, 129, 147, 176, 178, 182
RES, 31, 37
researchers, 116, 119, 120, 128, 129, 134
reserves, 96, 142
residuals, 116, 122
residues, 9, 12, 13, 14, 20, 69, 111, 112, 148
resilience, 75
resistance, x, 17, 47, 60, 71, 75, 105, 118, 139, 140, 141, 143, 144, 145, 149, 150, 155, 160
resolution, 29
resource allocation, 142
resources, xi, 143, 145, 148, 150, 152, 159, 160, 162, 173, 175
respiration, 153
respiratory rate, 132
response, 2, 29, 30, 52, 57, 63, 65, 71, 72, 73, 75, 81, 82, 88, 90, 91, 94, 95, 99, 114, 146, 151, 185, 186
responsiveness, 104
restriction enzyme, 9
restriction fragment length polymorphis, 173
restrictions, 144
retinoblastoma, 65, 66
revenue, 179
RH, 77, 105
ribosomal RNA, 70
ribosome, 69
risk(s), 136, 141, 148, 149, 150, 152, 155
risk factors, 136, 155
RNA(s), 16, 60, 63, 64, 65, 68, 69, 70, 72, 78, 80
RNA splicing, 60
rodents, vii, 1, 3, 5, 6, 9, 11, 32, 96

Romania, 186
Royal Society, 151, 152, 155
rules, 172

S

safety, 116
salinity, 153
saliva, 18, 117
salts, 123
savannah, x, 139
scavengers, 143
science, 76, 79, 98, 124, 141, 153
scope, 60
scrotal, 95, 96, 100, 101, 102, 103, 105
scrotum, 84, 95, 96, 102, 105
seasonal changes, 100
secrete, 87
secretion, 4, 17, 26, 30, 37, 38, 45, 46, 47, 49, 55, 85, 87, 88, 89, 90, 91, 92, 99
secretory leukocyte proteinase inhibitor, 37
seed, 93, 105, 106
selenium, 120
semen, ix, 83, 84, 86, 94, 95, 99, 100, 101, 102, 104, 106, 162, 169, 179, 181
seminal vesicle, 31
seminiferous tubules, 84, 85, 88
sensitivity, 43, 65, 99
sequencing, 12, 63, 64, 65, 68, 69, 74, 78, 80, 164, 167
serine, 12, 38
Sertoli cells, 85, 88, 89, 90, 91, 92, 98
serum, 4, 5, 9, 13, 17, 18, 19, 22, 30, 37, 54, 57, 90, 93, 94, 100, 102, 105, 106, 117, 118, 120, 121, 123, 124
services, 122
sex, 84, 87, 89, 93, 94
sex hormones, 84, 87
sexual behavior, 92
sexual development, 93
shape, 76, 81, 148, 176
sheep, vii, viii, 1, 5, 8, 9, 11, 12, 13, 18, 19, 20, 21, 22, 23, 25, 31, 33, 40, 45, 46, 48, 51, 52, 53, 55, 56, 57, 61, 153, 156
shelter, 95
shifting boundaries, 154
shock, 71, 73, 74, 81, 82
shortage, vii
showing, 47, 49, 51, 62, 71, 142, 164, 170
siblings, 104
side effects, 95, 141, 142, 155
SIGMA, 43
signal peptide, 26, 27

signaling pathway, 60
signals, 70, 88, 89
signs, 111, 118, 133
silica, 123
silicon, 117
simulation, 186
single chain, 104
single-nucleotide polymorphism, 80, 174
SKALP, 26, 37, 38
skin, 9, 26, 27, 35, 37, 38, 41, 45, 81, 85, 134
SLPI, 26, 27, 28, 29, 30, 31, 32, 35, 37, 38
small intestine, 5, 6, 18, 30, 35
SNP, 172
SNS, 14
social behaviour, x, 140, 150
social interactions, 146
social learning, 145
social relations, 152
social relationships, 152
social skills, 146
socialization, 147
society, 141, 149
sodium, 63, 78, 79, 92, 120, 121, 122, 123, 124
software, 32, 34, 38, 64, 66
solution, 112
somatic cell, 142, 156, 170, 176, 179, 181, 183, 185, 186
somatic hypermutations, vii, 1, 3, 5, 10, 12, 14
somatic mutations, 12
South Africa, 139, 142, 143, 151, 153, 156
South America, vii, x, 139, 140, 148
South Korea, vii
Southeast Asia, 161, 165, 168, 169, 170
soybeans, 94
species, vii, viii, ix, 1, 2, 3, 4, 5, 6, 8, 9, 10, 11, 12, 14, 15, 17, 22, 25, 31, 34, 35, 43, 45, 55, 61, 71, 77, 84, 85, 88, 89, 92, 95, 97, 98, 141, 143, 145, 146, 147, 149, 160, 172, 173
sperm, ix, 83, 84, 85, 86, 87, 88, 89, 90, 91, 92, 93, 94, 95, 96, 97, 98, 99, 100, 101, 102, 103, 104, 105, 106
sperm function, 103
spermatid, 85, 99
spermatogenesis, 85, 86, 88, 89, 90, 91, 92, 94, 95, 96, 98, 99, 100, 101, 103, 104, 105, 106
spermatogonial stem cells, 84, 85
spleen, 6, 7
Spring, 81
sputum, 26
SS, 19, 20, 21, 22, 23, 57
stability, 6, 60, 61, 75, 116
stabilization, 133
stallion, 84

standard deviation, 177, 178, 182, 183
standardization, 76
starch, 119
starvation, 40
state(s), 27, 72, 74, 81, 82, 95, 117, 136, 146, 147, 182, 187
statistics, 141, 172, 178, 179
stem cells, 63, 78
sterile, 134
steroids, 87, 91, 92
stillbirth, 184, 186
stimulation, 3, 44, 52, 88, 103, 104, 132
stock, 184, 185
storage, 85
strategy use, 146
stress, x, 47, 60, 69, 71, 72, 73, 81, 82, 94, 95, 97, 98, 105, 106, 127, 129, 135, 141, 143, 145, 148, 149, 150, 160, 176
stress factors, 129, 135, 141, 143
stress response, 71, 73
stressors, 71, 148
stretching, 109
structural changes, 61
structure, ix, x, 22, 25, 61, 63, 72, 74, 81, 99, 115, 116, 117, 127, 160, 162, 174, 178, 182
subgroups, 10
subsidy, 177
substitution(s), 8, 15, 141, 168
substrate(s), viii, 25, 26, 27, 31, 32, 38, 84
Sun, vi, 16, 17, 19, 20, 159, 169, 174
supplementation, 116, 117, 118, 122, 125
suppression, 67, 99, 105
surgical intervention, 109, 133, 134
surplus, 178, 179
survival, x, 71, 113, 139, 141, 143, 144, 145, 146, 147, 149, 151, 153, 155, 157, 188
susceptibility, 105, 141, 154
sustainability, 148, 149
sustainable development, 150
suture, 134, 136
sweat, 95
Sweden, 43
syndrome, x, 89, 115, 116, 120, 130
synthesis, 5, 17, 18, 61, 62, 63, 65, 66, 75, 91

T

T cell(s), 2, 5, 7, 18, 30
T lymphocytes, 5, 36, 37
tachycardia, 133
target, 13, 15, 68, 69, 70, 73, 79, 92, 94, 101
T-cell receptor, 30
TCR, 2, 30

techniques, 63, 140

technology(s), 63, 64, 74, 147, 148, 172

temperament, 155

temperature, x, 60, 72, 84, 95, 96, 101, 103, 106, 132, 133, 139, 140, 143, 144, 153

tension, 134

testicle, 98

testicular cancer, 104

testing, xi, 159, 160, 170, 171

testis, 84, 85, 86, 89, 90, 92, 93, 95, 100, 102, 103, 105, 106, 107

testosterone, 84, 85, 86, 87, 88, 89, 90, 91, 92, 94, 97, 98, 99, 102, 103, 104, 106, 107

therapeutic effects, 35

therapeutics, 15, 35, 77, 80

therapy, 87, 102, 103, 104, 110, 111, 112, 114

thermograms, 95

thermoregulation, 72, 94, 100, 101, 102, 105

thorax, 129

thymus, 7, 18

thyroid, 97, 101

Tibet, 160, 162, 164

tick-borne disease, 154

tissue, viii, ix, 5, 25, 28, 35, 45, 47, 51, 56, 61, 69, 96, 106, 109, 110, 128

TLR, 29

TNF, 27, 29, 30, 37, 69

TNF-alpha, 37

tonsils, 7

topology, 167

torsion, 128, 130, 134

total cholesterol, viii, 39, 47

toxic effect, 117

toxicity, 82

TP53, 63, 66, 67, 68, 79

trace elements, 121, 124, 135

trachea, 35

trade, 35, 77, 144

training, 148, 172

traits, ix, x, xi, 95, 105, 115, 122, 125, 139, 142, 144, 146, 155, 170, 171, 173, 175, 176, 177, 178, 179, 181, 182, 183, 184, 185, 186, 187, 188

transcription, ix, 59, 65, 67, 68, 70, 71, 72, 73, 74, 76, 77, 78, 79, 80, 81, 82, 94, 167

transcription factors, 67, 68, 71, 74, 81, 82

transcripts, 63, 69, 70

transformation, 67, 110

transforming growth factor, 90

transglutaminase substrate (TGS), viii, 25

transition period, 118, 119, 129, 135

translation, 68, 69, 73, 80, 81

transmission, 144

transplantation, 35

transport, 4, 17, 40, 49, 72, 84, 92, 97, 121, 178

transportation, 130, 160

trappin-2, viii, 25, 26, 27, 28, 29, 30, 31, 32, 33, 35, 36, 37

trauma, 89

treatment, ix, x, 35, 42, 45, 49, 50, 52, 53, 61, 62, 63, 64, 67, 68, 69, 70, 86, 92, 97, 101, 102, 105, 109, 110, 111, 112, 113, 115, 122, 124, 127, 128, 133, 134, 136, 180

trial, 42

triggers, 65, 71

trypsin, 28

tuberculosis, 36

tumor(s), 67, 71, 86, 89, 93, 101, 104

tumor cells, 71, 104

turnover, 92

twinning, 109

tyrosine, 68

U

ubiquitin, 29, 36

UK, 184, 187

ulcerative colitis, 35

ultrasound, viii, 39, 40, 41, 45, 55

ultrastructure, 88

underlying mechanisms, 98

underproduction, 97

uniform, 96

United, vii, 79, 144, 162, 174

United Nations, 162

United States (USA), vii, 25, 43, 59, 79, 113, 124, 144, 153, 169, 174, 176

untranslated regions, 69

urea, 56, 117, 123, 125, 143

urethra, 84

uric acid, 97

urine, 84, 109

USDA, 25, 35, 59, 77

uterus, ix, 109, 110, 111, 112, 130

V

vagina, ix, 109, 110, 111, 112

vaginitis, 109

variables, 44, 48, 136

variations, 49, 95, 143, 144, 147, 164

varieties, 149

vas deferens, 84

vasculature, 15

vector, 143, 144, 156

vegetation, 140

vein, 41, 42, 96, 134
vertebrae, 134
vertebrates, 2, 3, 16, 22
vesicle, 31
videotape, 41
viscera, 46
viscosity, 85
vitamin A, 121
vitamin D, 124
vitamins, 75, 121, 124, 135
volvulus, 133, 134, 136
vulnerability, 152

W

walking, 146, 154
water, vii, ix, x, xi, 42, 114, 115, 140, 141, 143, 146, 147, 153, 159, 160, 169, 174, 179, 181
water resources, 141
weight gain, 44, 154, 180, 183
weight ratio, 184
well-being, 75
Western blot, 62
whey acidic protein (WAP), viii, 25
wild animals, 145
wild type, 103
wildlife, 143

Wisconsin, 136, 153
withdrawal, ix, 76, 109
wool, 75
worldwide, ix, x, 109, 116, 120, 127, 128, 140, 153, 160

X

X chromosome, 60
xiphoid process, 129

Y

Y chromosome, 84, 161, 162, 174
yield, xi, 116, 122, 123, 124, 142, 156, 170, 173, 174, 175, 176, 177, 178, 179, 181, 182, 183, 185, 188
yolk, 6

Z

zeolites, ix, 115, 116, 117, 122, 123, 124, 125
zinc, 121, 123
zinc oxide, 123